Health Economics in Development

Human Development Network
Health, Nutrition, and Population Series

Health Economics in Development

Philip Musgrove, Editor

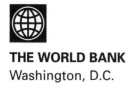

THE WORLD BANK
Washington, D.C.

Library of Congress Cataloging-in-Publication Data

Health economics in development / edited by Philip Musgrove.
    p. cm. — (Health, nutrition, and population series)
  Includes bibliographical references and index.
  ISBN 0-8213-5570-8
    1. Medical economics—Developing countries. I. Musgrove, Philip. II. Series.

  RA410.5.H4133 2003
  338.4'33621'091724—dc21

                              2003057155

Contents

Tables

Figures

Boxes

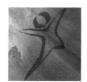

Foreword

My pleasure at being asked to write this foreword for Philip Musgrove's collected papers is both personal and institutional. The personal pleasure derives from my association with him and the respect I have developed for his thinking and work over the past 20 years. It was Philip who critically reviewed for me my first major address on the subject of health and development, and I remember with pleasure his providing me with a list of required reading on the subject and insisting that I read and reread Selma Mushkin's seminal work on health as investment.

The institutional pleasure arises because it was Philip who in my view introduced the appropriate line of thinking about health economics into the Pan American Health Organization in the decade of the eighties. I had been convinced that the majority of health economists were concerned mainly with the costs of health services and presenting to the developing countries various recipes for reduction of costs, including the employment of user fees. Philip Musgrove's early work that I recall was a critical analysis of the impact of the economic crisis of the eighties on the health services and health outcomes in Latin America and the Caribbean. It was partly from this work that he drew the conclusion, which is set out elegantly here, that public financing of health should be countercyclical. This very sensible view has yet to gain widespread acceptance.

I believe that one of the great virtues of this book, and Philip's papers in general, is that it is presented in eminently readable fashion and avoids the turgid writing that obfuscates rather than illuminates. This should be read by all health workers who are interested in the practical treatment of many of the problems that are usually dealt with by economists in the jargon of their guild.

It is gratifying to see the really difficult issues, such as the role of the state or the market, treated so clearly, avoiding the all-or-nothing thinking that unfortunately can be common among health workers. These two major actors in the organization and financing of health services are neither lionized nor demonized here. It is clear from Philip's papers that they both have their place even, or especially, in societies that are committed to equity in health outcomes as well as in the determinants of those outcomes, with emphasis on the role of the health services. Almost all of his conclusions need to be repeated to health workers and policy makers in all sectors, but the one that is likely to strike the loudest chord is his assertion that, except for the most inexpensive care, out-of-pocket spending is probably the worst way to pay for health services.

I hope that those who read this book *Health Economics in Development* will be convinced to abjure forever the loose thinking that goes into the expression "social sector." I appreciate that this will be difficult, but no one who reads his arguments can fail to be convinced of the naivety if not absurdity of the expression. This is not a matter of semantic jousting; experience shows that the public budget for health suffers in more ways than one when it is included in a fixed social sector budget, and governments studiously avoid discussing the merits of health spending in the distribution of public resources.

In his discussion on the cost benefit analysis of programs, Philip refers to the effort to establish the economic benefit from the program to eradicate poliomyelitis in the Americas. The outcome is now history, and for the past eleven years there has been no transmission of polio in the Western Hemisphere. There was never any doubt about the technical feasibility or the social desirability of the program, but when Philip demonstrated that it was also economically beneficial, the stage was set for the success of what has to be one of the most remarkable achievements of public health in recent times. That success led to the decision to mount a worldwide effort, which is now approaching its final goal of universal eradication of polio.

I hope this book will be well received and widely promoted, not only by financial institutions like the World Bank, where much of this material was produced, but also by institutions such as the Pan American Health Organization, where Philip first began to work on health. There is a need for critical and dispassionate thinking about all the issues he addresses. For those of us in the public health profession, there will be special interest in his treatment of the concept of equity and the possibility of equity in the

provision of health care in countries where health services are segmented—
to the detriment of the majority of the population and especially of the
poor.

I wish the book well and recommend it to you.

Sir George Alleyne
Director Emeritus
Pan American Health Organization
World Health Organization
Washington, D.C.

Acknowledgments

Numerous colleagues and friends, particularly at the World Bank but also at the Pan American Health Organization, the Inter-American Development Bank, and the World Health Organization, encouraged me in the only two beliefs that might justify this venture. One is that at least some of the papers included deserve a longer life and a wider audience than the original publications alone would provide; the other is that because of the development of certain ideas over the years and the connections between one piece and another, putting the papers together might create a whole greater than the sum of its parts. This collection owes its existence to Alexander Preker, who insisted on its potential when I doubted it, and to James Christopher Lovelace, who allowed me to devote to it the necessary time during my last months at the World Bank.

I have also accumulated debts, beginning more than twenty years ago, to all those who provided the environment and the experiences from which these ideas grew. These include a large number of government officials and scholars, especially in Argentina, Brazil, Chile, and Colombia, with whom I had the pleasure of working on empirical studies and health sector reform projects, and the many PAHO and World Bank colleagues who collaborated on those efforts. I trust they will forgive the failure to name them all individually. The acknowledgments for several chapters thank those whose help was particularly important in stimulating or improving a paper or in providing information and direction.

Turning a collection of papers into a book would have been impossible without Nicki Marrian's repeated guidance and encouragement. Daniel Cotlear, María Luisa Escobar, and Adam Wagstaff commented extensively on the first full draft, and contributed greatly to making it both leaner and more thoughtful. The final organization of the volume, and especially that of the Introduction, are due to their suggestions. Wagstaff also suggested the felicitous title. Olufumilayo Orisadipe undertook the tedious task of retyping papers written so long ago that there were no electronic files from which to work. Yvette Atkins and Sithie Naz Mowlana kept track of successive revisions. Rick Ludwick supervised the transformation of a manuscript into a book, with unfailing patience and efficiency.

A Note on Authorship

Five of these papers were written with co-authors, who in three cases deserve the lion's share of the credit. Chapter 13 derives from a much larger study by Dariush Akhavan for the World Bank. At the invitation of Alexandre Abrantes, who was the task manager for the Bank malaria control project, I condensed the study and developed the graphic and tabular presentations to emphasize how a change in strategy improved the cost-effectiveness of control efforts. The fourth co-author, Renato d'A. Gusmão, of the Pan American Health Organization, was responsible for the introduction of the new malaria control strategy into the World Bank project. Chapter 14 also derives from a larger study, by Osmil Galindo, undertaken for the Pan American Health Organization under my direction at the Fundação Joaquim Nabuco in Recife, Brazil. Besides overseeing Galindo's work, my contribution was to condense the study and put it into English (the original was in Portuguese). Dean T. Jamison and Joanne Leslie wrote the first version of Chapter 17, and later invited my help with reconstructing and interpreting the calculations and with the final writing. Chapters 3 and 19 are more conventional cases of co-authorship; I am most grateful to all the colleagues who shared in these efforts.

I had the satisfaction of contributing to two major publications that are not excerpted here. One is the World Bank's *World Development Report 1993: Investing in Health*, for which I wrote much of Chapter 3 and part of Chapter 2. The other report, for which I wrote Chapters 1 and 2 and also edited the rest of the text, is the World Health Organization's *World Health Report 2000–Health Systems: Improving Performance*. Both these reports were such joint products with several co-authors, from whom I learned a great deal, that it does not seem proper to appropriate any part of either one as my own work. Many of the key ideas in these two documents, which deal with the role of the state in health, with the use of cost-effectiveness analysis, and with how health is (or should be) financed, are either foreshadowed by, or subsequently developed in, several of the papers included here.

Introduction

The papers in this collection span 21 years of thinking and writing about health economics, first at the Pan American Health Organization (1982–1990) and then at the World Bank (1990–2002, including two years, 1999–2001, on secondment to the World Health Organization). They are divided into six general topics, which together touch on several of the major issues in this field. Chapters 1 through 3 concern the connection between health, particularly public health, and economics—a connection that has occupied much of my professional effort, in part because I started to work on the subject in an organization dominated by public health professionals, and only later moved to an organization dominated by other economists. Chapters 4 through 6 treat several different aspects of equity, while chapters 7 through 17 deal with effectiveness and efficiency, first in general terms and then with specific attention to communicable diseases and to malnutrition. Equity and efficiency are among the main issues in any branch of economics, and—as several chapters illustrate—they often cannot be sharply separated. Chapters 18 through 20 concern how health is, and how it should be, paid for—questions that involve both equity and efficiency.

Calling the collection *Health Economics in Development* conveys two meanings: that the science of health economics itself has been developing during the period covered, and continues to do so; and that the application of health economics contributes to development, broadly defined, both by improving health and by reducing the waste of resources devoted to health care. As to the first, health economics is a relatively young subdiscipline, roughly 40 years old and expanding rapidly. In 1982, the Pan American Health Organization (PAHO) sought to hire an economist with 10 years' experience in health issues in Latin America. That was a novel departure for PAHO, and it was resisted by a number of staff members trained in public health and deeply suspicious of economists and their ways of thinking. Moreover, there was probably no one alive who could meet the job requirements then. By the end of the century, the situation was quite different: PAHO not only employed several economists but promoted and published studies of the relations between health and development. This change of attitude reflects the growing realization that economic thinking is not inimical to the ethical concerns of health professionals, and that the expansion of health economics as a field of inquiry has made it steadily more relevant and more useful to health organizations. As to the second, there is increasing evidence that improvements in health, far from being a pure consumption good or even a luxury, often represent valuable investments in people's capacities to learn and to work, and are sometimes essential to rescue people from poverty or prevent their impoverishment (Ruger, Jamison, and Bloom 2001).

As is natural for papers written over a long interval on a variety of topics, these pieces originated in several different ways. The majority are responses to specific requests from supervisors or colleagues, or (in two cases) friends. This is the case for chapters 1 through 3 and 11 through 17, as well as chapter 19. Only chapters 4, 5, 7, 9, 16, 18, and 20 were completely unprovoked either by such requests or by criticism of previous work. Considering the time devoted at the World Bank to health projects, chiefly in Argentina, Brazil, Chile, and Colombia, it may seem odd that few papers resulted from those efforts. Only chapters 6 and 13 derived directly from Bank projects, in the former case as part of the design and in the latter from ex post evaluation. The kind of analysis and the style of writing required to develop projects do not often lend themselves to publication for a wider audience. In fact, the influence probably ran more often the other way, from the ideas in a paper to the way a project was conceived or conducted.

I am grateful to the publishers of the journals or other sources in which these papers first appeared for permission to reprint them here. Each publisher's approach to punctuation and the numbering of references and notes has been retained.

What is Peculiar About Health

There are two strongly connected issues in chapters 1 through 3: first, what it is that distinguishes health from other sectors of the economy, what makes it peculiar in economic terms; and second, what the consequences of those peculiarities are for the appropriate roles of the state and the market. That is, how far should governments interfere in the markets for health care and other determinants of health, to what ends, and with what instruments of intervention? This continues to be a contentious topic, both because the economics of health is complicated and because there is sometimes too much ideological rigidity, oversimplified theory, and mutual misunderstanding on both sides of the discussion. Health is emphatically a place where "market fundamentalism" is misguided, but what one might call "public health fundamentalism" can be equally mistaken.

Chapter 1 argues that it is valuable for health professionals to understand better how economists think in general, and how they approach issues in health in particular. A certain minimum understanding is desirable, but that understanding does not require any specific knowledge of many areas of economics. (Some public health specialist should perhaps write the mirror-image paper on the minimum that economists should know about health and medicine. Hsiao (2000) has provided an economist's view on what economists, particularly macroeconomists, not familiar with health issues should know about the subject.) Economists readily invade other professions' domains, in part because most microeconomics is about something particular and not just about "the economy," and also because economists travel light and carry relatively little baggage in the form of data or models specific to their subject (Hirschleifer 1985). Medical professionals, in contrast, must know a great deal of extremely detailed information, which makes them less prone to incursions into others' territory and often leads to a more defensive posture. These differences in the kind and amount of knowledge they need for their work help explain why the two professions often have trouble communicating with each other, to the detriment of how health systems function.

Chapter 2 is an excerpt from a much longer World Bank Discussion Paper, specifically about public and private roles in health. The empirical material in that piece, on health expenditure and relation to health outcomes, has been omitted, because chapter 19 includes more recent and reliable information. The theoretical or conceptual discussion has also been abbreviated, while trying to preserve the central ideas. Four of these, which can—I hope—be widely accepted, are worth mentioning here. The first is that all health interventions can be classified into just three groups, depending on how far they are public or private goods (in the economist's sense) and how much they cost. This classification links the characteristics of interventions to the question of who is to pay for them, emphasizing the importance of insurance or other forms of prepayment, including public financing. Second, the distinction between catastrophically costly interventions and those that consumers can afford to pay for out of pocket depends on people's incomes. Poverty greatly complicates the public/private distinction in the health sector, and becomes a justification for public spending on grounds of equity. The relation among income, costs of interventions, and public subsidy is treated further in several chapters, particularly 5 and 9. Third, delivering the right health interventions to the right people requires a coincidence among need, demand, and supply, which is why the task is so difficult. It is also the reason why most health systems are a mixture of the state and the market, each of which is prone to certain failures which the other can at least partially offset.

The fourth idea is that what really makes health peculiar is rooted in biology. The asset that health interventions exist to protect, *mens sana in corpore sano*, is unlike any nonhuman asset in several crucial ways, starting with the fact that one cannot separate oneself from the asset (Miller 1978). These differences are what make health insurance unlike any other form of insurance, and make health financing more complicated than the financing to protect any other type of asset. Table I.1 summarizes some of the most important differences, which carry numerous implications for both equity and efficiency.

There are of course other human assets than one's state of health, notably one's knowledge and skills, including those acquired through formal education. All these are forms of human capital, and as such have certain

Table I.1 Principal Differences between Health Insurance and Insurance for Nonhuman Assets

CHARACTERISTICS OF THE INSURANCE	TYPE OF ASSET		
	DWELLING	VEHICLE	BODY
Is the asset itself insured?	Yes	Yes	No
Does the asset have a well-defined market value?	Yes	Yes	No
Can the asset be replaced?	Yes	Yes	Only some parts
Can the asset be alienated?	Yes	Yes	Only some parts
Can a substitute be used while the asset is repaired?	Yes	Yes	No
Does the insurance cover catastrophic damage?	Yes	Yes	Yes
Is the owner responsible for maintaining the asset?	Yes	Yes	Only in part
Does the insurance cover ordinary wear and tear?	No	No	Yes
Is the insurance cost related to owner behavior?	No	Yes	No
Does the insurance pay directly to the owner?	Yes	Sometimes	Sometimes
Are there guarantees from the asset producer?	Sometimes, if new	Yes, if new	No
Does someone else pay for the insurance?	No	No	Often

features in common. Nonetheless, the peculiarities of health are such that no other sector is much like it, and in particular, it differs in several fundamental ways from education. These differences are partly intrinsic and partly socially determined; on balance, they make schooling and health care more unlike than similar. If schooling were really very much like health care, one would see attacks of ignorance whose sufferers were rushed to a university for specialized care; parents would seek to buy education insurance against such costly risks; nonemergency students would visit school only occasionally, and only chronic cases would spend much time there.

One crucial difference is that there is nothing in education corresponding to *referrals* in medical care. A sick or injured person can be referred "up" from a health center or physician to a hospital and referred "down" when hospital care is no longer required. There is a natural *hierarchy* of organizations and treatments in health care, but there is no natural *sequence* like primary education followed by secondary schooling followed by university or other higher-level training. If the health system worked the same way as education, no patient could get into a hospital until he or she had spent years at health posts, and then more years attending clinics. In schooling, the worse results are at one level, the harder it is to proceed to the next higher one; in health care the exact opposite is true. This is one of the reasons why health care costs increase more rapidly than educational costs: those who fail primary school are not sent, at great expense, to college. To emphasize these differences is to attack the common and rather imprecise idea that there is something called "the social sector" (Castro and Musgrove 2000), which is relatively homogeneous and is sometimes quite wrongly distinguished from "the productive sector." Lumping, on this logic, is more dangerous to clear thinking and sound public policy than splitting is. Table I.2 summarizes some of the key differences and similarities between the two sectors, noting that the similarities are greatest at the primary level, with increasing differences as emergencies and more complex levels of health care are considered.

The arguments in chapter 2 are illustrated by reference to several issues in the public/private balance, but no single issue is treated in detail. Chapter 3 applies some of the general ideas to one such issue, that of how far the state is justified in interfering with consumers' smoking habits. This is a much-disputed question, pitting public health views (actions bad for one's health should be suppressed) against those of consumer sovereignty (people should be free to decide for themselves whether to smoke). The only easy point of agreement between advocates of these different views is that people should be informed about the undisputed health risks of smoking. Simple-minded

Table 1.2 Principal Differences and Similarities between Education and Health

CHARACTERISTIC	HEALTH CARE IN GENERAL	PRIMARY HEALTH CARE	SCHOOLING
Responds to emergencies	Sometimes	Sometimes, often with referral	Never
Predictable demand	Only in part	More predictable than for health in general	Largely
Insurance market exists	Yes	Yes; less needed than for health in general	No
Nature of improvements	Episodic	Episodic, sometimes cumulative	Cumulative
Natural "good" state exists	Yes	Yes	No
Hierarchy of facilities	Yes	Yes	Yes
Referrals among facilities	Yes	Yes	No
Tendency to cost escalation	Strong	Less than for health in general	Slight
Concentrated early in life	No	Yes	Yes
Time-consuming	Sometimes	Sometimes	Always
Uniform treatment	Sometimes	More uniform than for health in general	Usually
Measurement of quality	Very difficult	Difficult	Relatively easy
Universal coverage	All services	Package of "basic" services	Up to some level
Gains from universal coverage	Nondecreasing	Nondecreasing	Decreasing
Public budgeting	Difficult	Less difficult than for health in general	Easy
Public finance	Quite variable	Quite variable	Always high
Relation to technical change	Technophilic	Less technophilic than for health in general	Technophobic
Externalities	Communicable diseases	Communicable diseases	General and diffuse
Concern for equity	Yes	Yes	Yes
Share of spending on the poor	Low	Higher than for health in general	Very low
Powerful providers	Yes	Less than for health in general	Yes

economic thinking would stop there, but chapter 3 develops several economic arguments why simply providing information, and relying on consumer rationality for the rest, is an inadequate response to the dangers of tobacco use. One of these arguments concerns the young age at which people typically start smoking, and illustrates the general idea from chapter 2 that children do not fit the model of *homo economicus*, able to take risks into account and make sensible decisions about them. The addictive nature of tobacco also undermines an overly market-oriented view of the issue. The attempt to reconcile smoking with the notion of a rational consumer leads to the "rational addiction" model, which is an oxymoron and is, in practice, hardly different from models of habit formation that do not include addiction. Economic science is not yet very good at incorporating aspects that undermine its own standard assumptions about how human beings behave.

Judging and Promoting Equity

Chapter 4 proposes a scheme for thinking about equity at each of several stages of an idealized or simplified episode of illness or accident. One may or may not become sick or hurt; receive treatment or not, when needed; be cured or at least benefit from treatment, or not; and recover without treatment, versus dying or continuing to suffer poor health. For a given illness episode, equity can be very different from one stage to another, and the amount of inequity (and the inequality from which it derives) depends on how the population is classified—by age, gender, income, location, or other characteristics. The conceptual scheme is filled in, so far as household and health system data allowed, with information from Peru. Where the health system is concerned, equity can also look very different depending on which resource—physicians, nurses, hospital beds, or money—or which activities—ambulatory consultations, hospitalizations, or immunizations—is studied. Given all these distinctions, it does not make sense to try to summarize equity in a single measure. Matters only become more complicated when one considers the equity of how health is paid for, since equity in finance can be interpreted in several different ways. Moreover, equity in finance is no assurance of equitable treatment, nor does financial inequity necessarily prevent equitable care.

Chapter 5 takes up one financing issue related to equity: it asks what prices consumers should pay for health care when payments do not have to cover costs because the services are publicly subsidized (and, often, publicly provided as well). The key assumption, which attempts to model how a government in a poor country might think, is that the Ministry of Health values both the quantity of services demanded and delivered and the revenue obtained from patients. The first element implies fees as low as possible, given that demand falls as prices rise; the second may justify substantially higher fees, if demand for health care is relatively inelastic. The model can also be complicated by allowing for price discrimination among consumers according to their incomes, and by trying to distinguish between necessary and frivolous demand. The accumulated empirical evidence concerning these issues strongly suggests that it is difficult to administer a user fee system so as to bring in significant revenue and at the same time to protect those least able to pay (Creese 1991; Newbrander, Collins, and Gilson 2000). It also seems clear that consumers' reactions to fees for health care do not follow a medically sound distinction between care that is more needed or justified and interventions that can be considered more frivolous or of low priority (Lohr et al. 1986). Prices or fees can certainly be used to *ration* health care, as with any other good or service, but not necessarily to *rationalize* its use, as is sometimes carelessly assumed. If the object is to promote needed care and discourage what is less needed, other means are required, and the burden of making that distinction should not fall primarily on patients.

Chapter 6 takes up a very different aspect of equity, the geographic distribution of resources to finance health care—specifically, how to allocate funds from a national government to state or provincial governments in a federal system in such a way as to compensate for differences in income, health needs, or capacity to raise revenue. Analytically, this question fits between a larger and a smaller issue. The larger issue is how *all* intergovernmental transfers are determined, including those that are not earmarked or that are designated for particular uses other than health. The net fiscal impact on a state or other subnational unit may be quite inequitable even if the health-specific transfer is equity-enhancing, and vice versa. Moreover, the net impact on the health of the state's population may differ from what the health transfers aim to achieve if other transfers facilitate or hinder spending by the state out of its own resources. The smaller issue is how the transfers specifically intended for health are actually used. A national government may preferentially distribute funds to a state or province because on average, its inhabitants are poorer or sicker than those of other states; but if the state then uses those funds primarily to benefit the richer or healthier part of its population, equity is hardly served.

The issue treated in chapter 6 is therefore far from a full exploration of how intergovernmental transfers promote equity in health or fail to do so. It is nonetheless ethically important to design those transfers to be equitable in their own right, and politically they can be of great importance in federal systems. The United States, Canada, and Brazil furnish three quite different examples of how federally organized countries have determined such allocations. All three schemes have two significant features in common. First, the formula for allocation contains only one arbitrary parameter, which has the advantage of concentrating political attention on a single decision. Second, the variables that go into the formula offer little scope for either level of government to take advantage of the other or to manipulate the outcome. These seem like valuable principles to follow in many different circumstances where resources have to be shared, so that what is judged technically to be equitable can also be readily understood and therefore accepted politically.

Costs and Outcomes: Effects and Efficiency

Chapters 7 through 10 are conceptual explorations of different aspects of effectiveness and efficiency. Chapter 7 asks the question of how to balance preventive and curative interventions when both are available to combat a given disease. Prevention is always preferable so far as pain, suffering, disability, and anxiety are concerned—"an ounce of prevention is worth a pound of cure" in those terms—but it does not follow that it is always the better choice once costs are taken into account. Assuming that the same final health outcome can be attained by prevention or by treatment, the marginal costs of the two alternatives determine the cost-minimizing mixture of activities. Under these circumstances—although *not* in general—the solution that minimizes costs also maximizes cost-effectiveness. Some very simple microeconomics leads to the conclusion that there is no general superiority to either prevention or treatment so far as efficiency is concerned. This idea is illustrated in detail in chapter 13, about combating malaria in the Amazon Basin of Brazil. A change in strategy developed by the World Health Organization, to focus preventive efforts more sharply and to give more emphasis to case treatment, greatly reduced the average cost of preventing a death. Preventive efforts, it turns out, can be extremely wasteful. Treatment at least has the advantage of not being applied to people who do not need it because they are not sick or hurt.

Chapter 11 considers a somewhat similar question—whether it would be economically justified to spend the considerable resources needed to eradicate polio in the Western Hemisphere, as the Pan American Health Organization concluded in 1985 was technically feasible. In this case the choice was not between prevention and treatment, but between a combination of immunization and treatment, with both continuing into the foreseeable future, and elimination of the disease so that treatment could stop. The answer from the empirical analysis was that eradication would be not only ethically preferable but actually cheaper than continuing to vaccinate some but not all the susceptible children and to treat those who contracted the disease. At that time, the choice was easy, and polio actually was eliminated in the Americas. The same logic—that elimination is cheaper as well as better than continuing to permit cases of the disease—has been followed in the near-elimination of polio in the rest of the world. However, it is no longer clear that eradication of the disease is possible, and there are now seen to be substantial risks of ceasing to immunize once the disease is eliminated everywhere (World Health Organization 2002). To choose the best course of action—how much to vaccinate, and with which of the two available vaccines—would now require a more thorough analysis than was necessary in the 1980s, and would have to take account of the uncertainties concerning the various risks of continued circulation of poliovirus and of future outbreaks in unprotected populations.

Both chapter 11 and chapter 13 illustrate ideal cases, in which it is possible both to improve health and to save money by a proper choice of strategy. Economic analysis can be decisive in such cases, without the need for questionable assumptions. Both chapters also deal with cases in which costs, or costs relative to effectiveness, can be analyzed without making comparisons across diseases. More often, the question is whether an additional health gain is worth the additional cost involved, relative to other ways of improving health or to nonhealth uses of the resources. In such cases, economic analysis is still helpful but depends more on assumptions and value judgments.

For polio, an effective vaccine existed and costs could be estimated rather well. When the vaccines needed to control diseases do not yet exist and the resources required to create and apply them cannot be known with any certainty, the question becomes, how large would the benefits need to be to justify the likely costs? Alternatively, how cheap would vaccination have to be for a program still to achieve benefits in excess of costs? This is an example of cost-benefit analysis, as distinct from the simpler cost-effectiveness analysis used in the study of malaria control. The benefits in this case could include the reduction in pain, suffering, disability, and death, rather than just the reduction in treatment costs that by itself justified the eradication of polio. Chapter 12 deals with these questions for a hypothetical immunization program considered by the Pan American Health Organization for the control of pneumonia, meningitis, and typhoid fever, including the development of vaccines. The analysis did not actually estimate the benefits: in fact, none of these papers presents a full cost-benefit analysis, because simpler analyses sufficed for the particular questions considered. This avoided the need to make assumptions about unobservable variables—the values or utilities different people attribute to different kinds of benefits.

The use of cost-effectiveness. Cost-effectiveness analysis is the common thread in chapters 8, 9, and 10, as well as chapter 13. Both chapter 8 and chapter 10 derive from the World Bank's *World Development Report 1993: Investing in*

Health (World Bank 1993), which used that analysis as a basis for recommending "essential" packages of health interventions to be given priority in low- and middle-income countries. More particularly, both these chapters derive from criticisms of the approach taken in that report. In the case of chapter 8, the criticism concerned how the "burden of disease" was calculated and used to help determine priorities (Paalman et al. 1998). In the case of chapter 10, the criticism, voiced by many World Bank economists during preparation of the *Report*, was that cost-effectiveness is a wrong, or even an irrelevant, criterion because it does not correspond to maximization of utility or welfare. Arguments continue over both these issues, especially the latter. Economists are trained to look for ways to maximize or at least improve welfare, which depends on many things besides health, while health specialists focus on health gains, often to the exclusion of any other consideration. Economists also differ among themselves on this issue. Some develop and employ cost-effectiveness analysis as a good approximation to cost-benefit analysis based on total welfare (Drummond et al. 1997; Gold et al. 1996), while others reject that approach or are uncomfortable with it.

As chapter 8 shows, some of the criticism of how burden of disease estimates were created and used results from simple misunderstanding. It remains true, however, that such estimates incorporate a number of unverifiable and subjective parameters, so that there is no right answer. Empirical applications of the method in different countries are often not comparable because of different choices about those parameters (Bobadilla 1998). In this respect such calculations violate the recommendation of chapter 6 that the number of arbitrary or subjective parameters should be held to a minimum, preferably to just one. It does not seem possible, however, to follow that rule once the health effects of interest take account of nonfatal disabilities and are therefore more complicated than just additional years of life. Progress in creating broader measures of health status or of the gains from health interventions therefore brings with it the necessity for assumptions that, ideally, reflect consensus about the damage from morbidity and disability.

The argument in chapter 10 was initially developed to justify the cost-effectiveness analysis in the *World Development Report* by starting from the economic theory of an individual consumer and moving toward a societal perspective. It begins by accepting that the health intervention an individual would choose to buy for him- or herself, in order to maximize utility, would not necessarily be the most cost-effective intervention against a particular disease or condition that he or she actually had or was exposed to. Still less would an individual care about the relative cost-effectiveness of interventions against *other* diseases or conditions he or she did not suffer or face a risk from. Nonetheless, when decisions about health interventions are socialized, whether through insurance or, even more clearly, through public finance, cost-effectiveness becomes relevant, as the total potential health gain for a group of people is considered relative to the total resources for purchasing the corresponding interventions. Rather than a right-or-wrong dichotomy, it appears that cost-effectiveness ranges from being largely irrelevant at the individual level—although both costs and effects matter, choices are not necessarily based on the ratio of the two—to being increasingly useful as a criterion for setting priorities as decisions are socialized and concentrated at a collective level.

This argument is more acceptable as one ignores distributional considerations, so that it does not matter *which* individuals gain additional or better years of life, and only totals or averages are considered. It is also more persuasive, as the resources necessary to achieve those gains can be transferred costlessly from one individual to another who can gain more from their use. It is therefore more acceptable, as there is a single agency making the allocation decisions and responsible to all the potential beneficiaries—a situation approximated by the health systems of some rich countries but not at all typical in poor countries. Somewhat paradoxically, then, cost-effectiveness is on firmest ground theoretically in high-income countries where most health care is financed collectively, while the potential gains from emphasizing cost-effective interventions are greatest in poor countries where the bulk of care is paid for out of pocket.

This line of argument, even if fully accepted, certainly does not mean that the cost-effectiveness of different interventions is the *only* criterion needed for choosing which of them to deliver or finance, as some public health professionals, eager to have the apparent support of economists, sometimes assume. Cost-effectiveness is one issue among several, even when the decision concerns only the use of public funds and not what individuals choose to spend out of pocket or on voluntary purchases of health insurance. Chapter 9 specifies no fewer than eight other criteria for public health spending, and shows how several of them are related to cost-effectiveness, sometimes being compatible with it and sometimes at least potentially in conflict. In particular, cost-effectiveness can easily be incompatible with both horizontal and vertical equity. For some interventions, especially those that are public goods, cost-effectiveness is an adequate criterion, whereas for those services that are private and not catastrophically expensive, cost-effectiveness may not affect priorities at all. The connections among such concepts as public goods, externalities, equity, poverty, catastrophic cost, and the proper role of insurance elaborate on some of the arguments in chapter 2. The logic of chapter 9 has been accepted and used in several other instances, including an analysis of the appropriate public sector role in mental health interventions (Beeharry et al. 2002; World Health Organization 2000). Nonetheless, the paper has also fueled continuing controversy about the legitimacy of cost-effectiveness analysis and in particular about whether cost-benefit analysis should always be used instead (Jack 2000; Musgrove 2000).

Beliefs and evidence about malnutrition. There was a widespread suspicion in Brazil in the 1970s and early 1980s that poor consumers were paying more for basic foodstuffs than better-off purchasers, and therefore needed a subsidy to prevent their being even worse off than they would be just because of low incomes. While this may have been true formerly, by the time of the study reported in chapter 14, food markets in the northeast of the country, where poverty is concentrated, were sufficiently competitive that the poor did not systematically pay more for their food. It also turned out that a government food subsidy program, based in part on the assumption of prices being higher for the poor, was not very successful at transferring the full amount of the subsidy to the intended beneficiaries. Policies and programs that are based on incorrect beliefs are less effective than they were intended to be.

Chapter 15 goes beyond the analysis of costs and prices and into cost-effectiveness, to judge whether four different food and nutrition programs in Brazil made any difference to the growth of young children who were the intended beneficiaries. The analysis is based on a number of detailed evaluations of one or more of the programs, conducted by Brazilian researchers. Comparisons among the programs emphasize the variability of outcomes—some children benefited and some did not, and many variables affected the result—and make it clear that malnutrition is due not only to poverty but also to illness and ignorance, so that programs need to address those causes as well. As in the case of tobacco, overly simple assumptions about consumer rationality do not hold up well; it is evident that the people who are supposed to benefit do not always behave as program designers expect. Arguments over which foods people would or should eat, and over whether they needed any assistance other than lower prices to improve their diets and their health, were sometimes quite ideological and based on little evidence (Castro 1985; Musgrove 1986).

Despite these limitations, there were many Brazilian studies that actually measured outcomes. This situation is, alas, quite unusual: In 18 other Latin

American countries, there were many food and nutrition programs in the 1980s but almost no evaluations of results (Musgrove 1993). The available data counted heads (of beneficiaries, or of malnourished children), money spent, and calories or protein distributed, but *not* who consumed the food or whether it made a difference to physical growth or other aspects of health. The amount being spent on the programs might have sufficed to eliminate most malnutrition, if it were better used. However, almost nothing can be concluded about which programs worked best, or how much malnutrition was being prevented or cured

Chapter 16 draws on cost-effectiveness analysis to justify fortification of basic foodstuffs with the three best-studied micronutrients: iron, iodine, and vitamin A. Relatively straightforward economic analysis does not provide any argument against the use of fortification to reach all of the population that suffers, or is at risk of, micronutrient deficiencies *and* that consumes purchased foods. (Households or communities that raise most of their own food are of course harder to reach in this way.) In particular, it is hard to see any reason to consider fortification less natural or less sustainable than other approaches to increasing micronutrient intake, such as promoting household gardens or otherwise changing what people eat. Taken together, the chapters on actual and potential food policies and programs tell a frustrating story—what is actually accomplished in improving child health seems to fall far short of the potential that has been well established by research (Allen and Gillespie 2001).

The research reported in chapters 14 through 17 mostly occurred in the late 1970s and early 1980s, which may give the impression that these matters are of no more than historical interest. However, recent increases in knowledge and changes in consumer behavior contribute to keeping some of these issues very much alive. For one thing, it appears increasingly that much conventional wisdom about diet, often codified into official advice, is seriously wrong (Willett and Stampfer 2003). Fat is not necessarily so bad for one's health, nor carbohydrates always so beneficial, as has been assumed; and it even appears that alcohol, while quite dangerous in excess, is so protective against heart disease that many adults would be better off drinking moderately than not at all (Klatsky 2003). And so far as growth is concerned, scarcity of protein is apparently more of a limitation than inadequacy of calories. Chapter 17 uses information from two surveys in China and a comparison among 41 populations for males and 33 populations for females, to show that availability of protein in the diet is strongly associated with adult heights, and sometimes with adult weights, while caloric availability is much less closely related to height or even to weight. Since growth in height is usually completed in adolescence, and seems to be strongly related to experience in the first few years of life; and since the data are aggregates rather than referring to individuals, it is "astounding" (Wray 2003) to find a clear association with *current* average food intake. This association is always found for males but not always for females; women do not, in many cultures, share equally in what protein is available, and when more protein is consumed on average, it appears that men account for most of the extra consumption. It is a matter of continuing controversy whether the result is due to protein alone or whether various micronutrients, found particularly in foods of animal origin that provide the highest quality protein also affect attained height. In any case, the composition of the diet, and not simply its energy content, appears crucial.

What is not in doubt is that underweight, short stature and micronutrient deficiencies together account for a large share, probably at least one-third, of the burden of disease in poor countries, a burden concentrated among young children but with effects on physical and cognitive development that can last a lifetime (Mason, Musgrove and Habicht 2003). At the same time, the definition of "malnutrition" is broadening beyond these traditional measures of deficiency, to include anthropometric states and health conditions associated with excess. In rich countries such as the United States, and even in middle-income Brazil, overweight children now outnumber those who are underweight, and obesity among adults is epidemic. Meanwhile, programs aimed at feeding poor children continue to operate on the assumption that they eat too little rather than too much (Besharov 2002). It is also clear now that markets can change people's eating habits thoroughly and rapidly, in contrast to the assumption in chapters 15 and 16 that such changes would be sluggish. Governments may need to play a major role in changing habits created or accelerated by the market, and not just traditional eating patterns, to ensure good nutrition.

Paying for Health

Paying for or "financing" health care can be thought of as consisting of three subfunctions: *funding*, or collecting revenues; *pooling* them so as to share risks among individuals and households; and using them for *purchasing* health-related goods and services (World Health Organization 2000, chapter 5). This distinction collapses in the case of out-of-pocket payments, because they are not pooled across households. The act of purchasing coincides with and determines, ex post, the corresponding amount of funding. All financing that is not out of pocket constitutes some form of *prepayment*, which includes all three subfunctions. Chapters 18 through 20 deal with only the first two subfunctions: funding and pooling. Purchasing involves decisions on what goods or services to buy, whom to buy them from, and how to pay the providers. Some of the issues involved are treated in chapter 9.

Funding, pooling, and purchasing are often described as if they followed a temporal as well as a logical sequence—funds are first collected, then allotted to one or more pools, and finally spent from those pools under various purchasing arrangements. This is a useful way to think of the *flow* of funds, which have to be collected somehow in order to go into a pool, but it does not always describe the *decisions* about those funds. For general revenue or "tax-based" financing, which can be considered *implicit insurance* because risks are shared among beneficiaries but there is no defined premium and there may be no defined benefits, a government first collects taxes and then determines what share of revenues to allocate to health. For any kind of *explicit insurance*, whether private or quasi-public (such as social security contributions), the causal relation is actually the other way around. The definition of the pool determines the nature of the funding and the way it is collected. Funds are collected—voluntarily or involuntarily—only because the pool exists, and the volume of funds is the product of the premium or mandatory contribution and the number of contributing members (or the sum of such products, if different insured members pay different premiums or contributions). Decisions that governments take affecting explicit insurance are in the first instance decisions about pooling, with funding as the consequence.

The argument for government to be involved in health financing turns on two facts. First, health needs are often unpredictable and can imply catastrophically high costs for individuals and households: hence the need for insurance rather than relying solely on payment out of pocket at the moment of need. Second, health insurance does not work like insurance for nonhuman assets, because the need for financial protection bears no relation to anyone's capacity to pay. Hence the need not only for subsidies or transfers from the healthy to the sick, parallel to transfers from the lucky to the unlucky in other forms of insurance, but also from the better-off to the worse-off. Pooling of funds is crucial, since it allows for sharing risks and therefore for the first kind of subsidy. Whether it also promotes the second kind depends on who belongs to which pool(s), how much revenue goes into the pool(s), and how the contributions to that revenue are distributed among the insured. Government decisions about health financing therefore typically are joint decisions affecting the sources of revenue and the number, size, and composition of pools and the relations among them.

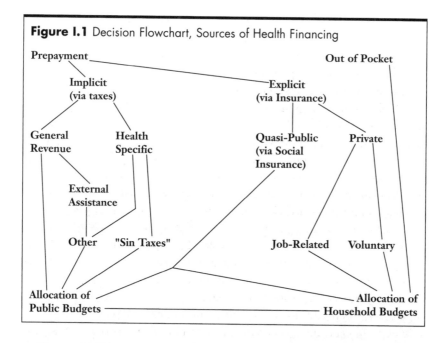

Figure I.1 Decision Flowchart, Sources of Health Financing

Figure I.1 illustrates some of the major choices about funding, starting with the fundamental distinction between prepayment and out-of-pocket spending, and continuing through different kinds of taxes and insurance arrangements to consider how these choices affect both government budgets and those of households (Musgrove 2001). At each stage in the figure, there are choices to be made about using particular taxes or social security schemes and promoting or inhibiting one or more forms of private insurance. Several of the issues related to these choices are not specific to health, since they concern the structure of a tax system and its relation to private sources of finance. What looks at first glance like a good way to raise resources for health may be quite ineffectual, or inequitable, when the entire financing system is considered. There is considerable naïveté on this point in the typical Ministry of Health, so it is worthwhile to create a better understanding of financing issues generally, rather than concentrating only on the size of the public budget or on particular taxes or other funds that are dedicated to health. Here, economic analysis can make a contribution that is independent of the specific epidemiological or medical issues considered in most other chapters. Partly for that reason, it may be easier to reach understanding between economists, whose specialty this is, and public health professionals.

Who pays for health care. Chapter 18 examines the pattern of household spending on health in Latin America three decades ago, using purely economic data that said nothing about health conditions or needs. The fundamental characteristic of the health systems generating the observed expenditures is that public and private health care facilities competed mostly on price, not on quality. As a result, consumers bought private care, which was more expensive but—at least in their opinion—better than subsidized public care as soon as they could afford it, leading to a very high elasticity of expenditure with respect to income. This effect was far from uniform, however; spending on drugs tended to rise quickly and then level off, whereas private hospital costs continued rising with income. This situation reflects the prevalence of self-medication among the poor and the fact that people often have to pay for drugs even if consultations are free or covered by insurance. Treating one input to medical care differently from the others makes little economic sense and merely exploits people's often desperate willingness to pay for medicines. (If what a patient needs are 15 minutes with a nurse or doctor and a bottle of pills, there is likely to be little gain from 30 minutes and no pills, or from no professional diagnosis or advice and two bottles of pills.) There is now much more information available about families' health spending, from household surveys that also ask about episodes of illness and care-seeking behavior; the analysis in chapter 4 is based partly on an early example of such surveys. However, some of the most undesirable features of health financing in poor countries continue largely unchanged.

Except for inexpensive care that presents no serious financial burden to the consumer, out-of-pocket spending is without doubt the worst way to pay for health services. Almost any form of prepayment is preferable. Chapter 19 looks at how health was actually financed in the mid- to late 1990s, using national health accounts estimates or less reliable approximations for all 191 member states of the World Health Organization. The strongest and most disturbing conclusion from that analysis is that out-of-pocket spending is relatively highest in precisely the poorest countries where people most need financial protection. Public spending is often only a small share of the total, and private prepayment is nearly nonexistent. Most spending directly by families is out of pocket, and the burden often falls chiefly on the poor and on rural dwellers who have little access to publicly subsidized care. Impoverishment for health reasons—because people cannot afford care and families lose their livelihoods to death, illness, or injury, or because they become poor paying for care—is a serious risk and a major impediment to poor people's acquisition of capital, whether human or material.

The two great failings of health finance. In static or cross-sectional terms, then, the way health is financed in poor countries is far from ideal. Too much spending is out of pocket, insurance of whatever sort is the privilege of the better off, and public health spending is often financed by dedicated taxes that may be unstable or inequitable and that in any case may not affect total expenditure because other sources are withdrawn in proportion. What is true in comparisons among countries is often true also when comparing how the health care of different population groups is financed. Those who least need prepayment, because they could afford all but catastrophic care, are the best protected, and sometimes also the best covered by public spending.

Dynamically, the situation is often even worse. In an economic crisis or even a downturn in incomes, the needs for health care are likely to rise just when people's capacity to pay for it declines because of lost income or employment and their financial protection weakens or disappears as they lose insurance or social security coverage. When that happens, only public expenditure can fill the breach—but it is usually cut back also, as public revenues fall. There is a strong argument for public spending on health to be counter-cyclical, an argument first made in 1984 (Musgrove 1984). Chapter 20 develops that argument and supports it with Latin American data on health expenditure and economic variables. A counter-cyclical health policy would of course require that planning for health expenditure be contingent on economic circumstances, with explicit decisions to protect health in downturns and to let private or social security spending meet more of the need in boom times. Such a policy would be compensatory through time, as the allocation policies discussed in chapter 6 are compensatory across space. That in turn would require long-term political agreements, including decisions as to which kinds of public spending to cut back when income and revenue fall. No government seems to have achieved such agreements—the political obstacles are daunting—and the response to economic crisis is often improvised. In these as in many other respects, there is still great room for improvement in health financing policies to promote both equity and efficiency.

Concluding Reflections

Economic analysis can lead to or support sound decisions to improve health: chapters 11 and 13, on polio eradication and malaria control, are clear illustrations of the potential benefits. Eventually the economic analysis of tobacco control in chapter 3 may prove of comparable value by overcoming some of the conceptual barriers to such control. And it may be hoped that the findings and arguments in chapters 14 through 17 will lead to more effective efforts to combat the huge problems of different kinds of malnutrition in poor countries. The contribution of health economics to development is potentially even broader than such instances suggest. Economic analysis, properly applied, can often help to clarify what the choices are for health policy, how to choose among different criteria, how to decide what to buy and how to pay for it, and how to evaluate the results. The indirect effects of good economic thinking, when dealing with such questions as the best use of taxes, insurance, and out-of-pocket payment, or the best way for governments to intervene in health, may affect a population's health and welfare more than decisions about how to combat particular maladies or risk factors. If it is true that "the ideas of economists and political philosophers, both when they are right and when they are wrong, are more powerful than is commonly understood" (Keynes 1965), then it is important to get those ideas right. This is especially so when the issues are increasingly complex and when ideology and misunderstanding, although on the decline, are still widespread.

Getting the ideas right is not easy, for those same reasons. The importance and peculiarities of health insurance, and the reasons why competitive private markets for it are likely to produce both inequity and inefficiency (Arrow 1963) are now widely understood. How to deal with these market failures without falling into equally dangerous government failures is a question still only partly settled. And while there is far more understanding and even rapprochement among economists and public health specialists concerning the state and the market than there was a few decades ago, the right balance of roles and the right choice of instruments continue to be debated, sometimes acrimoniously. Similarly, there is today much more understanding than formerly of how to relate the costs of health interventions to the various kinds of benefits they can yield, including their effectiveness in improving health. But controversy continues over the legitimacy and applicability of different methods, particularly when comparisons need to be made over different diseases or conditions, people with different health or economic prospects or cultural views, or completely different kinds of beneficial or harmful outcomes. Several of the chapters here try to develop better answers to these questions, or to provide persuasive counter-arguments to some wrong answers and mistaken views. The reader may judge how well this has been accomplished, and perhaps learn a little more about both the meanings of health economics in development.

References

Allen, Lindsay, and Stuart Gillespie. 2001. *What Works? A Review of the Efficacy and Effectiveness of Nutrition Interventions*. Manila: United Nations Administrative Committee on Coordination, Sub-Committee on Nutrition, and Asian Development Bank.

Arrow, Kenneth. 1963. "Uncertainty and the Welfare Economics of Medical Care." *American Economic Review* 53: 941–73.

Beeharry, Girindre, Harvey Whiteford, David Chambers, and Florence Baingana. 2002. "Outlining the Scope for Public Involvement in Mental Health." World Health Organization working paper. Geneva: World Health Organization.

Besharov, Douglas J. 2002. "We're Feeding the Poor as If They're Starving." *The Washington Post*, December 8, p. B-1.

Bobadilla, José Luis. 1998. *Searching for Essential Health Services in Low- and Middle-Income Countries*. Policy Background Study No. SOC-106. Washington, D.C.: Inter-American Development Bank.

Castro, Cláudio M. 1985. "Fubá, Formulados e Fundamentalistas." In Cláudio M. Castro and Marcos Coimbra, eds., *O Problema Alimentar no Brasil*. São Paulo: Almed Editora.

Castro, Cláudio M., and Philip Musgrove. 2000. "On the Non-Existence of 'The Social Sector,' or Why Health and Education Are More Different than Alike." Working Paper. Washington, D.C.: Inter-American Development Bank.

Creese, Andrew. 1991. User charges for health care: a review of recent experience. *Health Policy and Planning* (6)4: 309–319.

Drummond, Michael, Bernie O'Brien, Greg L. Stoddart, and George W. Torrance. 1997. *Methods for the Economic Evaluation of Health Care Programmes*. 2nd edition. Oxford: Oxford University Press.

Gold, Marthe R., Joanna E. Siegel, Louise B. Russell, and Milton C. Weinstein, eds. 1996. *Cost-Effectiveness in Health and Medicine*. New York and Oxford: Oxford University Press.

Hirschleifer, Jack. 1985. "The Expanding Domain of Economics." *American Economic Review*, 75, *Supplement*: 53–68.

Hsiao, William C. 2000. "What Should Macroeconomists Know about Health Care Policy? A Primer." Working Paper. Washington, D.C.: International Monetary Fund.

Jack, William. 2000. "Public Spending on Health Care: How Are Different Criteria Related ? A Second Opinion." *Health Policy* 54: 3.

Keynes, John Maynard. 1965. *The General Theory of Employment, Interest and Money*. First Harbinger Edition. New York: Harcourt, Brace and World, p. 383.

Klatsky, Arthur J. 2003. "Drink to Your Health?" *Scientific American* 288(2), February: 75–81.

Lohr, K. N., R. H. Brook, C. J. Kamberg, G. A. Goldberg, A. Leibowitz, J. Keesey, D. Reboussin, and J. P. Newhouse. 1986. "Use of medical care in the RAND health insurance experiment: diagnosis- and service-specific analyses in a randomized control trial." *Medical Care* 24 (supplement), 51–587.

Mason, John B., Philip Musgrove, and Jean-Pierre Habicht. 2003. "At Least One-third of Poor Countries' Disease Burden Is Due to Malnutrition." Disease Control Priorities Project Working Paper No. 1. Bethesda, Md.: Fogarty International Center, National Institutes of Health.

Miller, Jonathan. 1978. *The Body in Question.* New York: Random House.

Musgrove, Philip. 1984. "Health Care and Economic Hardship." *World Health,* October: 27–29.

———. 1986. "Ideología, Pesquisa y Realidad de la Situación Alimentaria y Nutricional del Brasil." *Cadernos de Estudos Sociais* (Recife, Brazil) 1(3), January–June: 329–348.

———. 2000. "Cost-Effectiveness as a Criterion for Public Spending on Health: A Reply to William Jack's 'Second Opinion'." *Health Policy* 54: 229–233.

———. 2001. "Choices in Health Financing." Draft paper for the World Health Organization. Geneva.

Newbrander, William, David Collins, and Lucy Gilson. 2000. *Ensuring Equal Access to Health Services: User Fee Systems and the Poor.* Boston: Management Sciences for Health.

Paalman, Maria, Henk Bekedam, Laura Hawken, and David Nyheim. 1998. "A Critical Review of Priority Setting in the Health Sector: The Methodology of the 1993 World Development Report." *Health Policy and Planning* 13(1): 13–31.

Ruger, Jennifer P., Dean T. Jamison, and David E. Bloom. 2001. "Health and the Economy." In Michael H. Merson, Robert E. Black, and Anne J. Mills, eds., *International Public Health: Diseases, Programs, Systems, and Policies.* Gaithersburg, Md.: Aspen.

Willett, Walter J., and Meir J. Stampfer. 2003. "Rebuilding the Food Pyramid." *Scientific American* 288(1), January: 64–71.

World Bank. 1993. *World Development Report 1993: Investing in Health.* Washington, D.C.

World Health Organization. 2002. Informal Consultation on Economics Research on Post-Certification Polio Immunization Policies. October 7–8, Geneva.

———. 2000. *World Health Report 2000—Health Systems: Improving Performance.* Geneva.

Wray, Joe, 2003. "Response to 'Malnutrition and dietary protein: Evidence from China and from international comparisons': Commentary." *Food and Nutrition Bulletin* 24: 291–5.

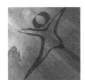

CHAPTER 1

What Is the Minimum a Doctor Should Know about Health Economics?

Acknowledgments

I must thank Bertoldo Kruse for inviting these reflections. Many colleagues and friends have contributed to these ideas, particularly those associated with the World Bank's Flagship Course in Health Reform. None of them bears any responsibility for what is said here.

Why Do Doctors Need to Know *Any* Health Economics?

The answer to this question is not obvious: after all, when a physician is actually practicing medicine there seems to be no room or need for economic understanding. In fact, it might get in the way, when what the doctor wants is to concentrate on the patient before him or her and bring to bear all his or her medical knowledge, which is typically much more detailed—and certainly more important at the moment of diagnosis or treatment—than what an economist typically knows or thinks about. And doctors have been treating patients, well or badly, for centuries without troubling themselves with economic concerns.

Economics perhaps has no place in the surgery, the consulting room or the laboratory, but that is not what matters. In each of those settings, resources are being used and a production process is under way, supposedly for the benefit of a consumer—and the use of limited resources to produce

Reprinted, with permission, from *Revista Brasileira de Saúde Materno-Infantil* 1(2), May–August 2001, (Recife, Brazil).

goods and services for intermediate or ultimate consumers is what economics is primarily about. How those resources are themselves produced, how they are combined, who chooses what to produce with them, who will pay for them, and what all that costs, create the setting in which the physician operates. Almost everything that happens prior to the encounter between the physician and the patient is relevant to the economist, even if the latter is kept outside of the medical practice itself. If there is something the doctor ought to know of health economics, it concerns those prior steps, including many of the factors that bring the patient to his or her attention in the first place.

There are at least three reasons why a physician might disregard this argument and suppose that economics has nothing useful to offer his or her profession. One is the fact that health economics is a relatively new subdiscipline. The seminal article explaining some of the subtleties that distinguish health from other sectors, particularly in relation to how it is financed, was published only in 1963 [1]. That opened the whole field of inquiry into risks and information that characterize health economics today and that has become steadily more important as more and more of health care is financed by insurance and the costs of it have risen. The *Journal of Health Economics*, the first publication devoted entirely to the subject, began to publish only in 1982; by now there is an entire two-volume *Handbook of Health Economics* [2] and a number of journals that publish on the subject. Economists are quick to "invade" fields they find interesting, and the practitioners of those subjects may take time to notice that they have become of economic interest.

A second reason is the mistaken supposition that economics is nothing more than accounting, and while accounts must be kept in medical practice as in other professions, the logic of the accounting is no different and the accountant has no special insights to offer. Much of economics does in fact depend on proper accounting: the creation of national accounts of income and product, starting more than a half-century ago, is the precursor of today's effort to create national health accounts [3] to show where the funds spent on health come from and where they go. But the interpretation of those flows does not follow only from their magnitude, but from economic theory about how doctors, patients, and financing agencies behave.

A third, even more mistaken reason, is summarized in the attitude that "health is not a business", or should not be one. Some doctors, and public health professionals in particular, often find it hard to accept that health care is financed, produced and delivered in a constellation of markets—as though markets or "business" were intrinsically inimical to human health. This argument usually rests on the claim that health care is a basic right or a basic need, and therefore too important to be left to markets. But food, which is a much more basic necessity than health care, is produced and delivered in markets, and there is nothing wrong with that. The question, in the case of health care, is whether those markets work in socially desirable ways, or whether they lead to situations in which some people cannot afford needed care, or the wrong kinds of care are produced, or at too high a cost, or something else goes wrong. Economics is, to a large extent, the science of how markets operate, so it is extremely relevant to markets in which failure may be a matter of life and death.

What Economics Does a Doctor *Not* Need to Know?

So it might be helpful for medical professionals to understand some economics, as it applies to medicine and health. Does that mean they need to comprehend all of economics, or would it be safe to ignore large areas of the subject? Fortunately, there is much that a doctor does not need to know, starting with the specific economic issues that arise in sectors very different from health. The frequent (and frequently loose) use of the adjective "social" to describe some sectors of the economy might suggest that medical professionals wanting to understand health economics need to know something about the economics of related sectors such as education. Fortunately, this is not the case: in economic terms these fields are much more different than they are alike [4], and although similar issues arise in both [5], it is more confusing than helpful to think of a general economics of "the social sector". The peculiarities of health economics mean that a doctor wanting to learn something about it need not try to understand the economics of any other sector in detail.

Currently there is great interest in what might be called "the macroeconomics of health", and a Commission on Macroeconomics and Health [6] has been created to study particularly the question of whether better population health contributes to economic growth, making health even more of a paying investment than it has traditionally been considered from an individual's perspective [7]. That is an interesting question, but health does not need to be subordinated to income or growth in order to be regarded as vitally important. (It is even dangerous to justify health investments by appealing to their effect on economic outcomes, since such investments may pay off best for young adults and thereby lead to discrimination against the very young and the very old.) And even if there is a strong connection, it does not mean that medical professionals need to know anything about macroeconomic theory in order to learn something useful for their own field. All that a doctor should know is that there are good macroeconomic policies and bad ones, that inflationary populism is a very bad policy and that poor macroeconomic management is bad for a country's health, particularly the health of poor people. Much of the criticism directed at "structural adjustment" and its supposed damaging effects on health really should be directed at the economic irresponsibility that sometimes made such adjustment necessary in the first place [8].

Of course, what economists think they know is often a mixture of what they know and what they only think, including their more ideological positions and beliefs. (The same is true of public health specialists, to be sure.) One reason that doctors are reluctant to learn more economics is that they reject some views as ideological—sometimes with good reason, sometimes mistakenly. For example, the claim by economists that most of the time, markets are an efficient mechanism for allocating resources to production and consumption may sound like ideology, but it is actually a strong empirical proposition. The history of efforts to control prices, dictate production or otherwise interfere with the normal working of markets, including particularly the sad history of Soviet-style economic management, offers abundant evidence. However, the claim by some economists that all markets are basically alike, and that in particular markets work just as well in health care as anywhere else, is not well supported either theoretically or empirically but includes a large dose of ideology. One needs to understand how markets work, without being taken in by "the mystique of markets" [9].

Doctors who have never talked much with economists—or who have had the misfortune to talk only to mediocre economists—often think that economists care only about efficiency and not at all about equity, equality, rights, or the suffering of the sick and the dispossessed. It is certainly true that in economic theory, it is easier to agree on what constitutes or leads to efficiency than to agree about equity; and it is also true that inefficiency means waste, which means less of something desirable for someone. But economic thought also includes a long and deep tradition of thinking about ethical issues, about what constitutes a just society, about rights and entitlements [10] and about the possible conflicts between equity and efficiency and the frequent necessity for choices among societal objectives [11]. Even for such a relatively narrow question as what health interventions to purchase with public money, there are no fewer than nine relevant criteria, of which at least three concern equity rather than efficiency [12]. The conclusion to draw from all this is that a doctor wanting or needing to learn some economics does not have to abandon his or her ethical principles or political views. What he or she should be prepared to do is to question those principles and views in the light of economics and see how well they hold up. Economic thinking can help to identify contradictions or poorly formulated opinions. It does not impose a set of ethical or political suppositions or preferences. (In fact, the economics of consumer behavior starts with an unquestioned respect for preferences.)

Understanding How Economists Think

More than knowing any particular conclusion of economics, a doctor needs to understand the way that economists think: incomprehension and conflict arise more from differences in the way the two professions approach questions, than from the specific answers to those questions. An economist does not, contrary to popular superstition, think only or primarily about money, even if he or she often tries to find monetary equivalents of other measures. Economists think about *resources*, and particularly about whether those resources have *prices* and if so, whether they are the right prices to assure efficiency or equity. Since resources have *costs*, whether those are recognized or not, economists want to know if the use of those resources produces *effects* (non-monetary) or *benefits* (usually monetized) sufficient to justify how they are used. Much work in economics is devoted to comparisons among these concepts, under the names of *cost-effectiveness analysis*, *cost-utility analysis* or *cost-benefit analysis* [13]. It is important for doctors to understand that while costs are the specialty of economists, the definition and estimation of effects or outcomes is the province of medical professionals: these analyses have to be joint efforts. Given an estimate of an effect (deaths averted, for example), economists often then go on to try to put a monetary value on the result, and such efforts can be questioned and rejected. What a doctor needs to understand is that while any particular kind of effect can be related to costs without monetizing the effect, there is no common currency besides money in which to compare different kinds of effects (health outcomes versus education, say), and that to avoid monetary valuations is to abstain from all such cross-sectoral comparisons.

As mentioned earlier, economists naturally think about markets, ideally without any prior assumptions about how well they work. To reject the idea of markets because some market outcomes are inefficient or inequitable or both, is to miss one of the main ideas that economists always carry with them. But markets are not simply theaters in which two characters called "supply" and "demand" interact, important as those two concepts are. Markets are places where people interact, in many different roles, as payers, investors, providers, patients, consumers and citizens; so economists concentrate on the *behavior* that occurs in markets, and in particular on the *incentives* that people face to behave one way or another. It is true that economists tend to talk mostly about financial or economic incentives, because they understand those best. That does not mean that other incentives—the desire to help others, professional pride, and so on—do not matter, only that economic analysis starts by taking those for granted, and then asks what happens to behavior when prices, means of payment, regulations or other incentives are modified. Particularly in the health sector, the economic incentives are often perverse, acting contrary to the desired outcomes, so it is crucial to analyze them and correct them if possible.

In considering the incentives and regulations to behave one way or another, economists have to assume that behavior is not simply a collection of responses to random impulses, but that people have some set of goals or objective function, that they are trying to get the most (or the least) of something out of their actions. It makes a difference, sometimes a great difference, what those objectives are. For example, a producer of a good or service will behave differently, depending on whether he or she aims to maximize profits, to maximize revenue, to assure a particular level of income, to capture a particular share of a market, to minimize risk, or to produce the highest possible quality of output. Since objectives are not always stated, and may not even be clearly known to the agent whose behavior is of interest, there is necessarily some speculation involved, and the confrontation of different assumptions with observed behavior. In this respect, economics has much more in common with psychology than with accounting or engineering. Incentives, to be effective, have to work on people's objectives; misunderstanding what they want or are trying to do can lead to perverse incentives and unwanted outcomes.

Finally, economists pay much attention to who has, and who needs, how much and what kind of *information*. People make all kinds of decisions based on the information they have (or think they have), and entire markets can work badly when information is incomplete (no one knows) or asymmetric (buyers know more than sellers, or vice versa), particularly if revealing information would damage the interests of the person who has it. Ignorance is obviously dangerous in the face of an epidemic, or for a person who faces a risk but is unaware of it or does not respond to information about it. Smoking is a marked example of this danger [14, especially chapters 7 and 8]. Some kinds of information lend themselves to accounting and standardized reporting (the basis of national health accounts and of much of epidemiology), but others do not, because they concern only individual actors or are costly to collect or interpret. Medical professionals also recognize the importance of information for detection, diagnosis, treatment and evaluation. What economic thinking adds is the emphasis on how information or the lack of it influences behavior, with economically important consequences [15].

Important Specifics of Health Economics

First, health is a very peculiar asset because unlike almost anything else, including even some other forms of human capital, it is almost entirely inalienable. One can donate blood or even a kidney to improve someone else's health, but "health" itself cannot be transferred, and one must have some state of health, however poor. Since health is subject to many random shocks of illness or accident, and since health care can be catastrophically costly, one needs insurance against financial risk as well as the protection against physical risks provided by good nutrition, exercise and a range of public health measures such as sanitation and immunization. But the character of health makes it harder to insure than other assets, especially since the value of one's health and the financial risk are not correlated with one's capacity to pay. Thus one of the principal obstacles to making a health system work properly, is the difficulty of financing it so as to provide a reasonable and affordable degree of protection to everyone, without creating incentives either to do without such protection or to over-use medical care because the cost is borne by others—and while assuring that subsidies flow in the desirable directions. This difficulty is independent of the amount spent on health.

The emphasis on *financing* in discussions of health economics is entirely justified, then; but a doctor also needs to understand that there are three parts to it. It matters not only how health is *funded*, that is, who pays for it and through what mechanisms (taxes, social security, voluntary insurance, charity, out of pocket payments) but also whether and how those funds are *pooled* to share risks among population groups, and how they are then used to *purchase* goods and services [16, chapter 5]. Each of these stages presents its own set of questions and difficulties, often with conflicts between economic efficiency and equity or fairness.

One important source of conflict is that what people *want* in the way of health care does not necessarily match what doctors think people *need*; and when needs and demands do not coincide, it is impossible for the *supply* of services simultaneously to satisfy both of them [17, pp. 23–24]. Several of the reasons why need, demand and supply do not automatically match up, go by the name of "market failure", meaning that while there is a working market for health care, it does not reach the kind of efficient equilibrium that a so-called perfect market would achieve. Doctors need to understand these reasons, which include standard economic concepts such as public goods, externalities, information failures, and non-competitive behavior. They also need to distinguish these problems from other reasons for unsatisfactory health outcomes which are just as important but which are not "failures" in the economist's sense—such as poverty, and inequality of risks or of income.

"Failure" is one word to which economists give a fairly exact meaning that may not match the commonsense notion doctors are likely to have, and it is important, as in any dialog, to develop a clear, shared vocabulary. Arguing over whose definition to use, or not recognizing that the same word may be used in two meanings, is wasteful: the best example of this is the difference between the economist's term "public good" and the medical sense of "public health". All public goods in health are part of public health, but the converse is not true, and the difference matters for public policy.

Purchasing, the last stage of financing health, involves two complex questions: what to buy, and how to pay the providers—doctors, hospitals, vendors of goods and services. The difference between need and want, and the enormous variation in costs of medical procedures, are crucial for the first choice, as is the definition of what one is trying to achieve. Maximal overall population health as an objective will lead to different choices than improving the health of the worst-off, or giving everyone something like the same chance to have his or her health problems resolved. And doctors need to understand that while the size of a health problem—for example, the burden of disease attributed to a particular disease or condition—is highly relevant to how much it might cost to deal with the problem, decisions about what interventions should have priority do not depend simply on the magnitude of the problem [18, 19]. A full evaluation of a health system draws on many different kinds of information [20]; some ways of using or combining different kinds of data are useful or legitimate, and some are not.

Incentives are crucially important to the second question, and deciding on the best way to pay providers is greatly complicated by a feature that is peculiar to health care—the practice of referral from one level or type of facility or professional to another. There does not seem to be one ideal way to pay all the different providers involved in a system, so a doctor needs to understand the virtues and deficiencies of different payment systems (fee-for-service, global budget, per bed-day, for diagnostic-related groups, and so on) and how they interact. Aligning incentives and creating a good institutional environment is most important for hospitals, the most complex organizations in the health system [16, chapter 3].

How to pay, as opposed to how much to pay, is an example of the importance of institutions and regulations in health economics: it is not a matter of costs, in the first instance, but it may have a large impact on both costs and health outcomes. More generally, doctors need to know that much of health economics is concerned with the rules of the game and not simply with the flows of money, goods and services. One particular issue of this sort is that of the right degree of autonomy for individual doctors and for the organizations in which they work and the organizations which purchase their services—which are not the same, when there is a "purchaser-provider split" between funding and purchasing agencies, and the producers of medical services. Too little autonomy, too much dictation from above or outside, is practically a guarantee of waste; too much freedom may be an invitation to abuse, low quality or excessive costs. As with many other issues, economics does not provide final answers, but it does offer a way of thinking about them that can facilitate better decisions and ultimately better outcomes.

Gains From Better Understanding

Suppose a medical professional accepts the need to understand some health economics, perhaps including the specific ideas just discussed. What can he or she hope to gain thereby? What is the likely pay-off for the effort involved in learning some new vocabulary, accepting new and different viewpoints, and possibly having to give up or modify some cherished ideas? The most obvious benefit is that it becomes easier to talk with economists, when one cannot avoid doing so—and as decisions about health care come to depend more and more on economic considerations, it becomes harder to keep economists out of the discussion. Doctors sometimes fear being crowded out of decisions over which historically they had full control. Perhaps the best way to assure that their knowledge and views continue to be respected is to learn something about the knowledge and views of the newcomers to the other side of the table. Reducing the level of incomprehension and antagonism that often characterizes such encounters at first, is worth some trouble.

Ideally, better mutual understanding between medical professionals and economists will actually improve the efficiency of health care, and maybe even its equity. By examining their own behavior and responses to incentives in the light of economics, doctors may see ways to be more effective or less wasteful of resources; and they should be better prepared to accept, and influence, reforms to how they work and how they are paid. There is nothing guaranteed, or easy, about reform processes in health, but they seem sure to work better when all involved have at least some knowledge of all the relevant factors. For society as a whole, a better working health system is clearly the greatest potential gain from a fuller understanding between the two professions.

Finally, at least for some medical professionals there can be a purely scientific or intellectual pleasure in exploring the thinking of another profession and thereby seeing one's own profession differently. Of course, this can lead to frustration, because the new ideas may be hard to put into practice and can lead to friction with one's own colleagues. This is especially likely when techniques of economic evaluation are stretched too far or their results conflict too strongly with perceived political imperatives [20, pp. 12–17]. But such stretching and conflict are often a necessary part of learning, and may ultimately be the basis for different political imperatives and reform opportunities.

References

[1]   Kenneth Arrow, "Uncertainty and the Welfare Economics of Medical Care". *American Economic Review 53: 941–73*, 1963.

[2]   Anthony J. Culyer and Joseph P. Newhouse, eds., *Handbook of Health Economics*. Volume 17 of *Handbooks in Economics*. Amsterdam: Elsevier, 2000.

[3]   Jean-Pierre Poullier and Patricia Hernández, "Estimates of National Health Accounts (NHA) for 1997", WHO/EIP Discussion Paper 27. Geneva: World Health Organization, 2000.

[4] Cláudio de Moura Castro and Philip Musgrove, "On the Nonexistence of 'the Social Sector', or why Education and Health are more different than alike". Washington, DC: Inter-American Development Bank discussion paper, 2000.

[5] Emmanuel Jiménez, *Pricing Policy in the Social Sectors: Cost Recovery for Education and Health in Developing Countries*. Baltimore: Johns Hopkins University Press for the World Bank, 1987.

[6] World Health Organization, Evidence and Information for Policy, *The Commission on Macroeconomics and Health (CMH): Overview*. Geneva: World Health Organization, 2000.

[7] William D. Savedoff and T. Paul Schultz, eds., *Wealth from Health: Linking Social Investments to Earnings in Latin America*. Washington, DC: Inter-American Development Bank, 2000.

[8] Michel Garenne and Eneas Gakusi, "Health Effects of Structural Adjustment Programs in sub-Saharan Africa". Paris: French Center for Population and Development Studies (CEPED) working paper, 2000.

[9] Sara Bennett, *The mystique of markets: public and private health care in developing countries*. London: London School of Hygiene and Tropical Medicine, Public Health and Policy Department Publication No. 4, 1991.

[10] Amartya Sen, *Poverty and Famines: an Essay on Entitlement and Deprivation*. Oxford: Oxford University Press, 1982

[11] Arthur M. Okun, *Equity and Efficiency: the Big Trade-Off*. Washington, DC: the Brookings Institution, 1975.

[12] Philip Musgrove, "Public Spending on Health Care: How are Different Criteria Related?" *Health Policy 47: 207–223*, 1999.

[13] Michael Drummond, Bernie O'Brien, Greg L. Stoddart and George W. Torrance, *Methods for the Economic Evaluation of Health Care Programmes*. 2nd edition. Oxford: Oxford University Press, 1997.

[14] Prabhat Jha and Frank Chaloupka, eds., *Tobacco Control in Developing Countries*. Oxford: Oxford University Press, 2000.

[15] Victor R. Fuchs, *The Health Economy*. Cambridge, MA: Harvard University Press, 1986.

[16] World Health Organization, *World Health Report 2000 – Health Systems: Improving Performance*. Geneva: WHO, 2000.

[17] Philip Musgrove, *Public and Private Roles in Health: Theory and Financing Patterns*. Washington, DC: World Bank discussion paper No. 339, 1996.

[18] Dean T. Jamison, W. Henry Mosley, Anthony R. Measham and José Luis Bobadilla, *Disease Control Priorities in Developing Countries*. Oxford: Oxford University Press for the World Bank, 1993.

[19] World Bank, *World Development Report 1993: Investing in Health*. Washington, DC: the World Bank, 1993.

[20] George E. Cumper, *The Evaluation of National Health Systems*. Oxford: Oxford University Press (Oxford Medical Publications), 1991.

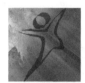

CHAPTER 2

Public and Private Roles in Health

Acknowledgments

This paper was written under the guidance of David de Ferranti, who also commented extensively on the first draft and made a valuable suggestion about the overall structure. Jacques van der Gaag, George Schieber and David Dunlop read early versions of the paper and provided immensely helpful information, suggestions and encouragement. Howard Barnum, José-Luis Bobadilla, Xavier Coll and Helen Saxenian also offered useful comments. Linda Kean edited the paper to take all these comments into account. The final version benefited from written review by Nicholas Barr, Ralph Harbison, Elizabeth King, Maureen Lewis, Samuel Lieberman, Paul Shaw and Verdon Staines, and verbal comments by Jeffrey Hammer. Any remaining errors or confusions are the author's sole responsibility.

Why the Public Role in Health Care Matters

Health care in about 1990 cost at least $1.7 trillion, or about 8 percent of world income [Murray, Govindaraj and Musgrove 1994], making it one of the largest industries in the global economy. On average, 60 percent of this is public spending. If this spending is excessive or otherwise inappropriate, the consequences for the economy and for health outcomes could be substantial. Governments also provide a large share of health services, sometimes as large as the share in spending, and often intervene in various ways in the private health care market. Since most health care is a private good, it is surprising that so much of it is provided, financed or regulated by the

Excerpted, with permission, from *Public and private roles in health: Theory and financing patterns*. World Bank Discussion Paper No. 339, 1996.

state. In contrast to what happens in many other sectors of the economy, this substantial public role is most pronounced in high income countries which are generally very market-oriented; the state usually finances a smaller share of health care in poorer countries. Does this pattern provide models for the future development of the health sector and the public role in it, for low-income countries? And is the variation among countries in the amount and kind of public intervention associated with differences in people's health, in what is spent on health care or in how well health systems function?

Besides consuming large resources, many health systems are regarded as inefficient or inequitable or both; they are often described as in "crisis", as needing "reform", or as having "failed". Are the supposed failures of health systems real? If so, they might be caused by misguided public intervention, so they could be corrected by a smaller or different public role and a greater reliance on private markets. Or governments might intervene for sound reasons, to correct or compensate for failings in those markets; that is, outcomes would be even worse if left entirely to the private sector. Is there an appropriate frontier between private and public action, and a best combination of instruments for the state to use when it intervenes? These and related questions must be confronted in any reform effort [Aaron 1994, Cutler 1994, OECD 1994]. It is relatively simple to conclude that governments should do certain things and should leave others to private activity; but often there is a variety of possible solutions and no obviously best approach. Theory does not always provide clear answers, and the empirical evidence is incomplete, extremely varied and difficult to interpret.

Choices for State Intervention

It matters not only *whether* governments intervene, but also *how* they do it: the second essential question is what the public sector should do, given that some problem in the private market appears to warrant some public action. This is particularly important because government failings in the health sector are also common, and often result from intervening in the wrong ways or with the wrong instruments. There are five distinct instruments of public intervention: arranged from the least to the greatest intrusion into private decisions, these are to—

- *inform*, which may mean to persuade, but does not require anyone to do anything. Governments do this when they publicize the health risks of smoking, or include health and basic hygiene education in public schools. These are examples of information directed at consumers, but governments also inform health care providers and suppliers of health care inputs, as by conducting research and disseminating information on disease patterns and on the effects and risks of medical procedures.

- *regulate*, which determines how a private activity may be undertaken. Governments sometimes regulate the medical profession by setting standards for doctors or accrediting hospitals, although these activities may also be undertaken by private bodies. And government regulation is common in the insurance industry, in the importation of medical equipment, drugs and supplies and in the protection of food and water quality. More generally, governments can influence private health care activity in many ways, often combining regulation with some financial incentives to offset the costs [Bennett et al. 1994] but without public financing. Regulation is usually pursuant to a law, and is often determined by an executive or administrative body.

- *mandate*, which obligates someone to do something and (usually, though not always) to pay for it. Compliance with regulations can also imply substantial private costs; but a mandated activity is different in that it *must* be performed, whereas a private producer can react to regulation by choosing not to undertake the activity. Mandates are usually specified in law, which may subsequently be adumbrated by regulation. The most important mandates, in financial terms, are the requirements that employers provide health services or insurance to their employees, or contribute to social insurance funds for that purpose. Governments can also impose mandates on individuals, as by requiring that children entering school be immunized.

- *finance* health care with public funds. Because mandated insurance is effectively paid for by an earmarked, involuntary contribution which is equivalent to a tax, "public" health expenditure is commonly defined to include such costs along with expenditures from public budgets. The obverse of spending public funds is to tax particular activities or goods, such as alcohol and tobacco, at least partly for health reasons. This issue is not treated here; while taxation which reduces consumption of specific goods may have substantial health effects, it is always limited to very few goods and is not used systematically to promote health. Finally, the state may—

- *provide* or deliver services, using publicly-owned facilities and civil service staff. This is what Ministries of Health in most poor countries do; so do various governmental bodies in many countries at all income levels.

Once a society has decided to finance health services with public funds, the choice arises of whether to provide them through public facilities or to pay private producers to provide them. The appropriate way to consider this choice is as a standard "make or buy" decision. The issues for a government are the same as for a private firm, and turn on costs—is it cheaper to produce something than to buy from an outside supplier?— and on the risks and difficulties of enforcing contracts and avoiding fraud when dealing with such suppliers [Coase 1988].

Because public financing requires public resources, it is perhaps the crucial choice about state action. However, all the instruments mentioned have costs; even information is not free. The benefits from any intervention have always to be weighed against these costs. In addition, sometimes two instruments overlap, or one requires the use of another: mandates imply regulation, and public provision usually implies at least partial public finance. (User fees or even private insurance payments to public facilities may cover part of the cost and could in principle cover all of it.) And two instruments can be alternatives: for part of the population, governments can either finance health care or mandate financing by employers or other private institutions. Differences in ability to pay make it natural to operate mixed systems of public intervention, such as mandated coverage for the non-poor and public finance for the poor. There are alternatives even within mandated coverage, such as "play or pay" arrangements in which employers can finance health care directly for their employees or pay into a social security scheme.

A Conceptual Basis for Public and Private Roles in Health

The health sector is sufficiently complicated, and the conditions of countries are sufficiently different, that economic theory by itself is an inadequate guide to where the frontier should be drawn between the private economy and state action, or to which state interventions should be undertaken, and in what degree. Nonetheless, theory is essential, particularly where two issues are concerned. Both of these refer to *market failure*, or circumstances in which private markets either cannot be expected to function at all, or can be expected to yield undesirable outcomes which appropriate public intervention might improve on. Some such failures may occur in any sector of the economy; traditional public finance theory [Musgrave 1959] explains these cases and provides guidance for public action. Other possible failures arise where insurance is involved, and for reasons specific to the health sector, present particularly acute problems for health insurance [Arrow 1963, 1985].

Since what the health care sector provides to consumers and beneficiaries are specific activities or *interventions*, it is useful to organize a conceptual basis according to distinctions among these activities. The next section provides this classification; three subsections elaborate on the peculiarities of each area.

The three domains of health care

While the activities that promote, protect or restore health are very heterogeneous, they fall into three natural domains, corresponding to *public goods*, to *low-cost private interventions* and to *catastrophically costly private goods*. These domains are constructed by classifying health-related activities along two dimensions, as shown in Figure 2.1: first by the degree to which they are private or public goods, and second, by how much they cost. Both dimensions refer only to characteristics of particular activities or interventions themselves, *not* to who consumes them or pays for them. As the descriptions of the three domains indicate, private goods are separated into low-cost and high-cost, whereas all public goods constitute one domain, regardless of their cost. The reason for this is that while the costs of public goods matter for deciding whether they should be produced, the issue of market failure related to such goods is independent of costs. With private goods, in contrast, some problems of market failure occur only with those services costly enough to be financed by insurance; and poverty, or the inability to buy even low-cost services, is a distinct reason for public intervention.

This classification of health-related activities does not reserve a place for "merit goods", interventions which everyone "ought to have". To exclude this category is not to deny the social or political importance of views about what people "have a right to". The difficulty is that there is no good way to define such goods *a priori*, and societies make different choices about them. Moreover, so far as these goods are supposed to justify public intervention, there are often other grounds for state financing, mandating or regulating of the goods or services regarded as meritorious. For example, it is widely believed that all children have a right to immunization, but public promotion of immunization can also be justified by the market failures involved.

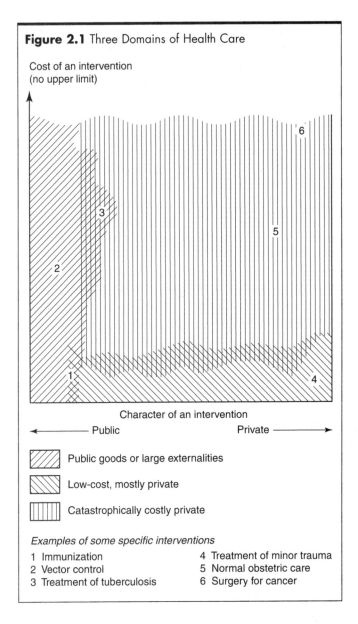

Figure 2.1 Three Domains of Health Care

Cost of an intervention
(no upper limit)

Character of an intervention

◄──────── Public   Private ──────►

Public goods or large externalities

Low-cost, mostly private

Catastrophically costly private

Examples of some specific interventions

1 Immunization   4 Treatment of minor trauma
2 Vector control   5 Normal obstetric care
3 Treatment of tuberculosis   6 Surgery for cancer

A particular intervention occupies a small space in Figure 2.1; to indicate how different interventions would be classified into the three domains, some typical health care activities are located approximately. The cost of an intervention can vary depending on many factors, such as how widespread the intervention is; there can also be variation in the public or private good nature of an activity. Because a health *system* produces a variety of interventions in all three domains, it is spread widely over the space. Figure 2.1 therefore does not serve to compare different systems.

Public goods are goods or services such that one person's consumption does not reduce the amount available for others to consume. Typically these are goods from which consumers cannot be excluded: if they are made available to anyone, they are available to all, at least locally or temporarily. Since people can consume such goods without having to pay for them, no one will produce them for sale to individual consumers. Therefore they will be produced only if government (or some other source such as a charitable organization) pays for their production. The notion of a public good is no different in health than in any other sector: wherever such goods or services are to be available, they must be financed by government or some other non-market alternative.

Control of disease vectors and protection of food and water safety are examples of (nearly) pure public goods in health. Individual action may be ineffective (if one's neighbor's house harbors rats or mosquitoes), costly (water purification) or virtually impossible (testing for food safety). Most activities in this category are preventive, but some curative actions are also partly public. And not all preventive interventions are public goods. For example, at low levels of coverage immunization confers some public good benefits—because the immunization of part of the population reduces the likelihood that un-immunized people will become infected—but it still produces mostly private benefit for the immunized individuals. However, as immunization coverage approaches 100 percent, the benefit becomes more and more public through the mechanism of "herd immunity": a lone un-immunized individual would be just as well protected as if he had been immunized, and could enjoy this protection without paying for it. When the disease can be *eradicated* by complete immunization coverage, a pure public good is created. This is an example of how the public or private nature of an intervention may depend on the degree of coverage. When smallpox was endemic, individuals had a strong incentive to be vaccinated, without regard for how many other people were also protected. Now that the disease has been eliminated, everyone benefits.

While the distinction between public and private goods is crucial, it does not by itself define the appropriate boundary between private and state action. Moreover, the boundary between public and private goods is not sharply defined, because some interventions provide substantial *externalities*. (Figure 2.1 treats such interventions as partly public and partly private, rather than locating them in a separate domain.) In these cases, individuals can and do buy an intervention and benefit from it, but they cannot prevent non-consumers from also deriving some benefit. Because the purchasers do not capture all the benefit, they may be unwilling to pay for all of it: in consequence, private markets can exist but will produce less of these interventions than would be optimal for society as a whole.

This problem arises most readily with communicable diseases, because the infected person puts others at risk. Curing one case therefore also prevents others. Tuberculosis control is a clear example: no victim of tuberculosis is likely to ignore the disease, so there is no problem of people undervaluing the private benefits of treatment. Rather, the cost of treatment—and the fact that they may feel better even though the disease has not been cured—may lead people to abandon treatment prematurely, with bad consequences not only for themselves but for others. The rest of society therefore has an interest in treating those with tuberculosis, and assuming at least part of the cost. Asymptomatic communicable diseases, such as some sexually transmitted infections, also create externalities; but because people may not realize they are infected, the demand for care is too low even when care is free (zero price). There is then an argument not only for subsidizing treatment, but for persuading those infected to seek care.

Most health care, however, is a (nearly) pure private good: Figure 2.1 reflects this by showing public goods as only a narrow band at the left-hand side, with private goods occupying most of the space. Largely or exclusively private activities include most curative care—especially for non-communicable diseases which pose no threat to others—and all rehabilitative care, and also some preventive or "pre-curative" care (such as well-baby visits, and screening for hypertension, cervical cancer, or glaucoma). They include home treatment, using health-specific purchased inputs, as well as medical or other professional care. This area shades into the myriad activities of daily behavior which also affect health, such as diet, exercise, safety precautions, sexual behavior, and the use of alcohol, tobacco or drugs. Among these activities, child-rearing is of crucial importance, both for the immediate effect on health—young children are especially vulnerable to infections and accidents—and for the formation of life-long habits. The health effects of these behaviors are usually small on a daily or episodic basis, but can be very large cumulatively.

Figure 2.1 distinguishes among private interventions according as they are cheap or costly. This is not a sharp boundary, because what is affordable for some people is out of reach for others. And activities which are individually not very expensive may have to be repeated often, creating large cumulative expenditures: renal dialysis and physical therapy are examples. Nonetheless it is crucial to distinguish interventions according to whether they can be paid for out-of-pocket, or financed from accumulated savings, or are so expensive as to represent a catastrophic burden. The cost of medical care is catastrophic if a family or individual can meet it only by selling assets, or taking on debt, to such an extent as to leave it permanently poor. As indicated above, it is initially assumed that no one is too poor to pay for interventions in the "low-cost" domain.

In any health system there is always some private out-of-pocket spending, corresponding to the band along the bottom of Figure 2.1. Before the modern understanding of disease and medicine, *all* health interventions were of this kind, and were paid for by consumers or by charity. Historically, health expenditure began in the lower right corner of the Figure and has expanded into public goods (to the left) and also into very costly private interventions (toward the upper right) as knowledge, wealth and institutional capacity have increased. While this pattern is general, countries have followed different paths in the expansion.

Interventions which are needed unpredictably, because disease strikes randomly, and are also too costly for households' ordinary budgets or savings to finance, define the domain of catastrophically expensive care. The only way to deal with the combination of high cost and uncertainty about needs is by risk-sharing, in which people finance health care collectively by contributions which are related to the expected expense in the group but not to any individual's (unknown) likely consumption of care.

Although the boundaries are blurred, the domain of risk-sharing is conceptually quite distinct from the other two. It normally does not extend into the many routine low-cost, health-related activities, because risk is unimportant there. (It is true that famine relief and other responses to unforeseen disasters amount to sharing the risk of inadequate food or other daily needs, but under normal circumstances it is impossible to buy food insurance.) And *explicit* insurance—a contract between the consumer who agrees to contribute, and someone else who agrees to pay for specified care—is simply not feasible for public goods. Of course, when the government or a private charity pays for public goods, it assumes the financial risk. This can be thought of as *implicit* insurance, and in this sense all publicly-financed health care is a form of insurance, even if there is no explicit contract and no payment of individual claims.

Risk-sharing presents the most numerous and complex issues for public policy. The growth in total health care costs is concentrated in this domain because it includes the catastrophically expensive activities. It also shows the greatest variety of institutional arrangements, including substantial participation by private but non-profit providers and financing institutions [Frank and Salkever 1994]. The reason is that while insurance is the natural solution to the risk of needing costly interventions, private insurance markets tend to fail in ways that affect both efficiency and equity, and different institutions represent different partial solutions to those failures. These problems are quite distinct from the inability of markets to deliver public goods or to assure the right level of production of goods with significant externalities. The question is how and how far governments can and should try to correct for the failings of the insurance market, and whether public finance is necessary or whether other instruments can be substituted for it. Because neither economic theory nor common sense provides as much of an answer as in the domains of public goods and low-cost interventions [Diamond 1992, Zeckhauser 1994], judgments in the domain of risk-sharing are more tentative and depend more on empirical information.

Intervention for public goods in health. By definition, public goods cannot be sold in private markets and so create a straightforward justification for collective action. However, the good or service also must be worth the required public expenditure: simply being a public good is an insufficient condition for state intervention. To take an extreme example, erecting giant fans to blow away polluted air would provide a public good, but would almost surely cost too much to be justified. The questions to answer then are, which goods are sufficiently public that private markets cannot provide them adequately? and how should they be valued to determine whether it is justified to pay for them?

As to the first question, governments usually try to provide such indisputably public goods as disease surveillance and sanitary inspection. They often err, however, by trying to cover too wide a range of interventions; Ministries of Health sometimes appear to regard all of health as a public good. An alternative explanation is that they regard all health care as a merit good; the belief that everyone has an unlimited or ill-defined right to free care is sometimes enshrined in legislation or national constitutions [Fuenzalida-Puelma and Connor 1989]. When public financing is insufficient to fulfill that promise, and particularly when public provision is poorly managed, the result is likely to be both inefficient and inequitable. Governments may err in another way, by recognizing that it can be efficient for the public sector to supply a service—the alternative being to regulate private provision—but subsidize it when most users could pay for it. Water supply and sanitation services are good examples [World Bank 1992a]; they generate large public health benefits but are nonetheless mostly private goods for which non-poor consumers are willing to pay.

Still, the state is not always wrong when it treats a largely private good as if it were entirely public. The most striking example is immunization. Had it been left to private markets during the last few decades, it is inconceivable that today some 80 percent of the world's children would be immunized against the six major vaccine-preventable childhood diseases [Geoffard and Philipson 1994]. Treating the Expanded Program of Immunization as a public good made possible high coverage even in very poor countries [EPI 1993]—often higher than in the United States, which has relied more on private finance and provision [EPI 1995, Haveman and Wolfe 1993]. This "mistake" doubtless imposed some costs, in the form of public expenditure which was unnecessary because some people would have paid for immunization privately, and in the distortions caused by the taxes to pay for the program. But such costs are negligible in comparison with the health gains. And the public intervention in organizing and largely financing the EPI did not crowd out, but probably stimulated, much private participation in both the financing and the delivery of vaccinations [van der Gaag 1995].

The second question is how to value a public-good health intervention. This is the natural domain of cost-effectiveness and cost-benefit analyses. If the only benefit from an intervention is improved health, it does not matter whether that is measured in health terms (lives saved, healthy life years gained) or monetized. When there are also significant collateral benefits, different approaches can lead to different rankings of interventions. This is the case for education, water supply and sanitation, and other activities which are valuable for health but also for other reasons—and which may not be justified for the health benefits alone [World Bank 1993b]. Cost-benefit or cost-effectiveness comparisons are also relevant to public intervention in the other domains of health care, but they are particularly important for public goods for which no private market prices exist.

The issues of which activities to consider public, and whether they deserve to be financed publicly, are difficult. Nonetheless, there are several reasons why this is the simplest domain in which to determine public policy. There is broad agreement on the substantial benefits from a few crucial interventions, which are extremely cost-effective [Jamison, Mosley, Measham and Bobadilla 1993]. Individual poverty is not a major source of problems, as it is with private goods: only society's overall capacity to pay matters. Individual ignorance or absence of demand is also of little importance. Finally, this area does not contribute much to the explosion of health care costs, and its financial importance declines as income rises.

The public role in low-cost private interventions. This domain includes so many different activities, which are undertaken repeatedly and usually have little health impact per episode, that continued, universal, direct public intervention is simply impossible. Governments cannot be responsible for everyone's daily life, and can probably contribute most by improving households' capacities to look after their own health. Promoting development generally—not only increased incomes but more education and access to all kinds of knowledge, goods and services—seems to be the best way to do this [World Bank 1993b, Chapter 2].

How far interference in people's ordinary behavior is justified, depends on whether the health benefits outweigh the curtailment or modification of individual choices, including non-health benefits. Apart from indefensible extreme positions—for example, that only health matters, and is worth any price; or that only people's private appreciation of their own utility matters, and should be treated as sacrosanct—there is no straightforward answer to this question. Public action cannot be justified simply because of a health improvement; neither can it be rejected just because individual liberty might be limited. Specific public intervention for improved health may be justified under three conditions: ignorance or incomplete knowledge, externalities, and the failure of adults to act as appropriate agents for children. Each of these involves some kind of market failure, or violation of the private market assumption that rational adults are making informed choices and paying the consequences of their decisions.

The first problem is *ignorance:* people might take better care of their health if they knew how. For example, vitamins are crucial to health but are not observable in food, and people may already believe untruths about diet that help cause vitamin deficiencies [Johns, Booth and Kuhnlein 1992]. In general, ignorance on the part of one or both parties to a transaction is a major source of failure in the health care market. Of course, "perfect decision making is not ever possible, so the real issue is when the government can or ought to intervene in the information market to improve the market's performance" [Beales, Crasswell and Salop 1981]. Moreover, information is not entirely free, and people do not always act on it. Thus while the cost-effectiveness of efforts to make behavior more efficient can be very high, it is also quite variable, and people's reactions to information are hard to predict.

Correcting ignorance is not simply a matter of telling people something new, but a larger question of changing beliefs and behavior. Where better knowledge alone does not lead to changed behavior, regulation or mandates may also be justified even though they imply more intrusive or coercive intervention. In all such cases, the difficult question is how far it is legitimate to try to change people's views of what they want or what is good for them. Information often complements these other instruments, to reduce opposition to them or improve their effectiveness. The interaction between information and other instruments of behavior change is seen clearly in the successful effort to reduce smoking in the United States [U.S. Dept. of Health and Human Services 1989, 1992].

This situation raises a second problem, of *externalities*, or interactions among presumably informed adults. Driving while drunk is an example, as is dumping feces or trash in communal water supplies. These activities impose both health damage and financial costs on others, and individual protection may be impossible or very costly. The chief instrument for public action is regulation, perhaps supported by mandates; these instances do not typically require public finance of health care activities. They may of course also require negative mandates, in the form of laws against certain activities or behaviors. In practice, there is no sharp boundary between this and the first problem, because some of the behavior that imposes costs on others may also arise from ignorance: thus reducing the harm from a particular behavior may require both information and monetary, legal or other incentives. It is more effective to criminalize drunk driving if people are also informed of the dangers, and the health damage can be limited by mandating the use of seat belts.

The third condition is an *agent-principal problem* [Stiglitz 1989] and, in contrast to the externalities just discussed, is intergenerational. Children are not yet informed, sovereign adults; they are vulnerable not just to accidents and disease but to the indifference and even sadism of their parents. This problem is somewhat similar to the situation of doctors acting as imperfect agents for their patients. However, patients often can choose and contract with the doctors who act as their agents, whereas children have no choice of who acts for them. (Similar problems arise for adults who are mentally retarded or incapacitated by some kinds of disease.) What should the state do when parents are inadequate agents for their children? Requiring that children be immunized is relatively easy, but it is harder to deal with child-beating or exposure of children to secondhand smoke, and still harder to confront parents' beliefs in such matters as sexual education. Where sexual behavior, vehicle use and consumption of alcohol, tobacco and drugs are concerned, these issues continue through adolescence.

This is an exceptionally contentious topic, where it is hard to draw the frontier between public and private responsibilities. Different societies have adopted different solutions, and there is often bitter disagreement within societies over the rights and duties of parents and the degree to which the state can or should interfere in family life. There are potentially very large health gains at stake in this debate: eight or nine of the ten worldwide leading causes of illness in young children are substantially correctable at low cost [World Bank 1993, Annex Table B.6], and four of these—diarrheal disease plus three nutritional deficiencies—can be largely controlled by the family, with little public expenditure. These diseases account for about 20 percent of young children's ill health; the total share of child health that depends on parental behavior is of course substantially larger.

In all these instances, the principal instruments of state action should probably be information and regulation. Mandates are justified *for* a few activities such as requiring schoolchildren to be immunized, or that foodstuffs be fortified, and *against* a few other activities. Substantial public finance, however, is usually justified only because some people are too poor to pay for health-related goods and activities, whether these involve medical care or such necessities as food.

Risk-sharing for catastrophically costly private goods. When risks cannot be fully controlled, and the associated costs may be catastrophic, the only solution is to share the risk. None of the features of this domain is unique to health care, but the magnitude and interaction of certain problems are especially important in health care markets. Moreover, the health risk is only partly associated with income or employment, and the financial risk is hardly associated at all with income or occupation.

Health insurance differs sharply from insurance for non-human assets such as homes or vehicles, where the value of the asset, and therefore the cost of insurance, is usually related to income. Another fundamental difference is that medical care allows for preventive maintenance and for repair, but not for complete replacement of the damaged capital, which in this case is a human body. Insurance for non-human assets operates in just the opposite way, protecting against the loss of the asset but not paying for its upkeep. Insurance may even cover the cost of a temporary substitute for the lost home or vehicle, which is impossible with health insurance. Risks are also harder to estimate for health insurance, both because of the inherently much greater complexity of the body than of non-human property and because there are often different possible treatments for a given health problem, with different costs, outcomes and risks. Insurance against health risks raises some well-known difficulties [Arrow 1985], leading to various kinds of market failure. One such problem arises because insurance is a contract by which someone other than the patient agrees to pay for his or her health care. As with all contracts, there is an incentive for the insured to behave differently because of the insurance; this is called *moral hazard* [Pauly 1968]. One consequence is that consumers who do not pay the full cost of health care will consume more of it. This is desirable, since the point of insurance is to let people consume health care they could not otherwise afford. It means, however, that the price must cover the increased demand that results from insurance, and not simply the care that people would otherwise want to buy out-of-pocket.

In theory, there are two potentially more worrisome problems associated with this moral hazard. The first is that people may not only consume more medical care generally, but care that costs too much relative to its effectiveness, yielding smaller health gains per dollar spent. The second risk is that people may take poorer care of their health via daily activities, because they pay the full cost of those, but only part or none of the cost of the resulting increased curative care. Both problems imply excess resources being dedicated to health care. They may also imply worse health, if increased curative care does not fully compensate for reduced prevention and protection. Some degree of moral hazard is intrinsic to all kinds of insurance, but it is more limited in the case of nonhuman assets because the insurance does not cover ordinary wear and tear. And cheating the insurer, by burning down one's house or abandoning one's car and reporting it stolen, is illegal, to prevent the insured person from fraudulently collecting cash. Such compensation is generally not possible under health insurance. (Cash payment for permanent disabilities is usually included with life insurance and represents compensation for the loss of part of a life. The only significant moral hazard for such insurance appears to be suicide, which is often specifically excluded from the causes of death for which compensation will be paid.) Moral hazard in health insurance is independent of how it is financed, so it does not by itself determine whether insurance should be paid for privately or publicly. A consumer who voluntarily buys private insurance ends up paying for the additional medical care consumed by other purchasers, and judges whether this cost is justified by his or her own greater access to care. When insurance is paid for by taxes or mandatory contributions, however, this choice cannot be made.

Moral hazard may then justify controls on what public money is used for, to avoid expenditure on interventions of little health value which consumers would not voluntarily agree to buy for other people [Musgrove 1995a]. There is scant empirical evidence on the importance of these problems, particularly as to whether insurance leads people to be *more* careless about their health than they would be if uninsured. As to the relation between insurance and less cost-effective medical care, the evidence in the United States is that higher out-of-pocket cost for medical care (higher co-payments or lower deductibles on insurance) does not make consumers choose more cost-effective services, and may even make poor consumers forego highly justified care [Lohr *et al.* 1986, Newhouse *et al.* 1993]. Except in the latter case, there is little evidence that making the consumer pay higher costs under insurance leads to worsened health. Inefficiency in a competitive insurance market also takes the form of *excess purchases of insurance*—that is, insurance for interventions which could be more efficiently financed out of pocket [Pauly 1974], or insurance which leads to needless or unjustified use of medical care. This is inefficient to the degree that it leads to excess administrative costs for handling numerous small claims, and because of the excess consumption of health care [Feldstein 1973]. Private insurers can only partly control this tendency through deductibles (which remove small risks from coverage, until out-of-pocket payments reach some limit). This problem arises partly because of ignorance: people tend to overestimate small risks and may buy too much insurance even when they pay its full cost. Moral hazard, however, is a greater problem: people who do not pay the full cost of insurance will buy too much of it, just as with medical services. Market failure in the form of over-insurance happens primarily through the tax system. Many governments allow private employers to treat insurance cost as an expense, but then—in contrast to salaries—do not treat the value of insurance as income to workers. Subsidy through the tax system is notorious in the United States [Pauly 1986], both for insurance for workers which is financed by employers and for part of the Medicare insurance for the elderly. It is estimated that employer-financed insurance would decline by one-sixth or more in the absence of this subsidy, and that in consequence the overall demand for medical services would fall by about five percent [Chernick, Holmer and Weienberg 1987].

Alternatively, governments directly subsidize social security health benefits (mandated insurance) out of general revenue. General revenues are used to support social security systems throughout Europe and Latin America [McGreevey 1990]. In Chile, payroll taxes can also be used to finance private insurance. All these direct and indirect subsidies to insurance are not only inefficient, but highly inequitable when only part of the labor force is covered. The poor typically benefit only when coverage is (close to) universal. When various profit-maximizing insurers compete to sell insurance, there are two further and closely related problems, of *adverse selection* on the part of consumers and of *risk selection* on the part of insurers. The former refers to selection of customers which would be adverse to the interests of insurers—fundamentally, it describes the danger of enrolling people who would cost more on average than the insurance could finance. This can happen because the amount of insurance coverage people want and are willing to pay for depends partly on their knowledge of their own health conditions and risks. People who expect to need little health care are unwilling to pay as much as those who expect to need much care, so a policy costly enough to cover high-risk people will lose out in the market to a cheaper policy adequate for low-risk people.

Universal coverage at the same price for everyone may therefore be impossible to achieve, or may not generate enough revenue to finance all the health care demanded [Summers 1989]. To protect themselves against the combination of low premiums and high potential costs, insurers engage in risk selection or "cream-skimming": they spend more on administration, or create barriers to enrollment, to screen out high-risk individuals (such as the aged) or conditions (such as cancer). Such "underwriting", as it is called, is particularly costly for individual applicants for insurance, and gives rise to large scale economies because when a large group is enrolled, the insurer needs to estimate only the average risk of needing care [Diamond 1992]. This practice is the natural market response to the problem of adverse selection. Inefficiency takes the form of increased administrative costs, and also increased health risks for those excluded from insurance. Particularly when pre-existing conditions are not covered, people with health problems who are insured by their employers cannot readily change jobs without losing their insurance; other differences in insurance coverage may also create "job lock" among workers. This labor immobility is another source of inefficiency, of unknown magnitude [Congressional Budget Office 1994]. One answer to the problems of adverse and risk selection is price differentiation according to risk, which is theoretically efficient in that it allows everyone to have the insurance he or she is willing to pay for. Such price variation is common to other forms of insurance: for example, rates for automobile insurance often vary by age and by the way a vehicle is used. Unfortunately, there are serious difficulties with letting the market create comparable differentials in health insurance. One is that some people are willing to pay only a small amount, because they expect to need little medical care. Faced with a price that would cover the cost of care for everyone, they will not purchase insurance. When they drop out of the market, the price of coverage for those who expect to need more care is driven up because the risk is spread over fewer and higher-cost people. Even if they are willing to pay more than those who anticipate needing very little care, the price of insurance may rise beyond their capacity to pay. They will be unable to buy insurance, despite a willingness to pay more than the average consumer. Such failures do not occur in other insurance markets because risks are more uniform or predictable, or more closely related to income.

Of course, people's willingness to buy insurance depends on their expectation about future needs for medical care, and they may guess wrong. People who are young and healthy today, and therefore unwilling to spend much on insurance, may when they are older want much more medical care than they now anticipate. But if they become willing to buy substantial coverage only late in life, the cost will be higher than if it were spread over a longer period, so they may be unable to pay for insurance once they recognize the need for it. The difficulty of predicting health care needs is exacerbated by the rapidity of technical change in this sector [Weisbrod 1991].

Another problem with differential prices is that despite the importance of many behaviors for specific health problems, rather little of total health risk is under the individual's control. People cannot be held personally responsible for much of their ill health since it is genetic in origin, or due to the actions of others. Often the best that people can do by controlling their own behavior is to postpone problems, which is very valuable but does not necessarily save money over a lifetime [Russell 1986]. Behavioral change may also take a long time to show effect on the burden of disease or the volume of treatment [World Bank 1994a]. Because so little health risk is under people's control, behavior-related prices—whether for health care or for insurance itself—are of only limited value in making markets work. One can charge people for smoking (by taxation) or for not wearing seat belts (by fines), or reward them for careful driving (by lower insurance rates), but prices are not feasible for most health-related behaviors. People have some choice of where to live and whether to drive a car, but no choice about inhabiting the body they were born with [Miller 1978]. Notions of fairness are involved in the choice of how far to allow or control price differentiation in health insurance, because people often do not think others should be punished financially, in addition to their physical suffering, for bad luck. In addition, the possibility of death or substantial permanent disability sometimes makes treatment urgent. Adverse selection is therefore a problem of equity as well as of efficiency.

The problems of moral hazard and adverse selection arise partly from the fact that consumers and insurers possess only *incomplete information*, which causes market failure in the sense that markets work perfectly only when both buyers and sellers possess full information [Arrow 1985]. Of course, insurance is wanted in the first place because people do not know what will happen to their health, and they agree to share risks when they do not know what will happen to others' health. A further complication is that of *information asymmetry:* information available to only one side of a market readily leads to market failure. For example, consumers who know their health risks have an incentive to conceal them from insurers so as to avoid higher premiums. They also know how they have modified their behavior, or mean to do so, because of insurance. Insurers, in contrast, generally know more than consumers about average risks and about costs of care; consumer ignorance of these matters can also lead to inefficiency.

Unfortunately, it does not follow that the problems of incomplete and asymmetric information could be corrected just by supplying information. Better knowledge on the part of consumers about health risks may lead to more efficient purchase and use of insurance. However, obtaining the information needed to restore symmetry would be impossible or very costly; too much is still unknown about how much people can control their health through behavioral choices. Even if it were symmetrically available to consumers, insurers and providers, more information might make it easier for insurers to practice risk selection and discriminate among customers, and thereby exacerbate inequity. In fact, in an unregulated market, this is the probable consequence of the increasing availability of information linking genetic endowment to the likelihood of developing specific illnesses or health problems [House of Commons 1995].

Information asymmetry also arises between patients and doctors, since the latter typically know much more about medical conditions and treatments. Patients may accept, or even demand, treatments they would not buy if fully informed, but which are advantageous, financially or otherwise, to medical professionals. There is however little firm evidence as to how much of this potential "supplier-induced demand" actually occurs [Pauly 1988]. In any case, this is not simply a problem of rich countries, where most people have insurance and therefore do not worry about costs; it has also been documented in poor societies where lack of education and information may make it particularly easy to exploit consumers [Bennett *et al.* 1994].

In summary, the consequence of these market failures is that in an unregulated, competitive private market in third-party insurance those with chronic conditions or high health risks will be under-insured, administrative costs will be higher than necessary because of insurers' efforts to screen out risks and the costs of processing claims in a market with many insurers and many providers, and procedures of low or questionable value will be performed because neither the provider nor the consumer pays for them. It is in these specific senses that "the market does not work" in health care; these are primarily failures of the insurance market rather than shortcomings of the market for health care itself.

Private markets have developed other forms of insurance which reduce, but do not eliminate, these problems, such as health maintenance organizations (HMOs). Under this arrangement, providers also act as insurers and assume the risk. Insofar as this controls costs by shifting the burden to suppliers of medical care rather than to consumers or third-party insurers [Ellis and McGuire 1993], it may allow more coverage of the chronically ill, and may reduce the utilization of relatively ineffective procedures. However, without some form of public intervention such arrangements will have little effect on the problems caused by poverty and adverse selection. The question remains which kinds and degrees of public intervention can best mitigate the problems inherent to private insurance markets without introducing worse inefficiencies or inequities.

Market Failure and Health Care Needs

Since the unregulated, unsubsidized private market is the extreme alternative to government intervention in health care, much of the debate as to appropriate public and private roles in the sector turns on whether, how, and how badly markets may fail. Market failure, as an economic notion, refers to possible mismatches or disequilibria between what the market supplies, and what fully-informed, rational consumers of health care would demand. It does not deal with the concept of *need* for health care, which is theoretically an unsatisfactory concept but is also difficult to do without [Culyer 1995]. People want health care not for any intrinsic utility but because they think they need it, that if care is not provided their health will deteriorate or fail to improve. In contrast, much of the criticism by both health care professionals and consumers of how health systems operate deals explicitly with needs.

Just as demand and supply may be out of balance, there can be imbalance between demand and need or between need and supply of services, as shown in Figure 2.2. Market failures in the narrow economic sense are among the reasons for these imbalances (these are indicated on the Figure by asterisks). Some failures result from barriers to the operation of competitive private markets in bringing supply and demand together. Others distort demand from what it would be if based on complete and symmetric information and if there were no public goods or externalities; this causes imbalance between demands and needs. While competitive private markets are generally the best way to bring demand and supply together, they are much worse suited to make either demand or supply match people's needs. Public intervention in the health market, in contrast, is aimed at satisfying those needs, and runs the corresponding risk of failing to take account of demand. Either a purely private or a purely public health care system is likely to control one of the three potential imbalances, at the cost of failing to control or even worsening one or both of the others [Musgrove 1995b]. This is a major reason why most health care systems are far from being all private or all public [Dunlop and Martins 1995].

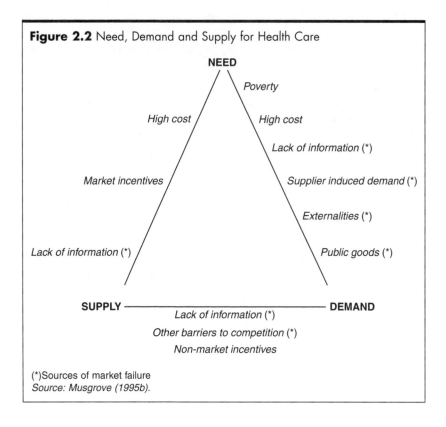

Figure 2.2 Need, Demand and Supply for Health Care

NEED

Poverty

High cost / High cost

Lack of information (*)

Market incentives / Supplier induced demand (*)

Externalities (*)

Lack of information (*) / Public goods (*)

SUPPLY ——————————— DEMAND

Lack of information (*)

Other barriers to competition (*)

Non-market incentives

(*)Sources of market failure
Source: Musgrove (1995b).

Dealing with poverty

In the discussion thus far, it has been assumed that no one is too poor to buy a variety of health interventions out of pocket. Similarly, it is assumed that no one is too poor to buy insurance against catastrophic health risks; people differ in income and in their assessment of risks, but everyone can afford some insurance. This means that the distinction between the "low-cost" domain in Figure 2.1 and the domain where insurance is needed is roughly the same for everyone.

A minimal state role in the absence of poverty. Under these conditions the state's role in the domain of private, inexpensive health-related activities would be limited mostly to information and regulation; there would be no reason to finance this kind of health care publicly if everyone could afford it out-of-pocket. (Mandates might still be justified to deal with some of the externalities mentioned above.) In the domain of risk-sharing, people who chose not to buy insurance, or bought too little of it, would have to pay for care out of pocket or do without it. Because doing without care would sometimes pose the risk of avoidable death, some kinds of care—emergency services, at least—are typically available even to the uninsured. People's willingness to let others suffer the consequences of imprudence does not usually include letting them die because they bought too little catastrophic protection. This kind of imprudence constitutes moral hazard, and unlike some behavior on the part of insured people, it cannot be dealt with by differential premiums. Motorcyclists who prefer not to wear helmets can in principle be charged more for their insurance, just as smokers can; the more difficult problem is how much care to provide for the uninsured cyclist whose injuries are worse because of failure to wear a helmet.

This situation provides a justification for enough public finance or mandated insurance to cover the cost of a few crucial services to which everyone would have access and for which everyone would have to pay through taxes [Summers 1989]. Except for these services, there would be no requirement for the government to subsidize insurance for anyone. If there were no poverty, then, the role of the state in the health sector might be relatively limited, and would—except for the minimum insurance requirement just described—concentrate on the adequate provision of public goods and the correction of market failure in the domain of risk-sharing. Whether in order to correct or compensate for that failure the state should mandate or finance insurance beyond that minimum of emergency care, is a question of the social efficiency of doing so, rather than leaving insurance to the private market.

The fact that insurance would not need to be subsidized—the removal of an equity justification for interfering in the insurance market—does not mean that governments should do nothing, because the efficiency failings of private voluntary insurance are as important as the inequities to which it gives rise.

How poverty complicates public roles. The existence of poverty, of people too poor to buy many "inexpensive" health activities or an "adequate" amount of insurance, complicates the question of what the state should and should not do in several ways. These complications are not limited to the domains of private goods, because problems of public health are often more severe among the poor. They are likely to be at particular risk from contaminated air and water and so to benefit more than the non-poor from public health interventions [World Bank 1992a, 1993b], and they often suffer more serious consequences from common illnesses. In general, imbalance between need and demand may be more important where the poor are concerned, because they have less knowledge on which to base their wants for health care as well as less resources with which to express demand.

Medical indigence is in most respects no different from poverty with respect to food and other basic needs, and, as with those needs, the rest of society may agree to subsidize the poor. The difference is that poverty relative to predictable, low-cost needs such as food can be dealt with either by transfers or subsidies in kind, or by supplementing income [Srinivasan 1994]. With health, the risk of needing very costly care generally makes it more efficient to deal with medical indigence by subsidizing insurance than through income transfers. However, there is little experience in most poor countries in subsidizing private providers or insurers to meet the health needs of the poor. This requires government administrative capacity and appropriate pricing mechanisms, to prevent excess provision and even outright fraud, which has been a major problem, for example, in Brazil [World Bank 1993c; Medici and Czapski 1995].

A public subsidy to private insurance, as an alternative to dealing directly with large numbers of providers, also requires premiums differentiated by age, sex or other conditions, to reduce the scope for risk selection and make it feasible to mandate universal coverage. In consequence, one of the most important effects of poverty is that it makes public provision, with all its typical problems, look attractive or even necessary in poor countries. Aside from the problems of regulation, it is financially difficult to provide the poor with the same level of services enjoyed by those already covered by private or social insurance. Even extending social security coverage to the poor, to replace the more limited services offered by Ministries of Health, would be very costly in many Latin American countries [Mesa-Lago 1992]. Public provision often means poor health care for the poor, but public financing of private services would not easily solve the underlying financial problem even if it led to improved quality of care. Finally, in countries where all public money now flows through government or parastatal facilities, shifting to public finance of private providers requires that public hospitals and clinics be privatized or at least given sufficient autonomy and capacity to manage themselves and compete for public funds against other providers. Such changes are potentially very valuable, but they are likely to be particularly difficult, since public facilities need to be exposed to some financial risk without the danger of collapse in publicly funded provision.

The difficulty of incorporating the poor into the same insurance schemes which cover the non-poor, whether by extending social security coverage or by subsidizing the purchase of private insurance, leads to efforts to create insurance specifically for the poor, typically at the community level. Any such scheme is intrinsically limited by the low incomes of participants, so it cannot finance very costly interventions and can only yield subsidies from the less poor to the more poor. It may nonetheless be appropriate when the insurance is meant to pay for only such health care as can also be provided locally and which therefore is not very costly—although perhaps still catastrophic for a poor family to finance. Unfortunately, the problems of moral hazard and adverse selection arise even in these circumstances. For example, if insurance is sold for short periods to accommodate families' fluctuations in income, then, as occurred in Burundi, people may buy the "health cards" entitling them to services only when they are already sick or can anticipate a medical need [McPake, Hanson and Mills 1993]. That effectively eliminates the difference between an insurance payment and a fee, and reduces the amount of money that can be raised by the scheme. These problems lead to complications such as rewarding people who use less (curative) health care by reducing the cost of their cards for the next period or by charging an additional fee or "fine" to those who pay for insurance only when ill [Chabot, Boal and da Silva 1991]. Such incentives work against moral hazard and adverse selection, but if they are large enough to have much effect they may greatly reduce the scheme's revenue or the demand for services. And administrative expenses may absorb a large share of revenue.

Poverty also creates or strengthens reasons for the state to intervene in low-cost, health-related activities, whether these are inexpensive medications and services or such non-medical items as food supplements. Some interventions can be accommodated by broadening public health services, for example by including micronutrient supplements or treatment for intestinal parasites. Others can be covered by financing private providers, such as the clinics which operate under "covenants" with the Brazilian social security system [World Bank 1993c]. However these activities are dealt with, poverty pushes governments to finance a wider range of low-cost interventions and to rely less on information and regulation. If this were the only force at work, it would lead to a larger public share of health expenditure in poor than in rich countries, simply because there are more poor people who cannot pay for those interventions. In the sum of health spending, however, this effect is overwhelmed by the tendency (and the capacity) of governments to mandate or finance more insurance for the non-poor, as income rises.

A third effect of poverty is to limit the use of prices to curtail demand or control costs. Being poor already greatly constrains demand, and poor people are necessarily more sensitive to prices for health care than the non-poor [Gertler and van der Gaag 1992]. This means both that user fees can raise relatively little revenue from the poor, and that unless there are offsetting improvements in quality, utilization may be sharply reduced [Lavy 1994, Litvack and Bodart 1993]. The experience with user fees has been extensively analyzed, notably in Sub-Saharan Africa in connection with the Bamako Initiative [Griffin 1987, Creese 1991, World Bank 1992, Vogel 1993, Makinen and Raney 1994, Nolan and Turbat 1994, Shaw and Griffin 1995]. There is evidence that—as might be expected—utilization declines, sometimes sharply, if fees are raised but nothing else changes. There is rather less information on service characteristics, such as whether user fees improve the availability of drugs. And almost nothing is known about the impact on health outcomes or on system efficiency or cost-effectiveness. Fees are sometimes set arbitrarily or with inconsistent criteria; charges low enough to have no effect on the poor may or may not be worth collecting; and targeting by exempting the destitute from fees does not have to be expensive [Grosh 1992], but there is a risk of high administrative costs and low net revenues. The same problems arise for collecting insurance deductibles and co-payments from the poor.

Not only does poverty increase the risk of ill health; sickness and disability can make or keep people poor. The relation between health and poverty is sometimes regarded as another reason for the state to invest in health, in order to raise productivity. However, the fact that some health care increases incomes is not a *separate* objective for government action. If health care made people so much more productive that the extra income could pay for the health care, then in perfect markets people could borrow against their future productivity. When capital market failures prevent such borrowing, and those failures cannot be corrected directly, then any public intervention—such as financing the health care or providing loans to consumers—that secures the health gains will also yield the increase in productivity.

Justifications and Risks of State Intervention

As the foregoing analysis shows, there are three distinct, independent arguments for governments to intervene in health care rather than leaving it entirely to private markets. One is to ensure the optimal level of production and consumption of public goods and goods which have a partly public character because of externalities. These can be health care services themselves, activities protective of health, or information that helps people take better care of their health and make better use of services. A second reason is to make insurance work more efficiently and more equitably, for those services which can be produced in private markets but for which risk-sharing is required because of high costs and uncertainty about needs. The third reason is to subsidize those too poor to buy insurance or even, sometimes, those inexpensive activities and services which the non-poor can afford out of pocket. These three reasons derive from the three domains of health care defined by cost and by the public or private nature of services. Market failures underlie two of these reasons, but in different ways. In the case of public goods and externalities, the failure arises from the nature of the good or service. In contrast, problems in insurance markets arise from the way the good is financed. None of the three reasons is unique to the health sector, but all are more important in this sector than in much of the rest of the economy.

The arguments for not leaving health care and health insurance to uncontrolled private markets are all arguments that efficiency or equity can be improved, if the state intervenes appropriately. They are not arguments that anything the public sector does, will improve matters. Just as there is a well-defined set of market failures typical of the health sector, there are consistent government failures, ways in which governments act to create worse outcomes than could be reached, and in some respects even worse outcomes than markets would generate. The most common and severe criticism of public action concerns provision [World Bank 1980 and 1987, Birdsall and James 1992]: especially in poor countries, governments offer medical care which is supposed to be free to users, on equity grounds, but which is centrally-controlled, under-financed and of poor quality in both medical and human terms. Because the budgets of public facilities often are unrelated to service output, and civil service rules make it difficult to fire, transfer or discipline unproductive staff, the costs of health gains may be very high even if salaries and other input costs are low. And the pervasive lack of incentives for efficiency means that capital is also bought in excess, not maintained, and under-utilized. The result is that even rather poor people, the supposed beneficiaries of the public system, often pay out of pocket for those private services they can afford. This makes them pay twice for some of their care, exacerbating the inequities arising from the tax system and from difficulties of access due to the geographic location of facilities.

Governments typically fail where provision is concerned, by trying to do too much and by competing with private providers only in price terms— that is, subsidizing provision rather than competing on quality and satisfaction. With respect to the other instruments of state action, failures are more varied, and often result from doing too little rather than too much. This is likely to be the case particularly for regulation and for the dissemination of information. Mandates show a very mixed pattern: middle-income countries in particular often mandate insurance for part of the population through social security schemes, but do not effectively mandate either insurance or care for everyone. Richer countries, in contrast, appear much less prone to government failure largely because they rely much more heavily on regulation and mandates, and much less on public provision. Where public facilities are important, as in some European countries, they operate under greater autonomy than in poor countries, and this is balanced by greater regulation of private providers. The result is to concentrate more on the right *roles* for public action, and less on dividing the health sector into disjointed private and public spheres. The distinction is particularly important because in many countries, the two sectors overlap greatly: the same professionals work part-time in each, private providers often use public facilities to treat private patients, and so on. To provide public goods and to subsidize health-related activities for the poor, two of the three main reasons for state action, both require public finance. In both these areas there is also room for the other instruments of state action; and the problems associated with risk sharing can lead to various combinations of interventions, which may or may not include spending public money. Societies therefore have much latitude in how much, and by what means, the government intervenes in health care markets, just as they have in deciding how much to spend on health in relation to income and to their health problems or needs.

The Appropriate Public Role in Health

As a first approximation, it is easier to say what governments *should not do* in health than to specify what they *should do*. That is, it is clear that certain actions are likely or certain to violate one or more of the objectives of a health care system to an important degree. To apply a topographic metaphor: such actions correspond to falling off a plateau of satisfactory outcomes, all somewhat different but none clearly dominating the rest, and into one of the surrounding chasms of one or another kind of failure. Four "don'ts" are discussed in what follows: they refer to the way the public is taxed, charged or exempted to pay for health care; the providers to which governments transfer public funds; the way providers are paid; and the services they are paid to provide.

What government should not do. The first thing governments should not do is to use the tax system, or any system of fees at public facilities, to make the poor subsidize the health care of the rich. Conceptually, subsidies are justified only for the poor, and broader financing of care through insurance is a question of efficiency rather than of equity. This is not only a matter of whether the rich use more of publicly-financed services than the poor do, although great inequities often arise because the rich have more access to those services. Financial equity also depends on who pays the taxes. More narrowly, governments should not contribute to social security financing from general revenues, unless coverage is universal, because when only part of the population is covered it is usually the poor who are excluded. And governments should not treat private insurance coverage as a cost to employers unless it is also treated as income to beneficiaries. Such practices are not only inequitable; they are also inefficient to the extent that they lead to excessive spending on health care, or reduce labor mobility.

Controlling inequitable subsidies does not mean that social security systems should be dismantled or must be made universal. Even when incomplete, such mandated insurance includes substantial progressive subsidies from high-paid to low-paid workers, and the mere fact that some people in society receive more generous health care is not necessarily a problem, so long as they pay for it. What matters is that governments not make everyone pay for what some are excluded *ex ante* from receiving. Perverse subsidies not only cause immediate inefficiencies or inequities, they also create interests that oppose subsequent health system reform. This is evident in the United States [Skocpol 1995] and Chile [Musgrove1995d], and it is the reason why the design of subsidies is a crucial part of any reform to extend or improve coverage for the poor. The second thing governments should not do is tie public finance to public provision. The choice of whether to provide care through public or parastatal facilities should be treated as a "make or buy" decision, subordinate to the larger decision about what to pay for. That does not necessarily mean eliminating public provision, which will sometimes be the best solution. It means rather that competition between public and private providers should be based on costs and on quality, and not on price to the consumer, as is commonly the case.

To achieve those goals, however, requires other changes in how public institutions operate, changes that probably cannot occur so long as public funds go automatically and exclusively to government facilities. This conclusion is most pertinent to poor countries where public systems are most likely to be inefficient and to be used only because they are free or nearly so. High-income countries with a large share of public provision, particularly in hospitals, suffer less from these problems.

A third thing governments should not do is pay for health care by fee-for-service, unless other mechanisms are used to control expenditures. This is seldom a problem with publicly provided services, but makes it hard to control costs when governments finance private providers. Even negotiating or controlling the fees is not enough, as the Canadian experience demonstrates, since providers can respond to fees they consider too low, by increasing output [Evans, Barer and Labelle 1988]. This helps explain why Canadian health expenditure has risen faster than that in European countries which rely on other payment mechanisms. European countries which pay for health care by fee-for-service also rely on global budgets, utilization reviews or other instruments of cost containment [OECD 1994, 1995]. Since expenditures equal prices times quantities, and since quantities of services respond to prices and are difficult to control directly, countries which pursue both macroeconomic and microeconomic efficiency in health spending usually control both prices and expenditures. In contrast to European and North American experience, Brazil applies this system to block grants for federal expenditure in states with relative financial autonomy; but in states where federal money is paid directly to providers, the federal government also controls one crucial quantity, the number of hospitalizations that federal money will pay for [World Bank 1994b]. In all cases, the government sets prices for services.

It also helps, in controlling expenditures, to define "services" as complete treatments for specific conditions rather than as all the individual components of such treatments, so they can be financed by mechanisms such as the Diagnostic Related Group (DRG) payments used in the United States and the provider can be required to assume part of the financial risk. Changing from a system based on overall budgets and on salaries for providers, to a fee-for-service system without offsetting the resulting incentives to overprovision can lead to an explosion of costs, as in the Czech Republic [Boland 1995]. Finally, if governments mean to pursue some combination of better health and lower costs, they should not—in fact they cannot—simply finance whatever people demand when care is free to consumers. This does not mean governments should not "subsidize demand" rather than "subsidizing supply" or providing services. It means only that there must be limitations on what will be paid for publicly. Such limitations are a particularly contentious matter, because both good health and cost containment may be opposed to consumer or provider satisfaction, which are also politically important objectives. Nonetheless, two empirical observations are germane to this decision. One is that private insurance always carries some limitations, either as to the services covered or as to cost-sharing. Except where poverty is important, so that cost-sharing is more difficult, there is no reason for public finance to be systematically more generous in this regard than private risk-sharing arrangements. The second observation is that, as the discussion concerning Figure 2.2 indicates, private markets will tend to supply what people demand, and public intervention typically acts to emphasize needs instead. In other forms of public subsidy, it is common to distinguish between wants and needs, and concentrate spending on the latter. This is the case, for example, with food subsidies, which are also very much health-related. Price subsidies are usually limited to "basic" foodstuffs, and food stamps cannot legally be used to buy alcohol or other non-necessities. This may be considered partly a matter of efficiency, assuring more health gain than would otherwise occur. But it is also a matter of equity: in contrast to actuarial private insurance, where every purchaser buys the expected value of the health services needed, public finance is involuntary. It comes from taxpayers who have a legitimate interest in meeting needs, and thereby getting value for their money, but not necessarily in paying for wants.

None of these "don'ts" is easy to implement, because some consumer or provider interests can be expected to oppose every one of them, in every country. But they are arguably the most important conclusions about where the public/private frontier should run in the health sector. It is notable that none of these conclusions depends solely on features unique to the health sector. The peculiarities of health matter most for the difficulty of distinguishing "needs" from wants, and—partly as a consequence—for the dangers of paying providers for whatever they choose to provide, without incentives to control costs. A system which avoided the problems described above would still present complex and difficult questions for the proper role of the state, but it would have more latitude to pursue improvements. And it would not matter so much, exactly what objectives the government pursued or which combination of instruments it applied.

What government should do. Beyond the prescriptions for how the state should deal with the problems of each of the three domains of health care, several "dos" appear to be generally valid for governments. If the objective is to minimize deadweight losses from public intervention and leave as much room as possible for private choices, then the first thing governments should do is to use each less-intrusive instrument to the point where a more intrusive intervention is justified, following the sequence of increasingly greater interference—inform, regulate, mandate, finance and provide services. That is, governments should regulate private activity when merely improving people's information is not enough, deliver services if it is infeasible to finance private providers equitably, and so on. Public finance is inescapable for some actions, but particularly in low- and middle-income countries much can probably be accomplished by better use of information and regulation. Failure to use these other instruments well, can increase the need for public finance.

Sometimes the problem is that governments exploit these instruments too little. They do not regulate private insurance when it first begins to expand, which makes subsequent regulation politically more difficult [World Bank 1994b; Musgrove 1995c]; or they do not initially react when health-damaging behaviors such as smoking become more entrenched. Sometimes the problem is inappropriate regulation, which needlessly restricts competition, or enforces inefficiency in the public sector by centralizing nearly all decisions. And poor countries in particular often get the worst of both worlds by paying for activities which should be, but are not, regulated: government subsidy of medical education without adequate control of quality or relation to needs is a common example. In the worst of cases, governments use all the available instruments in exactly the reverse order. They try to provide more health care than they can pay for, with the result that most services are under-financed and of poor quality; they try to finance services, some of which might be mandated and paid for by consumers or employers; they mandate care, as by social security systems, without adequately regulating it; and they do too little to inform the public and providers either of dangers to health or of how the health care system is actually working.

Much of the criticism of government failure in the health sector, especially in poor countries, describes the result of getting things backwards. These ideas are represented in Figure 2.3A, which shows the appropriate relation among the instruments by which the state can intervene in health care, and Figure 2.3B, which portrays the kind of inappropriate or imbalanced relation often found in poor nations. Figure 2.3A indicates that whatever is mandated, financed or provided publicly should also be regulated, and much else

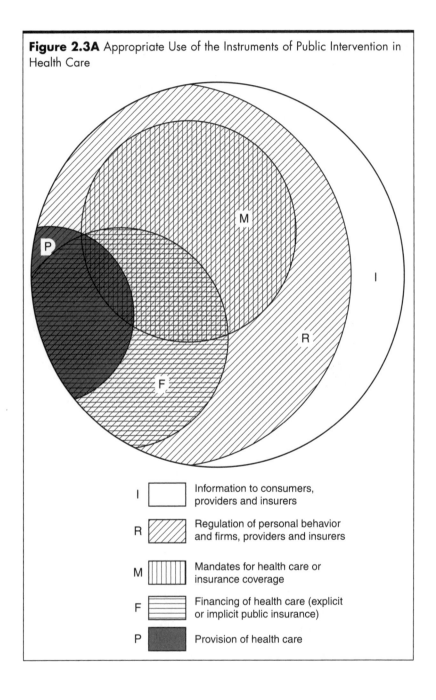

Figure 2.3A Appropriate Use of the Instruments of Public Intervention in Health Care

I — Information to consumers, providers and insurers

R — Regulation of personal behavior and firms, providers and insurers

M — Mandates for health care or insurance coverage

F — Financing of health care (explicit or implicit public insurance)

P — Provision of health care

Figure 2.3B Typically Inappropriate Use of the Instruments of Public Intervention in Health Care

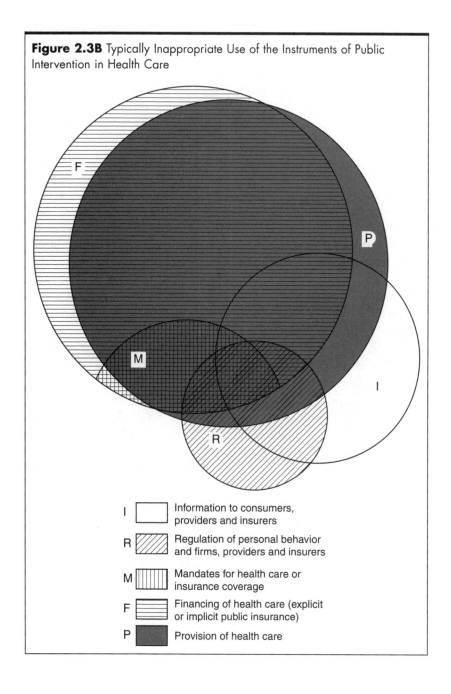

I	☐	Information to consumers, providers and insurers
R	▨	Regulation of personal behavior and firms, providers and insurers
M	▥	Mandates for health care or insurance coverage
F	▤	Financing of health care (explicit or implicit public insurance)
P	■	Provision of health care

besides. The state can finance some care that is not anyone's mandated responsibility, and can also mandate care or insurance coverage which is financed privately. And most if not all public provision should be fully financed by government, but possibly with much more scope for finance than for provision by the state. The largest sphere pertains to information, covering activities in which there is no other public interference with the market. In contrast, Figure 2.3B shows a much smaller effort to inform or regulate, very little use of mandates that are not also publicly financed, and a sphere of provision as large as, or even larger than, that of finance.

Of all the instruments of public action, regulation may be the most under-utilized. Brazil and Chile both provide examples of the resulting problems. In Brazil, the state finances three-quarters of medical care but directly provides only about one-quarter of it, so the instruments of finance and provision are used in the appropriate order. But there is very little regulation of the competence of medical professionals, of the quality of care, or of the rapidly-growing private insurance industry. The lack of regulation even interferes with financing the system, since private insurers sometimes send their customers to publicly financed facilities without paying for care, and until recently fraud was widespread [World Bank 1994b; Medici and Czapski 1995]. In Chile, the private insurance industry was created by public action, with essentially no regulation—but with a mandate allowing people to spend on private insurance, the tax contributions that formerly were used to finance the public system [World Bank 1994a]. The lack of regulation may not have affected medical quality, but it has worsened the financial situation of public facilities, raised administrative costs, and promoted risk selection. Even more serious failures to regulate have arisen in Eastern and Central Europe, as former state monopolies of health finance and provision have given way to competitive private provision.

A second thing governments should do is to stimulate competition in the *provision* of health care. This is largely a matter of promoting public/private competition, for the reasons described above, but it also includes removing any unjustified barriers to competition within the private sector, and between for-profit and non-profit providers such as non-governmental organizations. The lack of competition is usually less of a problem in the domain of low cost, health-related activities than in the domain of costlier activities requiring insurance. This recommendation extends *a fortiori* to non-medical components of health care such as the "hotel" services of hospitals. How far competition should be carried is not always obvious. For example, whether public facilities should make their own purchasing decisions for such inputs as drugs, depends on whether central bulk purchasing reduces costs while maintaining adequate supplies. Even in the latter case, there should of course be competition among suppliers for such purchases.

Except for the risk that providers will compete by offering more services rather than by raising quality or reducing costs—a risk that is greatest when payment is by fee-for service—competition appears to be beneficial in health care provision, just as in other industries. Competition is less desirable in health care *financing*, both because administrative costs are likely to be higher and because it is competition among insurers that leads to risk selection. Experience in OECD countries suggests that good results can be obtained with one or with many insurers, but only if they are closely regulated.

Third, governments should put as much of the incentive for cost containment as possible on the supply side of the market, rather than on consumers. This is almost a necessity where poor consumers are concerned, since their poverty already sharply limits what they can spend. But the evidence is that even non-poor consumers do not respond to higher prices by using health services more cost-effectively. It also appears that providers have considerable scope for controlling expenditure by limiting volume as well as unit costs. And theory indicates that an optimal payment system should use supply-side measures to control costs; reimbursing providers fully according to costs is never the best solution [Ellis and McGuire 1990, 1993]. As income increases and poverty declines, of course, it becomes easier to pass the burden of cost containment to consumers. However, it does not become medically any more effective or economically any more efficient to do so. Moreover, as income increases the capacity for supply-side responses by providers also increases, so it continues to be preferable to keep cost control incentives on the supply side of the market.

Finally, it is urgent to deal with the pervasive problem of government failure, and to improve the capacity to do whatever government ends up doing. This is especially important when market failures are so important that for the public sector to withdraw, on the ground that it also is subject to failure, would only make matters worse. Much of the criticism that governments, particularly in poor countries, try to do too much in health arises because of how *badly* they appear to operate, more than from any evidence that they have exceeded some optimum degree of state intervention. More skill and understanding, and fewer internal barriers to efficiency, make sense whether the state's role shrinks, as by leaving more provision to the private sector, or expands, to finance more coverage for the poor. One of the things governments generally need to do better, particularly in poor countries where much private medical practice may be of low quality, is to use regulation, mandates, training and other interventions to help the private sector function better. This is increasingly recognized as an essential component of almost any health sector reform, and the need for it will only increase as health systems become more expensive and complex. All five instruments of intervention—information, regulation, mandates, finance and provision—need to be used well, and using less of one instrument and more of another will not, in general, reduce the need for governments to perform capably.

References

Aaron, Henry J. 1994. Issues every plan to reform health care financing must confront. *Journal of Economic Perspectives.* Vol. 8, No. 3.

Abel-Smith, Brian. 1995. Assessing the experience of health financing in the United Kingdom. In Dunlop and Martins 1995.

Abel-Smith, Brian. 1984. Cost containment in 12 European countries. *World Health Statistics Quarterly.* Vol. 37.

Arrow, Kenneth J. 1963. Uncertainty and the welfare economics of medical care. *American Economic Review.* Vol. 53, No. 5.

Arrow, Kenneth J. 1985. Theoretical issues in health insurance. In *Collected Papers of Kenneth J. Arrow, Vol. 6, Applied Economics.* Cambridge: Harvard University Press.

Baker, Judy, and Jacques van der Gaag. 1993. Equity in health care and health care financing: evidence from five developing countries. In Van Doorslaer, Wagstaff and Rutten 1993.

Barnum, Howard, Joseph Kutzin and Helen Saxenian. 1995. Incentives and provider payment methods. The World Bank. HRO Working Paper 51.

Barr, Nicholas. 1992. Economic theory and the welfare state: a survey and interpretation. *Journal of Economic Literature.* Vol. 30, No. 2.

Beales, Howard, Richard Craswell, and Steven C. Salop. 1981. The efficient regulation of consumer information. *Journal of Law and Economics.* Vol. 24, No. 3.

Beaton, George H., R. Martorell, K. A. L'Abbe, B. Edmonston, G. McCabe, A. C. Ross and B. Harvey. 1993. *Effectiveness of Vitamin A Supplementation in the Control of Young Child Morbidity and Mortality in Developing Countries: Summary Report.* Toronto: University of Toronto.

Behrman, Jere. 1990. The action of human resources and poverty on one another: what we have yet to learn. Washington, D.C.: World Living Standards Measurement Study, Working Paper No. 74.

Bennett, Sara, George Dakpallah, Paul Garner, Lucy Gilson, Sanguan Nittayaramphong, Beatriz Zurita and Anthony Zwi. 1994. Carrot and stick: state mechanisms to influence private provider behavior. *Health Policy and Planning.* Vol. 9, No. 1.

Bitran, Ricardo, and D. McInness. 1991. Health care demand in Latin America: lessons drawn from the Dominican Republic and El Salvador. Washington, D.C.: World Bank, Economic Development Institute (processed).

Blendon, Robert J., Mollyann Brodie and John Benson. 1995. What happened to Americans' support of the Clinton Plan? *Health Affairs.* Summer.

Bobadilla, Jose Luis. 1996. Searching for Essential Health Packages in Low- and Middle- Income Countries. Washington, D.C.: World Bank (processed).

Boland, Vincent. 1995. Czech health minister sacked in costs crisis. *Financial Times.* 10 October.

Bovbjerg, Randall R., Charles C. Griffin and Caitlin E. Carroll. 1993. U.S. health care coverage and costs: historical development and choices for the 1990s. *Journal of Law, Medicine and Ethics.* Vol. 21, No. 2.

Chabot, Jarl, Manuel Boal and Augusto da Silva. 1991. National community health insurance at village level: the case from Guinea-Bissau. *Health Policy and Planning.* Vol. 6, No. 1.

Chernick, Howard A., Martin R. Holmer and Daniel H. Weinberg. 1987. Tax policy toward health insurance and the demand for medical services. *Journal of Health Economics.* Vol. 6.

Coase, Ronald. 1988. *The Firm, the Market, and the Law.* Chicago: University of Chicago Press.

Cochrane, A. L., A. S. St. Leger and F. Moore. 1978. Health service "input" and mortality "output" in developed countries. *Journal of Epidemiology and Community Health.* Vol. 32.

Congressional Budget Office, U. S. Congress. 1994. An analysis of the Administration's health proposal.

Creese, Andrew. 1991. User charges for health care: a review of recent experience. *Health Policy and Planning.* Vol. 6, No. 4.

Culyer, A. J. 1990. Cost containment in Europe. In Organization for Economic Cooperation and Development. 1990. *Health Care Systems in Transition: The Search for Efficiency.* Social Policy Studies No. 7. Paris: OECD.

Culyer, A. J. 1995. Need: the idea won't do - but we still need it. *Social Science and Medicine.* Vol. 40., No. 6.

Cumper, George E. 1991. *The Evaluation of National Health Systems.* New York: Oxford University Press.

Cutler, David M. 1994. A guide to health care reform. *Journal of Economic Perspectives.* Vol. 8, No. 3.

Diamond, Peter. 1992. Organizing the health insurance market. *Econometrica.* Vol. 660, No. 6.

Dunlop, David W., and Jo. M. Martins, eds. 1995. *An International Assessment of Health Care Financing: Lessons for Developing Countries.* Washington, D.C.: World Bank, Economic Development Institute.

Ellis, Randall P., and Thomas G. McGuire. 1990. Optimal payment systems for health services. *Journal of Health Economics.* Vol. 9.

Ellis, Randall P., and Thomas G. McGuire. 1993. Supply-side and demand-side cost sharing in health care. *Journal of Economic Perspectives.* Vol. 7, No. 4.

Elola, Javier, Antonio Daponte and Vicente Navarro. 1995. Health indicators and the organization of health care systems in Western Europe. *American Journal of Public Health.* Vol. 85, No. 10.

Expanded Programme on Immunization (EPI). 1993. *Newsletter.* Washington, D.C.: Pan American Health Organization. December.

Expanded Programme on Immunization (EPI). 1995. *Newsletter.* Washington, D.C.: Pan American Health Organization. April.

Evans, Robert G., Morris L. Barer, and Roberta J. Labelle. 1988. Fee controls and cost control: tales from the frozen north. *Milbank Memorial Fund Quarterly.* Vol. 66, No. 1.

Evans, Robert G., and Maureen M. Law. 1995. The Canadian health care system: where are we and how did we get there? In Dunlop and Martins 1995.

Feldstein, Martin S. 1973. The welfare loss of excess health insurance. *Journal of Political Economy.* Vol. 81.

Foldvary, Fred E. 1994. *Public Goods and Private Communities.* Cornwall, England: Hartnolls Limited.

Frank, Richard G., and David S. Salkever. 1994. Nonprofit organizations in the health sector. *Journal of Economic Perspectives.* Vol. 8, No. 4.

Fuenzalida-Puelma, Hernan L., and Susan Scholle Connor. 1989. *The Right to Health in the Americas: a Comparative Constitutional Study.* Washington, D.C.: Pan American Health Organization.

Geoffard, Pierre-Yves, and Tomas Philipson. 1994. Market structure and disease eradication: private versus public vaccination. Chicago: Department of Economics, University of Chicago (processed).

Gertler, Paul, and Jacques van der Gaag. 1990. *The Willingness to Pay for Medical Care: Evidence from Two Developing Countries.* Baltimore, Maryland: The Johns Hopkins University Press for the World Bank.

Govindaraj, Ramesh, Christopher J. L. Murray and Gnanaraj Chellaraj. 1994. *Health Expenditures in Latin America.* Cambridge: Harvard Center for Population and Development.

Griffin, Charles C. 1987. *User Charges for Health Care in Principle and Practice.* Washington, D.C.: World Bank Economic Development Institute. Seminar Paper No. 37.

Griffin, Charles C. 1992. *Health Care in Asia: A Comparative Study of Cost and Financing.* Washington, D.C.: World Bank.

Grosh, Margaret. 1992. *Administering Targeted Social Programs in Latin America: From Platitudes to Practice.* Washington, D.C.: World Bank.

Haveman, Robert, and Barbara Wolfe. 1993. Children's prospects and children's policy. *Journal of Economic Perspectives.* Vol. 7, No. 4.

Heysen, Socorro, and Philip Musgrove. 1986. Interdepartmental differences in life expectancy at birth in Peru as it relates to income, household drinking water, and provision of medical consultations. *Bulletin of the Pan American Health Organization.* Vol. 20.

House of Commons. 1995. Science and Technology Committee. Human Genetics: Minutes of Evidence. Wednesday 17 May. London: Her Majesty's Stationery Office.

Jamison, Dean, W. Henry Mosley, Anthony R. Measham and Jose-Luis Bobadilla, eds. 1993. *Disease Control Priorities in Developing Countries.* Oxford: Oxford University Press.

Johns, T., S. L. Booth and H. V. Kuhnlein. 1992. Factors influencing vitamin A intake and programmes to improve vitamin A status. *Food and Nutrition Bulletin* Vol. 14 No. 1.

Kim, Kwanrgkee, and Philip M. Moody. 1992. More resources better health? a cross national perspective. *Social Science and Medicine.* Vol. 34, No. 8.

Lachaud, Claire, and Lise Rochaix. 1993. France. In Van Doorslaer, Wagstaff and Rutten 1993.

Lavy, Victor. 1994. Household responses to public health services: cost and quality tradeoffs. Conference on social sector investments held at the World Bank, Washington, D.C., 18 May (processed).

Lazenby, Helen C., Katharine R. Levit, Daniel R. Waldo, Gerald S. Adler, Suzanne Letsch and Cathy A. Cowan. 1992. National health accounts: lessons from the U.S. experience. *Health Care Financing Review.* Vol. 13, No. 4.

Litvack, Jennie, and Claude Bodart. 1993. User fees and improved quality of health care equals improved access: results of a field experiment in Cameroon. *Social Science and Medicine.* Vol. 37, No. 3.

Lohr, K. N., R. H. Brook, C. J. Kamberg, G. A. Goldberg, A. Leibowitz, J. Keesey, D. Reboussin and J. P. Newhouse. 1986. Effect of cost-sharing on use of medically effective and less effective care. *Medical Care.* Vol. 24.

Makenbach, J. P. 1991. Health care expenditure and mortality from amenable conditions in the European Community. *Health Policy.* Vol. 19.

Makinen, Marty, and Laura Raney. 1994. *Role and Desirability of User Charges for Health Services.* Bethesda, Maryland: Abt Associates, Inc.

McGreevey, William. 1990. *Social Security in Latin America, Issues and Options for the Bank.* Washington, D.C.: World Bank Discussion Papers, 110.

McGuire, Alistair, David Parkin, David Hughes and Karen Gerard. 1993. Econometric analyses of national health expenditures: can positive economics help to answer normative questions? *Health Economics.* Vol. 2.

McPake, Barbara, Kara Hanson and Anne Mills. 1993. *Experience to date of Implementing the Bamako Initiative: a Review and Five Country Case Studies.* London: London School of Hygiene and Tropical Medicine.

Médici, André Cézar, and Cláudio André Czapski. 1995. *Evolução e Perspectivas dos Gastos Públicos em Saúde no Brasil.* Consultants' Report. Washington, D.C.: World Bank.

Mesa-Lago, Carmelo. 1992. *Health Care for the Poor in Latin America and the Caribbean* Washington, D.C.: Pan-American Health Organization and Inter-American Foundation.

Milgrom, Paul, and John Roberts. 1992. *Economics, Organization and Management.* Englewood Cliffs, New Jersey: Prentice Hall.

Miller, Jonathan. 1978. *The Body in Question.* New York: Random House.

Murray, Christopher J. L., Ramesh Gavindaraj and Philip Musgrove. 1994. National health expenditures: a global analysis. In World Health Organization 1994.

Musgrave, Richard A. 1959. *The Theory of Public Finance, A Study in Public Economy.* New York: McGraw-Hill.

Musgrove, Philip. 1986. Measurement of equity in health. *World Health Statistics Quarterly.* Vol, 39, No. 4.

Musgrove, Philip. 1995a. Cost-effectiveness and the socialization of health care. *Health Policy.* Vol. 32.

Musgrove, Philip. 1995b. Mismatch of need, demand and supply of services: picturing different ways health systems can go wrong. Washington, D.C.: World Bank, HCO Working Paper No. 59.

Musgrove, Philip. 1995c. Reformas al sector salud en Chile: contexto, lógica y posibles caminos. In Giaconi, Juan G., ed., *La Salud en el Siglo XXI: Cambios Necesarios.* Santiago, Chile: Centro de Estudios Públicos.

Navarro, Vicente. 1989. Why some countries have national health insurance, others have national health services, and the U. S. has neither. *Social Science and Medicine.* Vol. 28, No. 9.

Newhouse, Joseph P., *et al.* 1993. *Free for All? Lessons from the RAND Health Insurance Experiment.* Cambridge: Harvard University Press.

Nolan, Brian, and Vincent Turbat. 1995. *Cost Recovery in Public Health Services in Sub-Saharan Africa.* Washington, D.C.: The World Bank, Economic Development Institute.

Okun, Arthur M. 1975. *Equality and Efficiency: the Big Tradeoff.* Washington, D.C.: The Brookings Institution.

Organization for Economic Cooperation and Development (OECD). 1992. *The Reform of Health Care Systems: a Comparative Analysis of Seven OECD Countries.* Paris: OECD.

Organization for Economic Cooperation and Development (OECD). 1994. *The Reform of Health Care Systems: a Review of Seventeen OECD Countries.* Paris: OECD.

Organization for Economic Cooperation and Development (OECD). 1995. *New Directions in Health Care Policy.* Health Policy Studies No. 7. Paris: OECD.

Pan American Health Organization (PAHO). 1994. *Health Conditions in the Americas.* Washington, D.C.: PAHO.

Pauly, Mark V. 1968. The economics of moral hazard. *American Economic Review.* Vol. 58.

Pauly, Mark V. 1974. Overinsurance and public provision of insurance: the roles of moral hazard and adverse selection. *Quarterly Journal of Economics.* Vol. 88.

Pauly, Mark V. 1986. Taxation, health insurance, and market failure in the medical economy. *Journal of Economic Literature.* Vol. 24.

Pauly, Mark V. *et. al.* 1988. Issues related to volume and intensity of physician services. Report prepared for the U. S. Health Care Financing Administration. Baltimore.

Pelletier, David, L. 1994. The relationship between child anthropometry and mortality in developing countries: implications for policy, programs and future research. *Journal of Nutrition.* Vol. 124, No. 10S.

Poullier, Jean-Pierre. 1992. Administrative costs in selected industrialized countries. *Health Care Financing Review.* Vol. 13, No.4.

Ricklefs, Robert E., and Caleb E. Finch. 1995. *Aging: a Natural History.* New York: W. H. Freeman, Scientific American Library.

Russell, Louise B. 1986. *Is Prevention Better Than Cure?* Washington, D.C.: The Brookings Institution.

Schieber, George, Jean-Pierre Poullier, and Leslie M. Greenwald. 1992. U. S. health expenditure performance: An international comparison and data update. *Health Care Financing Review, International Comparison of Health Systems.* Vol. 13, No. 4.

Schieber, George, Jean-Pierre Poullier, and Leslie M. Greenwald. 1994. Health System Performance in OECD Countries, 1980-1992. *Health Affairs.* Fall.

Skocpol, Theda. 1995. The rise and resounding demise of the Clinton Plan. *Health Affairs.* Spring.

Shaw, R. Paul, and Charles C. Griffin. 1995. *Financing Health Care in Sub-Saharan Africa through User Fees and Insurance.* Washington, D.C.: World Bank, Directions in Development.

Shea, Dennis G., and R. Patrick Stewart. 1995. Demand for insurance by elderly persons: private purchases and employer provision. *Health Economics.* Vol. 4.

Srinivasan, T. N. 1994. Destitution: A Discourse. *Journal of Economic Literature.* Vol. 32.

Stiglitz, Joseph. 1989. Principal and agent. In Eatwell, John, Murray Milgate and Peter Newman, eds. *The New Palgrave: Allocation, Information and Markets.* New York: W. W. Norton.

Summers, Lawrence H. 1989. Some simple economics of mandated benefits. *American Economics Association Papers and Proceedings.* Vol. 79, No. 2.

Tresseras, R., J. Canela, J. Alvarez, J. Sentis and L. Salleras. 1992. Infant mortality, per capita income, and adult illiteracy: an ecological approach. *American Journal of Public Health.* Vol. 82, No. 3.

U. S. Department of Health and Human Services. 1989 *Reducing the Health Consequences of Smoking: 25 years of Progress. A Report of the Surgeon General.*

Rockville, Maryland: Prepublication Version, DHHS Publication Number (CDC) 89-8411.

U. S. Department of Health and Human Services. 1992. *Smoking and Health in the Americas.* Atlanta, Georgia: DHHS Publication Number (CDC) 92-8419.

Van der Gaag, Jacques. 1995. *Public and Private Initiatives: Working Together for Health and Education.* Washington, D.C.: World Bank, Directions in Development.

Van Doorslaer, Eddy, Adam Wagstaff and Frans Rutten. 1993. *Equity in the Finance and Delivery of Health Care: an International Perspective.* Oxford: Oxford University Press.

Vogel, Ronald J. 1993. Financing Health Care in Sub-Saharan Africa: A Policy Study. Silver Spring, Maryland: Basic Health Management, Inc. for the African Development Bank.

Weisbrod, Burton A. 1991. The Health Care Quadrilemma: An Essay on Technological Change, Insurance, Quality of Care, and Cost Containment. *Journal of Economic Literature.* Vol. 29, No. 2. pp. 523-552.

Wolfe, Barbara L. 1986. Health status and medical expenditures: is there a link? *Social Science and Medicine.* Vol. 22, No. 10.

World Bank. 1980. *Health: Sector Policy Paper.* Washington, D.C.: World Bank.

World Bank. 1987. *Financing Health Services in Developing Countries: An Agenda for Reform.* A World Bank Policy Study. Washington, D.C.: World Bank.

World Bank. 1991. *World Development Report: The Challenge of Development.* Washington, D.C.: World Bank.

World Bank. 1992a. *World Development Report: Development and the Environment.* Washington, D.C.: World Bank.

World Bank. 1992b. *China: Long-Term Issues and Options in the Health Transition.* Washington, D.C.: World Bank.

World Bank. 1993a. *Argentina: Public Finance Review—from Insolvency to Growth.* Washington, D.C.: World Bank. Report No. 10827-AR.

World Bank. 1993b. *World Development Report: Investing in Health.* Washington, D.C.: World Bank.

World Bank. 1993c. *The Organization, Delivery and Financing of Health Care in Brazil.* Washington, D.C.: World Bank. Report No. 12655-BR.

World Bank. 1994a. *Chile: The Adult Health Policy Challenge.* Washington, D.C.: World Bank. Report No. 12681-CH.

World Bank. 1994b. *Private Sector and Social Services in Brazil: Who Delivers, Who Pays, Who Regulates.* Washington, D.C.: World Bank. Report No. 13205-BR.

World Bank. 1995. The World Bank in the Health Sector. Washington, D.C.

World Health Organization. 1994. *Global Comparative Assessments in the Health Sector: Disease Burden, Expenditures and Intervention Packages.* Geneva: World Health Organization.

Zeckhauser, Richard. 1994. Public finance principles and national health care reform. *Journal of Economic Perspectives.* Vol. 8, No. 3.

CHAPTER 3

The Rationale for Government Intervention in the Tobacco Market

Acknowledgments

I am grateful to all those colleagues at the World Bank who provided the opportunity to work on this subject, including those whose criticisms required sharpening the arguments; among the latter, Michael Walton deserves particular mention.

Introduction

There is no doubt that prolonged smoking is an important cause of premature mortality and disability worldwide. Strictly on health terms, then, there is a strong reason to intervene to reduce this damage.

However, smoking is voluntary and is not illegal for adults, so the existence of an enormous health problem is not, *prima facie*, sufficient to justify interference with people's choice to smoke. An *economic* rationale for such intervention requires that failures in tobacco markets are sufficiently large to justify the costs of such interference. Despite the strong consensus that smoking harms health, there is much debate about proper government roles, if any, in reducing smoking (see, for example, *The Economist* 1997).

Co-authored with Prabhat Jha, Frank Chaloupka, and Ayda Yurekli. Excerpted and reprinted, with permission, from "The Rationale for Government Intervention", in Prabhat Jha and Frank Chaloupka, eds., *Tobacco Control Policies in Developing Countries*. Oxford: Oxford University Press for the World Bank and the World Health Organization, 2000.

We explore the economic rationale for government intervention in tobacco markets. We first discuss the two key market failures that justify government intervention on efficiency grounds: first, consumers' incomplete information about the risks of addiction and disease; and, second, external costs. We do not deal with supply side market failures, such as the monopoly power of the tobacco industry. Next, we discuss which interventions are available to governments to correct these market failures, noting their specificity and effectiveness and their economic costs. We focus in this section on interventions that would protect children and adult non-smokers, and that would inform adult smokers. Third, we discuss whether government intervention in tobacco markets is appropriate to reduce inequity between rich and poor.

This exploration will take account of particular epidemiological features of the tobacco epidemic that are relevant to the economic arguments. The first of these is the early age at which people typically start smoking, which, in high-income countries at least, is during the teen years. The risk of lung cancer is far higher in individuals who start smoking at age 15 and smoke one pack a day for 40 years than among those who start at age 35 and smoke two packs a day for 20 years (Peto 1986). Therefore, the early age of onset has a direct bearing on individuals' health risks. From the standpoint of economics, the early typical age of onset is also relevant because the standard economic concept of consumer sovereignty, which holds that the consumer knows what is best for him or her, may not apply so forcefully to adolescents as to adults. The second key epidemiological feature of the tobacco epidemic is that fully half of smoking related deaths occur in productive middle age (defined as 35–69 years) (Peto et al. 1994). This is relevant to the economic debate about smoking, since it dispels the notion that smoking kills people mostly in old age, when the economic losses (as well as the health losses) are small.

Inefficiencies in the Tobacco Market

Smokers clearly receive benefits from smoking; otherwise they would not pay to do it. The perceived benefits include pleasure and satisfaction, stress relief (presumably derived in part from the nicotine content of the smoke), peer acceptance, and a sense of maturity and sophistication (most important for adolescent smokers, and derived from the act of smoking as such). An additional important benefit for the addicted smoker is the avoidance of nicotine withdrawal. There is little that economics can say about the preferences that determine smoking, except to try to understand how the addictive nature of cigarettes influences subsequent consumption. As with other addictive behaviors, the decision to start and the "decision" to continue are quite different, and different economic arguments may be relevant to each. The private costs to be weighed against those benefits include money spent on tobacco products, damage to health, and nicotine addiction. Defined this way, the *perceived* benefits evidently outweigh the *perceived* costs for at least 1.1 billion people who smoke today. Economic theory assumes that the consumer knows best and that privately determined consumption will most efficiently allocate society's scarce resources. Thus, *if* smokers know their risks and internalize all their costs and benefits, there is no justification, on the grounds of inefficiency, for governments to interfere (Pekurinen 1991).

However, these assumptions may not hold for several reasons, leading to market failures. (Note that even efficient markets do not necessarily achieve equity, and that inequity is not normally classified as market failure. We discuss equity issues later in the chapter.) Below, we analyze three failures in the tobacco market. The first is incomplete information about health risks. The second is incomplete information about addiction, specifically the complex issue of children's tendency to under-estimate the addictive potential of smoking (and therefore the costs of quitting). The third failure consists of costs imposed on others.

Incomplete information about health consequences

Incomplete information about the risks of smoking leads to behavior that smokers would not otherwise choose for themselves. Poorly-informed smokers often underestimate the risks of their action (Weinstein 1998). Since people usually react to known risks by reducing the risky consumption, incomplete information means more smoking than would otherwise occur. There are two principal reasons why smokers tend to be inadequately informed. The first is that the market, far from providing information, has actually hidden or distorted it. The second is the long delay between starting to smoke and the onset of obvious disease, which has obscured the link between the two. Each of these are discussed in turn. The tobacco industry, like other industries, has no financial incentive to provide health information that would reduce consumption of its products. On the contrary, the industry has consistently hidden product information on the ill effects of smoking or actively misinformed smokers about risks (Sweda and Daynard 1996). Notably, the industry has used advertising and promotion to promote its products as 'safe' despite internal evidence that all types of smoking are harmful. For example, the industry has tried to advertise filter cigarettes as 'healthier' (USDHHS 1989). The industry has also used advertising to reach young smokers (Institute of Medicine 1994). Other tactics of the industry to leave smokers uninformed or misinformed include dissuading lay journals from reporting on smoking's health effects (Warner *et al.* 1992), and sponsoring biased scientific research (Bero *et al.* 1994). Internal industry documents uncovered in recent lawsuits in the United States confirm such practices (Glantz *et al.* 1995).

Second, consumers derive information on the costs and benefits of smoking primarily from their own experience and what happens to their peers, as well as from studies largely financed by the public sector. However, the obvious health damage from smoking usually emerges at least 20–30 years after exposure. This differs from most other risky behaviors, such as fast driving, where the costs and benefits are more readily and immediately appreciated.

The long delay between exposure and effect has also impeded the growth of scientific knowledge. In the United States, the 1960s evidence suggested that only one in four smokers died from smoking. When risks were reassessed decades later, when the epidemic had matured, the evidence showed that the risks were actually much higher: one in two long-term smokers die from smoking (see Doll *et al.* 1994; Peto *et al.* 1999). Anyone who considered starting or continuing smoking 20 or 30 years ago in high-income countries would, therefore, have under-estimated the risks, even if he or she had based the decision on the best available information. Moreover, as the list of diseases and conditions associated with smoking expands, smokers continue to under-estimate the risks. Most developing countries still do not have estimates of the health hazards of smoking for their own populations. It is, therefore, not surprising that even respectable journals, such as *The Economist* (1997), reveal their confusion about the scale of the true risks or the high proportion of smokers who die in middle age:

> ". . . most smokers (two-thirds or more) do not die of smoking-related disease. They gamble and win. Moreover, the years lost to smoking come from the end of life, when people are most likely to die of something else anyway."

As Kenkel and Chen (2000) discuss, there are two key features of consumers' incomplete information: first, in low-income and middle-income countries, absolute awareness of the health risks is still comparatively low. For example, in China, about two-thirds of adult smokers surveyed in 1996 believed that cigarettes did them "little or no harm" (Chinese Academy of

Preventive Medicine 1997). Second, consumers in all countries may not clearly internalize the risks, even when they have been informed about them, nor may they accurately judge the risks of smoking relative to other environmental exposures, such as 'stress' or radiation.

Children and teenagers generally know less about the health effects of smoking than adults. A recent survey of 15- and 16-year-olds in Moscow found that more than half either knew of no smoking-related diseases or could name only one, lung cancer (Levshin and Droggachih 1999). Even in the United States, where young people might be expected to have received more information, almost half of 13-year-olds today think that smoking a pack of cigarettes a day will not cause them great harm (National Cancer Policy Board 1998).

In addition, teenagers—even those with good understanding of the risks of smoking—may have a limited capacity to use information wisely. Teenagers behave myopically, or short-sightedly. It is difficult for most teenagers to imagine being 25, let alone 55, and warnings about the damage that smoking will inflict on their health at some distant date are unlikely to reduce their desire to smoke.

In developing countries, there is less awareness of the hazards of smoking at all ages, including among adults, for several reasons. Education levels are lower, and, since education leads to more rapid and thorough absorption of information, it is reasonable to conclude that less-educated populations will be less receptive to health information.

There are fewer local data on the hazards of smoking and less dissemination of existing data on health risks. Governments less often regulate industry information practices, such as advertising and promotion. For all these reasons, it is unlikely that current smokers and potential smokers in low-income and middle-income countries have adequate knowledge from which to make informed decisions.

Inadequate information about addiction

The second major information failure in the tobacco market involves inadequate information about nicotine addiction. Smokers acquire *psychological addiction* to the act of smoking itself, and *physical addiction* to nicotine (Kessler *et al.* 1997). Psychological addiction to cigarettes is hardly different from habit formation with respect to other products or practices. Nicotine addiction, however, is not simply a matter of choice or taste reinforced by repetition, such as choosing to listen to certain music or keeping company with dangerous friends. Of course, as with all biologically addictive goods, many people can change their behavior and quit using nicotine, as the decline in smoking among adults in high-income countries demonstrates. However, the costs of quitting are significant, so much so that some people find quitting virtually impossible. Most smokers who quit have to make several attempts before they succeed, and former smokers remain vulnerable to resuming smoking at times of stress (USDHHS 1990).

Is addiction alone reason enough for governments to intervene against smoking? If children had full information about the likelihood of becoming addicted and understood the long-run implications of their addiction, they might conceivably become 'happy addicts' who are maximizing their own welfare by smoking. For example, the teenager might argue that it would be 'better to suffer lung cancer at age 60 than to suffer Alzheimer's disease at age 80'. Models of so-called 'rational addiction' (Becker and Murphy 1988) assume that individuals maximize utility over their lifetime, taking into account the future consequences of their choices. However, the key assumptions of the model are that people are fully rational, that they are far-sighted about their choices, and that they have full information on the costs and benefits of their choices. These assumptions are not satisfied in the case of smoking. Children are more myopic, or 'short-sighted', than adults, and they typically have less information. Recent extensions to the rational addiction model by Orphanides and Zervos (1995) take some of this into account when looking at youthful 'decisions' to become addicted. In their model, imperfect information about addiction early in life can result in seemingly rational decisions that are later viewed with regret.

Other recent theoretical work emphasizes the role of 'adjustment costs' for addictive goods (Suranovic et al. 1999). The presence of these adjustment costs, in the context of less than fully rational behavior, implies that smokers may continue to smoke while regretting this decision, given that the costs of stopping are greater than the costs of continuing. In this context, rather than providing benefits, continued smoking for an addicted smoker is the lesser of two evils. Some might interpret the differences between the short- and long-run price elasticities of demand for an addictive good as reflecting the magnitude of these adjustment costs. That is, much of the difference between the long-run and short-run consumer surplus may be thought to reflect the adjustment costs. Assuming a linear demand curve, and given the evidence that the long-run elasticity for cigarette demand is about double the short-run elasticity, this suggests that as much as half of perceived consumer surplus (based on short-run demand) reflects the adjustment costs associated with addiction.

Perhaps most importantly, there is clear evidence that young people under-estimate the risk of becoming addicted to nicotine, and, therefore, grossly under-estimate their future costs from smoking. Among high-school seniors in the United States who smoke but believe that they will quit within five years, fewer than two out of five actually do quit. The rest are still smoking five years later (Institute of Medicine 1994). In high income countries, about seven out of ten adult smokers say they regret their choice to start smoking and two-thirds make serious attempts to quit during their life (USDHHS 1989). In sum, it is the combination of imperfect information about addiction and myopia that results in significant under-estimation of the risks of future health damage. In the absence of addiction, teenagers could more easily quit later, when they become aware of the health risks, as they tend to do where other risky behaviors are concerned. We discuss this further below. The risk that young people will make unwise decisions is recognized by most societies and is not unique to choices about smoking, although in the case of smoking it is compounded by addiction and inadequate information. Therefore, most societies restrict young people's power to make certain decisions. For example, most democracies prevent their young people from voting before a certain age; some societies make education compulsory up to a certain age; and many prevent marriage before a certain age. The consensus across most societies is that some decisions are best left until adulthood. Likewise, many societies consider that the freedom of young people to choose to become addicted should be restricted.

It might be argued that young people are attracted to many risky behaviors, such as fast driving or alcohol binge-drinking, and that there is nothing special about smoking. However, few other risky behaviors carry the high risk of addiction that is seen with smoking, and most others are easier to abandon or modify, and are abandoned or modified in maturity (O'Malley *et al.* 1998; Bachman *et al.* 1997). For example, teenagers often binge drink, but most grow to be responsible moderate drinkers later in life. Driving motor vehicles is risky, but most young drivers survive long enough to learn to drive more responsibly. With smoking, there is no comparable way to behave more prudently, except to quit; even cutting back somewhat on consumption does not reduce the risks proportionally. Also, compared with other risky behaviors, such as alcohol use, new recruits to smoking face a very high probability of premature death. These factors combined create a probability of addiction and premature death that is higher than for other risk behaviors. Using estimates from Murray and Lopez (1996) and WHO (1999), and studies in high-income countries, we estimate that of 1000

15-year-old males currently living in middle-income and low-income countries, 125 will be killed by smoking before age 70 if they continue to smoke regularly. By comparison, before age 70, 10 will die because of road accidents, 10 will die because of violence, and about 30 will die of alcohol-related causes, including some road accidents and violent deaths.

The tobacco industry has a clear incentive to subsidize or to give away free cigarettes to potential smokers, especially young people, in order to induce them to smoke and become addicted to nicotine (Becker *et al.* 1994; Ensor 1992). The same incentive applies to creating addiction among adults in low-income and middle-income countries by manipulating price.

Thus, at best, nicotine addiction greatly weakens the argument that smokers should exercise consumer sovereignty. Given the myopia of young consumers and the likelihood of information failure for all smokers, it is inappropriate to regard an addiction-induced demand as representing genuine welfare gains to the smoker.

External costs

Consumers and producers in any transaction may impose costs or benefits on others, which are known as externalities. The costs—or benefits—imposed by smokers on others are of three types. First are the direct physical costs for non-smokers who are exposed to others' smoke. Second are the financial externalities that cause monetary loss (or gain) for non-smokers, whether or not they are exposed to smoke. Last (and most difficult to assess) are the so-called 'caring externalities' or 'existence value' effects of smoking, whereby non-smokers suffer emotionally from the illness and death of smokers unrelated to them personally.

Physical externalities. Physical externalities from smokers involve both health effects for non-smokers, such as a higher risk of disease or death, and other effects, such as the nuisance of unpleasant smells, physical irritation, and smoke residues on clothes, and the greater risks of fire and property damage. The health effects are briefly summarized. They include, for children born to smoking mothers, low birth weight and an increased risk of various diseases (USDHHS 1986; Charlton 1996), and an increased risk of various diseases in children and adults chronically exposed to environmental tobacco smoke either at home or in the workplace (Environmental Protection Agency 1992; Wald and Hackshaw 1996). Importantly, the list of diseases and conditions associated with environmental tobacco smoke is expanding (California Environmental Protection Agency 1997).

Financial externalities. Financial externalities are costs that are imposed by smokers but at least partly financed by non-smokers. In countries where there is an element of publicly financed healthcare, these include medical costs, among them the costs of treating the newborns of mothers who smoke during pregnancy. Non-smokers also help to pay for the damage from fires and the higher maintenance costs of workplaces and homes where smokers are present. Here we briefly summarize the key arguments related to healthcare costs and to pensions.

In high-income countries, the overall annual cost of healthcare that may be attributed to smoking has been estimated to be between 6% and 15% of total healthcare costs. In most low-income and middle-income countries today, the annual costs of healthcare attributable to smoking are lower than this, partly because the epidemic of tobacco-related diseases is at an earlier stage, and partly because of other factors, such as the kinds of tobacco-related diseases that are most prevalent and the treatments that they require. However, these countries are likely to see their annual smoking related healthcare costs rise in the future as the tobacco epidemic matures (World Bank 1992).

For those concerned with public spending budgets, it is vital to know these annual healthcare costs and the fraction borne by the public sector, because they represent real resources that cannot be used for other goods and services. For individual consumers, on the other hand, the key issue is the extent to which the costs will be borne by themselves or by others. As the following discussion shows, the assessment of these costs is complex, and therefore it is not possible yet to draw definitive conclusions about whether or how they may influence smokers' consumption choices.

In any given year, on average, a smoker's healthcare is likely to cost more than that of a non-smoker of the same age and sex. However, because smokers tend to die earlier than non-smokers, the *lifetime* healthcare costs of smokers and non-smokers in high income countries may be fairly similar. Studies that measure the lifetime healthcare costs of smokers and non-smokers in high-income countries have reached conflicting conclusions. In the Netherlands (Barendregdt *et al.*1997) and Switzerland (Leu and Schwab 1983), for example, smokers and non-smokers have been found to have similar costs, while in the United Kingdom (Atkinson and Townsend 1977) and the United States (Hodgson 1992), some studies have concluded that smokers' lifetime costs are, in fact, higher. Part of this confusion stems from the fact that it is relatively easy to make actuarial estimates of the potential for smokers' earlier deaths to bring savings in public health or pension expenditures. In contrast, the external financial costs of smoking are more difficult to measure reliably, and may be considerably under-estimated (Chaloupka and Warner, 2000). Recent reviews that take account of the growing number of tobacco-attributable diseases and other factors conclude that, overall, smokers' lifetime costs in high-income countries are somewhat greater than those of non-smokers, despite their earlier deaths (Chaloupka and Warner, 2000). There are no such reliable studies on lifetime healthcare costs in low-income and middle-income countries.

Clearly, for all regions of the world, smokers who assume the full costs of their medical services will not impose costs on others, however much greater those costs may be than non-smokers'. In developing countries, higher proportions of healthcare costs are borne by private individuals, rather than by the public system (Bos *et al.* 1999). Nonetheless, even in low-income countries, a significant percentage of medical care, especially that associated with hospital treatment, is financed either through government budgets or through private insurance. To the extent that taxes, co-payments, or social insurance premiums are not differentially higher for smokers, the higher medical costs attributable to smokers will be at least partly borne by non-smokers. To the extent that private business healthcare costs are passed on to consumers in the form of higher prices, or to workers in the form of lower wages, any costs incurred by workers who smoke will similarly be partly passed on to non-smokers. However, such costs are small in low-income and middle-income countries (Collins and Lapsley 1998). Out-of-pocket payments and risk-adjusted insurance schemes do not burden non-smokers with some of the costs of smokers. For private insurance, where premiums for non-smokers are lower than for smokers, there may be little economic justification for public intervention. In reality, however, most health insurance plans are increasingly group-based and contain no risk-adjustment for smoking.

In low-income and middle-income countries, intra-household transfers of income or welfare may be as important a source of externalities as formal, extra-household transfers (James 1994). Manning *et al.* (1991) and others argue that intra-household transfers are irrelevant, since adults' decisions to smoke are made on behalf of a whole household, and reflect the preferences of all family members. This is implausible, since adults are likely to become smokers before marrying or having children. They are likely to find it difficult to quit later—even if spouses or children urge them to. Furthermore, very young children, who may be the most severely affected by exposure to others' smoke, have no voice in such decisions.

Spouses may, in deciding to marry, have taken into account the addiction of their partner, and may, therefore, be said to acquiesce in the decision; but that is not the same thing as helping to make the decision or approving of it.

In high-income countries, public expenditure on health accounts for about 65% of all health expenditures, or about 6% of GDP (Bos *et al.* 1999). If smokers have higher net lifetime healthcare costs, then non-smokers will subsidize the healthcare costs of smokers. The exact contribution is complex and variable, depending on the type of coverage and the source of taxation that is used to pay for public expenditures. If, for example, only the healthcare costs of those over 65 are publicly funded, then the net use of public revenues by smokers may be small, to the extent that many require smoking-related medical care and die *before* they reach this age. Equally, if public expenditure is financed out of consumption taxes, including cigarette taxes, or if third-party private insurance adjusts smokers' premiums because of their higher health risks, then their costs may not be imposed on others. Once again, the situation differs in low-income and middle-income countries, where the public component of total healthcare expenditure is on average lower than in high-income countries, at around 44% of the total, or 2% of GDP (Bos *et al.* 1999). However, as countries spend more on health, the share of total expenditure that is met by public finance tends to rise too (World Bank 1993).

While it is difficult to assess the relative healthcare costs of smokers and nonsmokers, the issue of pensions has proved at least as contentious, and has attracted some popular debate. For example, an editorial in *The Economist* (1995) expressed the view that smokers 'pay their way'. It continued:

> ". . . what they cost in medical bills, fires and so on, they more than repay in pensions they do not live to collect."

This assertion is based on analyses from high-income countries that suggest that smokers contribute more than non-smokers to pension schemes, because many pay contributions until around retirement age and then die before they can claim a substantial proportion of their benefits (Manning 1989; Viscusi 1995). There are several problems with this assertion. First, there is an ongoing academic debate over definitions of the social costs of smoking, and particularly the extent to which 'savings' from not collecting pensions should be included. Depending on differing assumptions, other studies (see, for example, Atkinson and Townsend 1977) have not found net costs for smokers to be lower. Second, the issue is not currently relevant to many of the low-income and middle-income countries where most of the world's smokers live. In low-income countries, only about one in ten adults has a public pension, and in middle-income countries the proportion is between a quarter and half of the population, depending on the income level of the country; private pension plans are less common (James 1994). Finally, and perhaps most importantly, most of these studies have followed traditional notions of economic externalities, and have not placed any value on life *per se*. Even if smokers do reduce the net costs imposed on others by dying young, it would be misleading to suggest that society is better off because of these premature deaths. To do so would be to accept a logic that says society is better off without its older adults (Harris 1994).

Caring externalities. The third group of externalities that we consider are those that are the most difficult to assess: they are known as 'existence value' or 'caring' externalities (Krutilla 1967). There is evidence that people are willing to pay for another's well being, even if they do not know the person and even if they do not benefit directly themselves. Public spending on health partly reflects such externalities. Existence value is most readily applied to children, whom society typically protects more than adults. In contrast, caring externalities for adults almost directly contradict the notion of consumer sovereignty. Clearly, caring externalities differ across cultures and countries, depending among other things on the importance society assigns to individual sovereignty. Nonsmokers may be willing to subsidize efforts to prevent people taking up smoking or efforts to help smokers quit. They may also be prepared to contribute towards the care of sick smokers, even when these represent a financial burden. However, their attitudes may change over time as knowledge about the health effects of smoking becomes more widespread and non-smokers' tolerance for smokers may decline (Gorovitz et al. 1998). In any case, there is little solid information of such willingness, so it is difficult to use it to formulate public policies.

In sum, there are clearly direct costs imposed by smokers on non-smokers, such as health damage. There are probably also financial costs, although it is more difficult to identify or quantify these.

Government Responses to Market Failure: What, For Whom and at What Price?

Given that, as we have argued, the markets for tobacco products suffer efficiency failures that result in premature death and illness, and costs imposed on others, it is appropriate to ask if government intervention can correct them. Here we ask whether governments have interventions available to correct these failures, and discuss the costs and effectiveness of these interventions.

Below we describe briefly those interventions that respond to, or deal with, each of the types of inefficiency in the tobacco market that we have described above. Governments can use information, regulation, taxation, or subsidies to address these market failures.

Government responses to *incomplete or erroneous information* include, specifically, mass information campaigns, warning labels, and publicly-financed research to create more, or better, or more easily assimilated, information. All are public goods, which the market is unlikely to provide adequately. Public responses to existing addiction in adults include, specifically, incentives to quit, such as cessation programs (with or without pharmacological therapies) offered free or at subsidized prices, and education campaigns that raise awareness of the risks of smoking and the benefits of cessation. In addition, governments can encourage deregulation of the market for nicotine replacement therapy. Public responses to preventing new addiction in children (discussed in more detail below) include education campaigns about the danger of addiction, restricting children's access to tobacco products, bans on the advertising and promotion of tobacco products, and taxation. Increased taxation will also increase cessation rates among adults.

Government responses to *direct physical externalities* include education campaigns emphasizing the right of non-smokers to a smoke-free environment, restrictions on smoking in public places and workplaces, and taxes. Government responses to *financial externalities* may include risk-adjusted health or pension premiums, or anything that restricts tobacco consumption, whether or not in the presence of non-smokers. These may include taxation, information campaigns, and restrictions on where people can smoke.

Government responses to *'existence value'* externalities also include any intervention that restricts consumption and thereby reduces the health damage from smoking. Concern for smokers at highest risk—those already addicted who have smoked for many years—would lead to specific subsidies for cessation programs, the deregulation of nicotine replacement markets, and information campaigns emphasizing the dangers of long-term smoking. However, in reality, governments do not always aim interventions directly at the sources of market failures themselves, but to particular constituencies or population groups affected by those market failures. In the case of the tobacco market, government intervention is often designed to protect children.

We turn now to a discussion of the appropriateness of the various available interventions.

Choosing 'first-best' and 'second-best' interventions

Government intervention in the tobacco market is most easily justified to deter children and adolescents from smoking and to protect non-smokers. But it is also justified for the purposes of giving adults all the information they need to make an informed choice. Ideally, government interventions should address each identified problem with a specific intervention tailored to solve that particular problem and none other. These may be thought of as first-best interventions. However, a neat one-to-one correspondence between problems and solutions is not always possible, and some interventions may have broader effects. We discuss first-best interventions, their effectiveness, and their limitations, first for protecting children, then for correcting the physical and financial costs imposed by smokers on others, and lastly for informing adult smokers. A common theme emerges: the use of taxes, though a second-best and more blunt instrument, is more effective.

Protecting children. Several economists have suggested that protection of children is the most compelling economic argument for higher taxes (Warner *et al.* 1995). Governments can choose to protect children for several reasons. First, childhood is when nicotine addiction is likely to begin. Second, children are not yet sovereign adults making informed choices, so the principal argument for not intervening does not apply to them as strongly as to adults. Third, there is evidence that the tobacco industry targets children with glamorous advertisements and promotion. Fourth, compared with many consumer goods that may appear desirable to children, such as automobiles, cigarettes are generally affordable and accessible: thus the market does not spontaneously protect children from them. Finally, children have no way to become better or safer smokers as they mature, except by quitting.

A priori, parents would ideally always be willing and able to protect children from tobacco themselves. If this happened, there would be little need for governments to duplicate such efforts (Musgrove 1999). Perfect parents, however, are rare. Adults may smoke themselves, thereby modeling this behavior for their children, and, even though few would actually encourage their children to start smoking, they may also fail to educate them about the risks. Parents' responsibilities on the question of smoking are not comparable to, say, their responsibilities to ensure their children are immunized. In the latter case, the parent or caregiver has a defined responsibility to protect the child through a fairly simple action, and the child's lack of information is irrelevant.

The next best public or non-parental interventions would be to try to educate children, restrict advertising and promotion targeted to children, and to restrict their access to tobacco products. As discussed above, information campaigns have had an important impact on overall declines in smoking in high-income countries. But information campaigns targeted at children are likely to be less effective than those targeted at adults, because children discount the future more, and have difficulty considering consequences of today's behavior that may not take effect for three or four decades. Individual youth-centered programs, including school health programs, have often been found ineffective (Reid 1996).

For a specific campaign aimed at children, governments would need to ban advertising and promotion of tobacco products in the media that children are most often exposed to, such as television or radio. Empirical evidence (Saffer 2000) suggests that partial bans cause the tobacco industry to shift to other media, including promotional goods (such as free samples), and sponsorship of sports events, which do influence children (Charlton et al. 1997). Finally, efforts to restrict young people's access to tobacco products in shops, restaurants, and bars appear to have had mixed success to date, given that the enforcement of bans is difficult. Moreover, youth restrictions have relatively high administrative costs (Reid 1996).

In contrast to these measures, there is ample evidence that tax increases are the single most effective policy measure for reducing children's consumption of tobacco products. Young people are more sensitive to price changes than older people. Estimates suggest that a tax increase of $2 per pack in the United States would reduce overall youth smoking by about two-thirds (National Cancer Policy Board 1998). To the extent that low-income and middle-income countries have younger populations than high-income countries, tax increases would be expected to be effective in these countries too.

In theory, if cigarette taxes are to be used mainly to deter children and adolescents from smoking, then the tax on children should be higher than any tax on adults. Such differential tax treatment would, however, be virtually impossible to implement. Yet a uniform rate for children and adults, the practical option, would impose a burden on adults. Societies may nevertheless consider that it is justifiable to impose this burden on adults in order to protect children. Moreover, if adults reduce their cigarette consumption, children may smoke less, given evidence that children's propensity to smoke is influenced by whether their parents, and other adult role-models, smoke (Murray et al. 1983).

Physical costs imposed on non-smokers. Governments can choose to protect non-smokers from the health effects of exposure to environmental tobacco smoke, including the effects on children and babies born to smoking parents. The externalities of maternal smoking for infants are less clear than for other non-smokers exposed to others' smoke, at least where mothers are assumed to have rights over fetuses, including the right to submit them to risks. However, the literature on the attitudes of pregnant women to their own health and that of their fetuses suggests that those who are informed about healthy behaviors are more likely to act to protect their fetuses' health (Charlton 1996).

Costs to non-smokers' health would appear, *a priori*, to be easily reduced through bans on public and workplace smoking. These 'clean-air' restrictions have the advantage that they limit the conditions under which people can smoke, without directly addressing the choice of whether to smoke. It should be noted that direct physical externalities do not by themselves justify widespread government interventions, such as advertising and promotion bans, and tax increases, since what matters is not how much people smoke, but whether others are exposed to tobacco smoke. As discussed by Woollery *et al.* (2000), restrictions in high-income countries on smoking in public places and private workplaces reduce both smoking prevalence and average daily cigarette consumption. Data from developing countries are much less complete, but experience from South Africa suggests that restrictions do reduce smoking (Van der Merwe 1998). Such restrictions are clearly weakened where there is a lack of enforcement, or a reliance on self enforcement. However, a more significant problem with this approach is that the vast majority of exposure to environmental tobacco smoke is in homes, and this is where children are also more likely to be exposed. (Mannino *et al.* 1996; NCI 1999). In contrast to clean-air restrictions, tax increases, by significantly reducing smoking in all settings, could lower this cost to children.

Financial costs borne by non-smokers would, *a priori*, be best reduced through adjusted risk premiums on health services or pension services. Financial costs could be calculated over short intervals, but lifetime medical costs for today's young smokers are more unpredictable. Private insurance markets sometimes include such price differentials, without requiring regulation; publicly-financed insurance seldom or never does. As the administrative costs for adjusting risk premiums are high, a less precise but more efficient method would be to simply tax cigarettes at the source. Note that in contrast to physical externalities, financial externalities would justify such general consumption-reducing measures, since what matters is how much people smoke rather than where they do it.

Giving adult smokers information. Governments can use a number of measures to protect adult smokers' health by inducing them to quit or to smoke less, but this most directly conflicts with the assumption of consumer sovereignty, except in the case of smokers who want to quit but find it difficult because they are already addicted. Public policy responses include information about the health risks, subsidization of cessation programs and tax increases. Only the last of these conflicts with permitting individuals to make risky decisions (such as playing dangerous sports, or associating with dangerous friends) on the assumption that individuals know their risks and bear the costs of their choices. Providing information, and helping individual smokers who want to quit, are not in conflict with the principal of consumer sovereignty.

Publicly financed information campaigns and research on the health risks of smoking for adults are justified as a 'first-best' intervention. As Kenkel and Chen (2000) elaborate, such information has had a powerful impact on smoking in high-income countries, although the effects take time to appear. Statutory warnings on tobacco products and regulations on tar and nicotine content are also common throughout the world, but few countries use strong and varied warning labels that convey meaningful information on the hazards of smoking (WHO 1997). An extension of information measures are bans on advertising and promotion. Such bans can help smokers to quit or to avoid starting again (USDHHS 1990). As discussed above, historically the tobacco industry has used advertising to make misleading claims about the health risks. Thus, bans on advertising and promotion are justified as a more intrusive but effective intervention.

Governments may also deregulate nicotine replacement, finance, or provide cessation advice, or even subsidize cessation treatment. As discussed by Novotny *et al.* (2000) and Gajalakshmi *et al.* (2000), an individual's risk of premature mortality drops sharply on quitting, especially at younger ages (Doll *et al.* 1994). Note that nicotine replacement products are not public goods, and are in fact provided by the private market: smokers wanting to quit can buy private cessation-help programs and nicotine-delivering patches to ease withdrawal. The argument for public intervention is only that the private market's response may be sub-optimal, partly due to regulation that restricts the public's access to cessation aids.

Taxation is also an effective intervention. Cigarettes are taxed in nearly all countries, sometimes heavily, but mainly because of the administrative ease of collecting tobacco taxes and the relatively inelastic demand. Adults are less price-responsive than children to increases in tobacco tax.

The economic costs of intervening

Given that the effective interventions do not neatly correspond to the market failures they were designed to correct, an important consideration is whether they also generate further economic costs that may be worse than the original market failure. This specifically applies to taxes, given that they are the most blunt, and also most effective, measure to protect children. Below we discuss the key economic costs of intervening, including the costs of foregone pleasure from smoking. Unfortunately, there are few empirical studies of the economic costs of intervening (Warner 1997). We focus on the conceptual framework of costs from various interventions, emphasizing the costs to individuals. We do not discuss costs to producers. Estimates by Peck *et al.* (2000) suggest that consumer satisfaction is the lion's share of any plausible estimate of benefits from smoking, with producers' benefits being much smaller. Ranson *et al.* (2000) provide estimates of cost-effectiveness from the perspective of the public sector. Control measures would cause regular smokers to forego the pleasure of smoking, or incur the costs of quitting, or both. A priori, this loss of consumer surplus would appear to be the same as it would be for bread or any other consumer good. However, tobacco is not a typical consumer good with typical benefits. For the addicted smoker who regrets smoking and expresses a desire to quit, the benefits of smoking are largely the avoidance of the costs of withdrawal. If tobacco control measures reduce individual smokers' consumption, those smokers will face significant withdrawal costs. Furthermore, the costs would differ between current smokers and potential smokers who have not yet begun.

Clean-air restrictions impose costs on smokers by reducing their opportunities to consume cigarettes, or by forcing them outdoors to smoke, raising the time and discomfort associated with smoking, or by imposing fines for smoking in restricted areas. Such restrictions raise the individual's costs relative to his or her benefits, and prompt some smokers to quit or cut back their consumption. For non-smokers, however, restrictions on smoking in public places will bring welfare gains. Given that most regular smokers express a desire to quit but few are successful on their own, it seems likely that the perceived costs of quitting are greater than the perceived costs of continuing to smoke, such as damage to health. By making the costs of continued smoking greater than the costs of withdrawal, higher taxes can induce some smokers to quit. However, smokers who quit or cut back would face withdrawal costs from higher taxes. The extent of the loss depends on levels of tax already paid, price responsiveness, and other factors (see Chaloupka and Warner, 2000, for a related discussion on the distributional impacts of taxes).

In considering economic costs to smokers, it is important to distinguish between regular smokers and others. For children and adolescents who are either beginners or merely potential smokers, the costs of avoiding tobacco are likely to be less severe, since addiction may not yet have taken hold and, therefore, withdrawal costs are likely to be lower. Other costs may include, for example, reduced acceptance by peers, less satisfaction from the thwarted desire to rebel against parents, and the curtailment of other pleasures of smoking.

Bans on advertising and promotion might be expected to increase the costs for smokers of obtaining information about their preferred products. However, to the extent that tobacco advertising focuses more on establishing brand loyalty among the new smokers it attracts rather than on providing information of value to current smokers, even established adult smokers would suffer little information loss or search costs if advertising and promotion were banned (Chapman 1996).

In sum, interventions in the smoking market vary by specificity to the market failure and groups most affected. It is obvious that some interventions are fairly specific to particular problems. This is notably the case for bans on smoking in public places, which are intended to control physical externalities. It is also the case for measures to make smokers pay any additional medical costs due to their behavior, which are intended to control financial externalities. But measures that are aimed at reducing cigarette consumption, rather than controlling where it occurs or who pays the associated costs, are much more general. Taxation and information campaigns are both measures of this type. When it comes to protecting or affecting particular population groups, there is similarly a mixture of more specific and more general connections between an intervention and the group(s) it is meant to affect.

Government Interventions to Protect the Poor

Aside from government interventions to correct for market failures, intervention to protect the poor is a well-recognized government role (Musgrove 1999). Investing in health is one method, but another is to reduce poverty or alleviate its consequences (World Bank 1993). We examine next the issues of how smoking burdens are distributed and the equity implications of some of the interventions analyzed above.

In most countries of the world, tobacco consumption is highest among poorer socioeconomic groups, and, accordingly, so is the incidence of tobacco-related disease. Comparison between countries reveals that the poor have higher death rates from smoking-related diseases. Moreover, the poor spend a considerable amount on tobacco as a percentage of their household income, which adversely affects household consumption of items beneficial to children's health (Cohen 1981; World Bank 1993). To some extent, the market failure of incomplete information is more pronounced among the poor (Townsend et al. 1994).

Government interventions to reduce the impact of smoking among the poor include taxation, information, and subsidizing access to cessation advice or nicotine replacement therapies (NRT). Differences in the relative importance of different problems imply that the optimal combination of interventions should probably be different for poor and non-poor populations. Several studies suggest that information is less effective in reducing smoking among poor groups than among richer groups (see, for example, USDHHS 1989; Townsend 1998). Smoking prevalence has declined much faster among higher socio-economic groups than among lower groups. The provision of information (such as mass information campaigns and warning labels), and bans on advertising and promotion are justified on efficiency grounds. There is little doubt, however, that the poor would use such information less, or less quickly, than would the rich. Another strategy would be to finance or provide cessation advice and cessation aids to help the poor quit smoking if they could not afford to pay for them (Musgrove 1999), provided the effects justify the costs. Delivering these services may be costly or difficult, however, since the poor tend to have less access to basic health services than the rich, and the costs of expanding these services to reach the poor might be considerable.

In contrast to information, tax increases on tobacco reduce consumption more among the poor and less educated than among the rich and more educated. Evidence from the United Kingdom and the United States (CDC 1998; Townsend 1998; Chaloupka 1991) suggests that price elasticities in the lowest income groups are significantly higher than in the highest income groups. Tobacco taxation would thus narrow the difference in consumption between rich and poor (Warner et al. 1995). In high-income countries, the poor usually spend a larger share of their incomes on tobacco than do the rich. Thus, a tax on tobacco is necessarily regressive *among those who continue to smoke*. Whether the overall effect of tax increases is regressive, depends on what share of each group, poor and non-poor, would react to the higher price by quitting. If more of the poor quit, then the tax effect could even be progressive. Tobacco taxes, like any other single tax, need to work within the goal of ensuring that the entire system of tax and expenditure is proportional or progressive (Townsend 1998; Chaloupka and Warner, in press). Studies of tobacco taxation in the United States and the United Kingdom suggest that tax increases are less regressive than presumed, and may even be progressive. In contrast to the taxation of other goods, when the poor reduce their consumption of tobacco they gain a health benefit in return for the tax burden they continue to pay. Finally, the poor may benefit in another way from increased tobacco taxes, if health and social services are targeted to the poor and financed by those taxes (Saxenian and McGreevey 1996; WHO 1999).

It might be argued that taxes and other tobacco control measures would impose bigger costs on poor individuals. But if this is true for tobacco, it is not unique in public health. Compliance with many health interventions, such as child immunization or family planning, is often more costly for poor households. For example, poor families may have to walk longer distances to clinics than rich families and may lose income in the process. Yet health officials do not hesitate to argue that the health benefits of most interventions, such as immunization, are worth the cost, provided the costs do not rise so high that poor individuals are deterred from using services.

In summary, the fact that the poor devote relatively more of their income to tobacco does not provide any strong equity-based argument against the tobacco control measures analyzed here.

Conclusion

We have described specific failures in the tobacco market: first, inadequate information about the health risks of smoking; second, inadequate information about the risks of addiction (and particularly the youthful onset of use of an addictive product); and, third, the external costs of smoking. We argue that because of these market failures, government intervention is justified on economic grounds. However, the interventions themselves are often non-precise and impose costs on even informed adult smokers. What then do these findings imply for public policy?

First, the public health arguments and the economic arguments for tobacco control differ on goals. Public health goals would, rationally, be to eradicate smoking if possible, given that tobacco hazards increase with increasing exposure and overwhelm any possible beneficial effects on health. In contrast, the economic arguments suggest that the socially optimal level of consumption of tobacco would not be zero. Ideally in economic terms, children would not smoke, but adults who knew their risks and bore their costs entirely themselves could smoke (Warner 1998).

Such a situation would involve considerably less smoking than at present, but would stop well short of eradication. Preventing children from smoking could, in theory, eventually lead to the epidemic disappearing. In reality, slightly older cohorts may take up smoking, and it is unlikely that the recruitment of new smokers would cease. Several of the interventions discussed here, particularly those designed to prevent smoking in youth, protect non-smokers from externalities, and leave smokers better informed.

However, a major problem for the 'economically optimal' view of smoking is the fact that nicotine is addictive. This undermines the consumer-sovereignty argument against intervention, because all evidence suggests that the conditions for a rational choice to become addicted are not met, and the addicted smoker is to some degree a different person from the one who decided to start smoking. If addiction is taken into account, a 'middle-ground' rationale that is justifiable by both economic and public health arguments becomes feasible. It still falls short of eradication, but is more realistic and justifiable than a purely economics-led view that defines adult consumers as rational and informed. The economic rationale for intervention described here largely involves information and regulation, and not direct public finance or the provision of private goods, except perhaps to the poor. As such, it leaves much room for private choice.

As with other areas of public policy, governments have to make choices, drawing here on economics, epidemiology, and public health. Even limited reductions in the prevalence of smoking, achieved as the result of interventions to correct market failures, would, by any measure, constitute an enormous public health victory, avoiding millions of deaths per year.

References

Atkinson, A. B. and Townsend, J. L. (1977). Economic aspects of reduced smoking. *Lancet*, 2(8036), 492–5.

Bachman, J. G.,Wadsworth, K. N., O'Malley, P. M., Johnston, L. D., and Schulenberg, J. (1997). *Smoking, drinking, and drug use in young adulthood: The impacts of new freedoms and new responsibilities*. Mahwah, NJ: Lawrence Erlbaum Associates.

Barendregt, J. J., Bonneux, L., and van der Maas, P. J. (1997). The health care costs of smoking. *New England Journal of Medicine*, 337(15), 1052–7.

Becker, G. S. and Murphy, K. M. (1988). A theory of rational addiction. *Journal of Political Economy*, 96(4), 675–700.

Becker, G. S., Grossman, M., and Murphy, K. M. (1994). An empirical analysis of cigarette addiction. *American Economic Review*, 84(3), 396–418.

Bero, L. A., Glantz, S. A., and Rennie, D. (1994). Publication bias and public health policy on environmental tobacco smoke. *JAMA*, 13, 133–6.

Bos, E. R., Hon, V., Maeda, A., Chellaraj, G., and Preker, A. (1999). *Health, Nutrition, and Population Indicators: A Statistical Handbook*. Washington, DC: World Bank.

California Environmental Protection Agency (1997). *Health Effects of Exposure to Environmental Tobacco Smoke: Final Report*. Office of Environmental Health Hazard Assessment (OEHHA). http://www.oehha.org/scientific/ets/finalets.htm

Centers for Disease Control and Prevention (CDC) (1998). Response to increases in cigarette prices by race/ethnicity, income, and age groups–United States, 1976–1993. *Morbidity and Mortality Weekly Report*, 47(29), 405–9.

Chaloupka, F. J. (1991). Rational addictive behavior and cigarette smoking. *Journal of Political Economy*, 99(4), 722–42.

Chaloupka, F. J. and K. E. Warner (2000). The economics of smoking. In *The Handbook of Health Economics* (ed. J. Newhouse and A. Culyer). Amsterdam: North Holland. (In press.)

Chapman, S. (1996). The ethics of tobacco advertising and advertising bans. *Br. Med. Bull.*, 52(1), 121–31.

Charlton, A. (1996). Children and smoking: the family circle. *Br. Med. Bull.*, 52(1), 90–107.

Charlton, A., While, D., and Kelly, S. (1997). Boys smoking and cigarette-brand-sponsored motor racing. *Lancet*, 350(9089), 1474.

Chinese Academy of Preventive Medicine (1997). *Smoking in China: 1996 National Prevalence Survey of Smoking Pattern*. Beijing: China Science and Technology Press.

Cohen, N. (1981). Smoking, health, and survival: prospects in Bangladesh. *Lancet*, 1(8229), 1090–3.

Collins, D. and Lapsley, H. (1998). Estimating and disaggregating the social costs of tobacco. In *The Economics of Tobacco Control: Towards an Optimal Policy Mix* (ed. I. Abedian, R. Van der Merwe, N. Wilkins and P. Jha), pp. 155–78. Cape Town, South Africa: Applied Fiscal Research Centre, University of Cape Town.

Doll, R., Peto, R., Wheatley, K., Gray, R., and Sutherland, I. (1994). Mortality in relation to smoking: 40 years observations on male British doctors. *British Medical Journal*, 309(6959), 901–11.

The Economist (1995). An anti-smoking wheeze: Washington needs a sensible all-drugs policy, not a 'war on teenage smoking'. 19 August, pp. 14–15.

The Economist (1997). Tobacco and tolerance. 20 December, pp. 59–61.

Ensor, T. (1992). Regulating tobacco consumption in developing countries. *Health Policy and Planning*, 7, 375–81.

Environmental Protection Agency (1992). *Respiratory Health Effects of Passive Smoking: Lung Cancer and Other Disorders*. EPA, Office of Research and Development, Office of Air and Radiation. EPA/600/6–90/006F.

Glantz, S. A., Barnes, D. E., Bero, L., Hanauer, P., and Slade, J. (1995). Looking through a keyhole at the tobacco industry. The Brown and Williamson documents. *Journal of the American Medical Association*, 274(3), 219–24.

Gorovitz, E., Mosher, J., and Pertschuk, M. (1998). Pre-emption or prevention?: lessons from efforts to control firearms, alcohol, and tobacco. *Journal of Public Health Policy*, 19(1), 36–50.

Harris, J. E. (1994). *A Working Model for Predicting the Consumption and Revenue Impacts of Large Increases in the U.S. Federal Cigarette Excise Tax*. Working paper no. 4803. Cambridge (MA): National Bureau of Economic Research.

Hodgson, T. A. (1992). Cigarette smoking and lifetime medical expenditures. *Milbank Quarterly*, 70(1), 81–125.

Institute of Medicine (1994). *Growing Up Tobacco Free*. Washington, D.C.: National Academy Press.

James, E. (1994). *Averting the Old Age Crisis: Policies to Protect the Old and Promote Growth*. Oxford and New York: World Bank and Oxford University Press.

Kessler, D. A., Barnett, P. S., Witt, A., Zeller, M. R., Mande, J. R., and Schultz, W. B. (1997). The legal and scientific basis of FDA's assertion of jurisdiction over cigarettes and smokeless tobacco. *Journal of the American Medical Association*, 277, 405–9.

Krutilla, J. V. (1967). Conservations reconsidered. *American Economic Review*, 57, 776–86.

Leu, R. E. and Schaub, T. (1983). Does smoking increase medical care expenditure? *Social Science and Medicine*, 17(23), 1907–14.

Levshin, V. and Droggachih, V. (1999). *Knowledge and Education Regarding Smoking Among Moscow Teenagers*. Paper presented at the workshop on Tobacco Control in Central and Eastern Europe. Las Palmas de Gran Canaria. February 26.

Manning, W. G. (1989). The taxes of sin: do smokers and drinkers pay their way? *Journal of the American Medical Association*, 261(11), 1604–09.

Manning, W. G., Keeler, E. B., Newhouse, J. P., Sloss, E. M., and Wasserman, J. (1991). *The Costs of Poor Health Habits*. Cambridge, Mass.: Harvard University Press.

Mannino, D. M., Siegel, M., Husten, C., Rose, D., and Etzel, R. (1996). Environmental tobacco smoke exposure and health effects in children: results from the 1991 National Health Interview Survey. *Tobacco Control*, 5(1), 13–18.

Murray, C. J. L. and Lopez, A. D. (eds.) (1996). *The Global Burden of Disease: a Comprehensive Assessment of Mortality and Disability from Diseases, Injuries, and Risk Factors in 1990 and Projected to 2020*. Cambridge, Mass.: Harvard School of Public Health.

Murray, M., Swan, A. V., Johnson, M. R., and Bewley, B. R. (1983). Some factors associated with increased risk of smoking by children. *Journal of Child Psychology and Psychiatry*, 24(2), 223–32.

Musgrove P. Public spending on health care: how are different criteria related? *Health Policy* 1999, 47(3):207–23.

National Cancer Institute (NCI) (1999). *Health Effects of Exposure to Environmental Tobacco Smoke*. The Report of the California Environmental Protection Agency. Smoking and Tobacco Control Monograph no. 10. Bethesda, MD. US Department of Health and Human Services, National Institutes of Health, National Cancer Institute, NIH Pub. No. 99–4645.

National Cancer Policy Board (1998). *Taking Action to Reduce Tobacco Use*. Washington, DC: National Academy Press.

O'Malley, P. M., Bachman, J. G., and Johnston, L. D. (1988). Period, age and cohort effects on substance use among young Americans: a decade of change, 1976–86. *American Journal of Public Health*, 78(10), 1315–21.

Orphanides, A., and Zervos, D. (1995). Rational addiction with learning and regret. *Journal of Political Economy*, 103(4), 739–58.

Pekurinen, M. (1991). *Economic Aspects of Smoking: Is There a Case for Government Intervention in Finland?* Helsinki: Vapk-Publishing.

Peto, R. (1986). Influence of dose and duration of smoking on lung cancer rates. In *Tobacco: a Major International Health Hazard*. (ed. R. Peto, and D. Zaridze), pp. 23–34. International Agency for Research on Cancer, 1986 (IARC Scientific Publications, no. 74).

Peto, R., Lopez, A. D., Boreham, J., Thun, M., and Heath, C. Jr. (1994). *Mortality from Smoking in Developed Countries 1950–2000*. Oxford: Oxford University Press.

Peto, R., Chen, Z. M., and Boreham, J. (1999). Tobacco: the growing epidemic. *Nature Medicine*, 5(1), 15–7.

Reid, D. (1996). Tobacco control: overview. *British Medical Bulletin*, **52**(1), 108–20.

Saxenian, H. and McGreevey, W. P. (1996). *China: Issues and Options in Health Financing*. World Bank Report No. 15278-CHA,Washington, DC.

Suranovic, S. M., Goldfarb, R. S., and Leonard, T. C. (1999). An economic theory of cigarette addiction. *Journal of Health Economics*, 18, 1–29.

Sweda, E. L. Jr. and Daynard, R. A. (1996). Tobacco industry tactics. *British Medical Bulletin*, 52(1), 183–92.

Townsend, J., Roderick, P., and Cooper, J. (1994). Cigarette smoking by socioeconomic group, sex, and age: effects of price, income, and health publicity. *British Medical Journal*, 309(6959), 923–27.

Townsend (1998). The role of taxation policy in tobacco control. In *The Economics of Tobacco Control* (ed. I. Abedian, R. van der Merwe, N. Wilkins, and P. Jha), pp. 85–101. Cape Town, South Africa: Applied Fiscal Research Centre, University of Cape Town.

US Department of Health and Human Services (1986). *The Health Consequences of Smoking For Women*. Rockville, Maryland: US Department of Health and Human Services, Public Health Service, Office of the Assistant Secretary for Health, Office on Smoking and Health.

US Department of Health and Human Services (1989). *Reducing the Health Consequences of Smoking: 25 Years of Progress. A Report of the Surgeon General*. Rockville, Maryland: US Department of Health and Human Services, Public Health Service, Centers for Disease Control, Center for Chronic Disease Prevention and Health Promotion, Office on Smoking and Health. DHHS Publication No. (CDC)89–8411.

US Department of Health and Human Services (1990). *The Health Benefits of Smoking Cessation: A Report of the Surgeon General*. Rockville, Maryland: US Department of Health and Human Services, Public Health Service, Centers for Disease Control, Center for Chronic Disease Prevention and Health Promotion, Office on Smoking and Health. DHHS Publication No. (CDC) 90–8416.

Van der Merwe, R. (1998). The economics of tobacco control in South Africa. In *The Economics of Tobacco Control* (ed. I. Abedian, R. van der Merwe, N. Wilkins, and P. Jha), pp. 251–71. Cape Town, South Africa: Applied Fiscal Research Centre, University of Cape Town.

Viscusi, W. K. (1995). Cigarette taxation and the social consequences of smoking. In *Tax Policy and the Economy*. (ed. J. M. Poterba). Cambridge, MA, MIT Press. 9, 51–101.

Wald, N. J. and Hackshaw, A. K. (1996). Cigarette smoking: an epidemiological overview. *British Medical Bulletin*, 52(1), 3–11.

Warner, K. E., Goldenhar, L. M., and McLaughlin, C. G. (1992). Cigarette advertising and magazine coverage of the hazards of smoking. A statistical analysis. *New England Journal of Medicine*, 326, 305–9.

Warner, K. E. (1997). Cost-effectiveness of smoking cessation therapies: interpretation of the evidence and implications for coverage. *PharmacoEconomics*, 11, 538–49.

Warner, K. E. (1998). The economics of tobacco and health: an overview. In *The Economics of Tobacco Control* (ed. I. Abedian, R. van der Merwe, N. Wilkins and P. Jha), pp. 55–75. Cape Town, South Africa: Applied Fiscal Research Centre, University of Cape Town.

Warner, K. E., Chaloupka, F. J., Cook, P. J., Manning W. G., Newhouse, J. P., Novotny, T. E. *et al.* (1995). Criteria for determining an optimal cigarette tax: the economist's perspective. *Tobacco Control*, 4, 80–6.

Weinstein, N. D. (1998). Accuracy of smokers' risk perceptions. *Annals of Behavioral Medicine*, 20(2), 135–40.

World Bank (1992). *China: Long-term Issues and Options in the Health Transition.* Washington, DC.

World Bank (1993). *The World Development Report 1993: Investing in Health.* New York: Oxford University Press.

World Health Organization (1997). *Tobacco or Health: a Global Status Report.* Geneva, Switzerland.

World Health Organization (1999). *The World Health Report 1999: Making a difference.* Geneva, Switzerland.

Zatonski, W. (1996). *Evolution of Health in Poland Since 1988.* Warsaw: Marie Skeodowska-Curie Cancer Center and Institute of Oncology, Department of Epidemiology and Cancer Prevention.

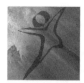

CHAPTER 4

Measurement of Equity in Health

Equity, according to the Plan of Action of the Pan American Health Organization (1), is one of three essential qualities of a system of health services, efficiency and effectiveness being the other two. None of these concepts is simple to define or measure, so it is not surprising that no indicators of progress towards them have been adopted, in contrast to the situation for a number of more specific goals such as high life expectancy or low infant mortality. However, a number of simple indicators can be used to tell something about equity, even if there is no single measure of it. This article discusses the logic behind various such indicators, drawing on recent data from Peru for empirical illustration.

Equity as Equality of Treatment

The fundamental idea of equity is that of equal treatment for all the population. The intention is to assure good health for all, and as far as possible, equally good health, to be pursued through preventive or curative treatment. Equity cannot simply be identified with equality in general, because of differences in needs, but it can be judged by considering certain kinds of equality. The idea may be "to provide 100% of the population with access to health services" (1), but the crucial notion is that whatever the level of access, it should be the same for all. Inequity results from *differences* in the ability to obtain health care, whatever the reasons may be, that prevent some people and not others from getting medical assistance (2). Since illness and accident are randomly and non-uniformly distributed, it cannot be expected that

Reprinted, with permission, from *World Health Statistics Quarterly 39* (4), 1986.

everyone will see a doctor equally often, or that spending per person on health care will be the same for all groups in the population. Treatment and resources should go where they are most needed. It is to be expected, however, that if the health-care system is equitable, certain *probabilities* will be equal across population groups for a given set of health problems.

Probabilities of illness, treatment and recovery

This idea is shown schematically in Fig. 4.1. Within a given interval of time, a person may or may not become sick or hurt; he or she may receive treatment or may not; and there may or may not be a cure as the result of treatment, or a recovery in the absence of treatment. The complete passage from an initial state to a final state (health, illness, disability or death) can be described by just four probabilities, indicated by the bold arrows in Fig. 4.1. These are:

P(S)   the unconditional probability of needing medical care
P(T/S)   the conditional probability of receiving treatment, given the need for it
P(C/T)   the conditional probability of being cured by treatment
P(R/T*)   the conditional probability of recovering without treatment

If the chance of being treated when there is no need for it—shown by the dashed arrow—is excluded from consideration, then every other probability, including those of final good health and ill health, P(H) and P(H*), is just some combination of these four basic probabilities (3).

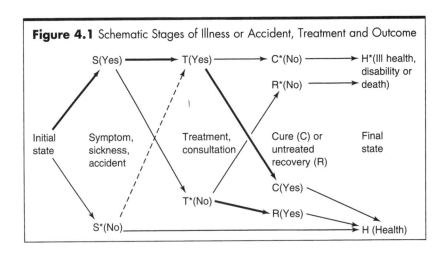

Figure 4.1 Schematic Stages of Illness or Accident, Treatment and Outcome

Different Dimensions of Equity

This scheme simplifies a great deal, but it serves to emphasize several issues to consider in attempting to judge the equity of a health service system. Among these are:

Which stage of the sequence is analyzed. The system might, for example, provide roughly the same chance of being cured to all patients who receive treatment, but be inequitable in reaching some people for treatment much more readily than others.

The difference between prevention, which acts on P(S), and curative treatment, which involves P(T/S) and P(C/T). Some differences in the likelihood of getting sick or hurt should not be considered inequitable, since they are associated with age or other risk factors largely outside the control of the health care system. Other differences in P(S)—for example, in the chance of getting diphtheria or poliomyelitis—are inequitable because prevention is within the power of the system and can be applied equally to virtually the entire population.

The particular condition, illness or need, studied. A health care system may provide everyone with the same chance of emergency care after a motor-vehicle accident, but maintain marked inequalities in the treatment of cancer or tuberculosis.

The level or quality of treatment. Does equity require the same type of care for everyone who is treated for a particular condition? Or should the system be regarded as equitable if every patient gets at least a minimal adequate level of care, even though some receive more elaborate, prolonged or expensive treatment (3)? A similar issue arises in analyzing the distribution of income: does equity require equality of incomes, or is what matters a decent minimum income for everyone? This issue becomes particularly important when analyzing expenditure on medical care.

The interaction of supply (physical availability of services) and demand (individual perception of need) in determining who does and who does not get treatment. For example, is it fair to describe a system as inequitable if it provides relatively little care to a cultural group which is more stoic than average, or more likely to rely on home remedies or traditional healers? How much responsibility falls to the government to change such cultural patterns so as to relate medical need and individual demand in the same way for the whole population?

All these questions show clearly why there cannot be a single measure of how equitable a health care system is: the same system may be quite fair by some indicators, and grossly inequitable according to others. It is no more possible to judge a country's health services as to equity by just one number than it is to summarize the population's health status in one indicator.

Finally, there is one important issue which is not clear from Fig. 4.1. In order to estimate and compare probabilities, the population must be divided into groups on some basis. How this is done may greatly affect the apparent inequality. Just as income typically is distributed more unequally among educational classes than among geographical regions, the health care system may look much more equitable in one dimension than in another. An adequate evaluation will probably require that the population be divided in more than one way, for example, by socioeconomic criteria as well as by geographical location.

Several of the issues discussed above can be illustrated by recent data from Peru. These include the usual administrative data collected by the Ministry of Health and analyzed by the country's Central Reserve Bank[1], household level information obtained in the 1984 National Health and Nutrition Survey, and analyses conducted as part of the 1985-1986 National Health Sector Analysis by various public and private agencies in Peru, with financing from the United States Agency for International Development (USAID)[2].

Not all the possible measures of equity can be computed—there are, for example, no data on the probability of cure or of spontaneous recovery—but a variety of indicators is available.

Distribution of health-related resources

In comparing different countries, it is common to refer to the share of the population which has access to safe water or sewerage connections, or to compute the ratio of population to such health care resources as physicians or hospital beds. The same analysis can be carried out within a country, as illustrated in Table 4.1. This comparison shows that physicians are very highly concentrated, especially in the department of Lima, which has just over a quarter of the population but two-thirds of all the physicians in Peru. Nurses are much more equally distributed, although still tending to concentrate in the same departments as physicians. Hospital beds are slightly more equally distributed, and access to safe water still more so. In general, expensive resources seem to be more concentrated than cheaper ones (physicians vs. nurses, and sanitation vs. water supply).

These rather easy indicators, which need no information about the population except place of residence, suffer three important limitations as

Table 4.1 Measures Related to Equity in Health Care, Peru, 1982: Health Care Resources and Sanitation Services (Percentages of National Total)

DEPARTMENT	POPULATION	RESOURCES PHYSICIANS	NURSES	HOSPITAL BEDS	DWELLINGS TOTAL	WITH WATER	WITH SEWERAGE
Amazonas	1.5	0.0	0.1	0.3	2.4	0.6	0.4
Ancash	4.8	1.2	3.4	2.7	5.1	4.5	3.7
Apurímac	1.9	0.1	0.5	0.7	2.2	0.5	0.2
Arequipa	4.2	5.3	8.2	6.8	4.3	5.7	6.0
Ayacucho	2.9	0.2	1.3	0.9	2.6	1.5	0.7
Cajamarca	6.1	0.5	0.6	0.9	6.3	2.0	1.4
Callao	2.7	6.3	4.5	4.9	2.3	4.4	5.3
Cuzco	4.9	1.0	2.2	2.9	5.4	2.6	2.1
Huancavelica	2.0	0.1	0.4	0.7	2.4	0.6	0.4
Huánuco	2.8	0.6	0.6	1.5	2.9	1.0	0.9
Ica	2.5	2.8	3.8	3.7	2.5	3.1	2.4
Junín	5.0	1.5	4.0	4.5	5.3	4.3	3.1
La Libertad	5.6	4.9	5.5	4.9	5.5	6.5	6.1
Lambayeque	4.0	2.6	5.4	3.8	3.5	4.5	4.3
Lima	28.1	66.6	50.7	48.4	26.4	45.1	52.8
Loreto	2.6	0.8	0.7	1.5	2.2	2.0	1.8
Madre de Diós	0.2	0.1	0.1	0.2	0.2	0.0	0.1
Moquegua	0.6	0.7	0.2	1.1	0.2	0.7	0.7
Pasco	1.2	0.6	1.2	1.7	1.3	0.8	0.6
Piura	6.6	2.3	2.7	3.2	6.1	5.2	4.2
Puno	5.2	0.5	1.5	1.6	6.4	1.5	0.8
San Martín	1.9	0.2	0.5	0.8	1.7	0.9	0.3
Tacna	0.9	0.6	1.3	1.4	0.9	1.5	1.4
Tumbes	0.6	0.2	0.3	0.3	0.5	0.1	0.1
Ucayali	1.2	0.3	0.3	0.6	1.0	0.4	0.3
National total	100.0	100.0	100.0	100.0	100.0	100.0	100.0
Gini coefficient of inequality		0.51	0.38	0.34		0.32	0.41

Source: [Health map of Peru]. Lima, Central Reserve Bank of Peru, 1984.

measures of equity. Firstly they are restricted to geographical comparisons; without knowing who actually consults the physicians, one cannot know their distribution according to other dimensions of the population, such as income. Secondly, it is implicitly assumed that needs are uniformly distributed. This is probably a reasonable assumption for sanitation facilities, but is questionable for health needs. The incidence or prevalence of health problems may differ substantially from one region to another, so that an equitable distribution of resources would in fact be unequal, not uniform. Third, it is presumed that the resources or facilities analyzed answer the needs of the population. Again this is a more reasonable assumption for sanitation facilities, although the health effects of safe water may differ considerably depending on the pattern of illness in a region and the hygienic behavior of the population. For health care the assumption is still more questionable: treatment by a physician may not be necessary in many cases; many physicians may be engaged in teaching or research; patients with more difficult problems may travel to other departments for treatment; etc. Thus while these measures say something about equality in the distribution of resources, and consequently in expenditure or health care, they should not be assumed to be the only or the best indicators of the equity of the system.

Probabilities of need and of treatment

A principal weakness of the resource vs. population comparisons in Table 4.1 can be overcome by referring to the morbidity and utilization data obtained from a large sample of the Peruvian population in the 1984 survey, and given in Table 4.2. With one dramatic exception, among the urban population of the country's mountainous central region, the probability of presenting with some illness or symptom was fairly uniform, at

Table 4.2 Measures Related to Equity in Health Care in Peru, 1984: Morbidity and Medical Attention

AREA	PREVALENCE (%) OF SYMPTOMS				PERCENTAGE SEEKING MEDICAL ATTENTION WITH SYMPTOMS			
	ALL KINDS	RESPIRATORY DISEASE	PARASITIC INFECTION	TOTAL	ALL AGES	UNDER 1 YEAR	1-4 YEARS	OVER 4 YEARS
Coast	34.89	16.11	0.21	12.67	30.86	51.41	30.68	28.64
Urban	34.87	16.34	0.20	13.36	31.54	55.74	32.69	29.96
Lima	36.57	17.68	0.15	14.88	33.49	59.43	35.87	31.62
Slums	37.32	16.85	0.19	14.14	32.05	64.84	32.85	29.78
Rural	35.00	14.38	0.28	7.50	18.76	27.14	16.52	18.71
Mountains	30.05	11.95	0.16	5.53	15.89	24.13	15.47	15.49
Urban	21.50	9.88	0.11	7.38	28.20	41.33	25.63	28.09
Rural	33.75	12.84	0.18	4.73	12.49	19.32	12.33	12.10
Jungle	36.03	12.06	1.78	7.65	18.39	27.33	17.20	17.94
Urban	33.72	11.59	1.36	10.36	25.59	42.63	22.34	24.97
Rural	37.35	12.32	2.02	6.11	14.69	18.42	14.46	14.41
National total	33.31	14.20	0.36	9.60	24.18	38.89	23.83	23.35
Urban	32.51	14.93	0.26	12.15	30.77	52.64	30.90	29.46
Rural	34.62	13.01	0.53	5.45	14.01	20.55	13.51	13.69

Source: National health and nutrition survey, Peru, 1984 (unpublished).

about one-third, during the two-week reference period. The unconditional probability of seeking medical care (including a visit to a pharmacy,
but excluding home care), however, ranged from almost 15% in Lima
down to less than 5% in rural mountainous areas. Consequently, the conditional probability P(T/S) ranged from over one-third in Lima to 12.5% in
the rural mountainous areas. If equity means equal likelihood of attention—
not necessarily the certainty of attention, since many illnesses and symptoms do not require more than home care—then the Peruvian health care
system shows dramatic geographical inequity.

Several other features of these estimates merit consideration. For one
thing the "geographical dimension" has several possible meanings. The data
in Table 4.2 are presented according to the survey area, in order to bring out
urban/rural differences. For Peru as a whole, P(T/S) is more than twice as
high in urban areas as it is in rural areas. The results could instead be shown
according to the "health regions" of the Ministry of Health, which are used
in Table 4.3. Neither of these classifications matches the departmental
boundaries used in Table 4.1, although the health regions correspond
approximately to departments or combinations of them.

Table 4.3 Measures Related to Equity in Health Care in Peru, 1984
Consultations, Hospitalizations and Expenditures (Percentages of National Total)

HEALTH REGION	POPULATION		MINISTRY OF HEALTH		
	TOTAL	WITH SYMPTOMS	CONSULTATIONS	HOSPITALIZATIONS	PATIENT-RELATED EXPENDITURES
Ancash	4.92	7.26	3.25	7.25	3.57
Arequipa	4.33	2.19	7.63	5.98	6.07
Cajamarca	4.48	5.08	1.57	1.38	1.80
Chiclayo	7.30	7.71	3.62	3.40	2.79
Cuzco	7.00	2.64	3.64	5.70	4.42
Huancayo	7.07	3.95	4.01	5.46	7.30
Huánuco	4.75	4.52	2.67	4.64	2.65
Ica	3.40	2.58	4.04	5.16	4.55
Iquitos	3.01	2.95	1.88	2.84	2.06
Lima	32.12	35.81	52.79	41.25	46.71
Moyobamba	2.00	3.30	2.18	2.20	2.51
Piura	7.44	10.28	4.29	4.81	3.90
Puno	5.09	5.26	1.36	2.13	2.81
Tacna	1.51	1.39	1.880	2.27	3.03
Trujillo	5.59	5.08	5.33	5.51	5.83
National total*	100.0	100.0	100.0	100.0	100.0

*Excluding the Ayacucho health region; percentages have been adjusted to 100% over
the rest of the country.

Differences by illness and by age. The relative uniformity of total morbidity hides larger variations for specific illnesses or symptoms. Respiratory disease affected from under 10% to over 17% of the population, while parasitic diseases, although unimportant overall, were extremely frequent in the jungle, and especially in rural areas. Conditional probabilities of treatment can be calculated separately for different causes such as these. Table 4.2 also shows that P(T/S) varies considerably by age, because infants under 1 year have a much higher likelihood of receiving medical care than do older children. This presumably reflects the greater risk of a serious illness in the first year of life. Inequality, however, appears to be worse where treatment of infants is concerned: for example, the urban/rural differential in the probability of care is greater for infants than for other age groups. Thus higher overall coverage or utilization of services need not imply greater equity or less inequality.

Equity in vaccination coverage. As the comparison of infants and older children emphasizes, illnesses and symptoms differ in danger or severity, and this may account for much of the variation in the likelihood of obtaining medical care. Not all such differences can be interpreted as indications of inequity. In order to control for this source of variation, it may be advisable to study equity with respect to a single well-defined need or condition. This is done in Table 4.4, for vaccination against the six target diseases of the Expanded Programme on Immunization, for all children under 5: first by type of vaccine and then according to the schooling of the child's mother. (This is one of the few analyses so far prepared using a socioeconomic classification; eventually the survey data will allow classification by income, or a proxy variable for it, as well as by educational level.)

Comparison across the four types of vaccines shows clearly that as the total coverage drops, the inequality of coverage increases. For BCG vaccine, the urban/rural differential is less than 2:1, reaching about 2:1 for measles vaccination and close to 4:1 for protection against poliomyelitis, diphtheria, whooping cough and tetanus. This national pattern is repeated within the mountain and jungle regions of the country. The differential is considerably less in the relatively favoured coastal region. Of course, as the national coverage approaches 100%, inequality necessarily disappears; but the great inequity occurring in rural areas when coverage is low reflects the very poor protection against these diseases in those areas.

Table 4.4 Measures Related to Equity In Health Care in Peru, 1984: Vaccination Coverage (%) of Children under 5.

AREA	BCG	POLIO	DPT	MEASLES	ALL TYPES
			BY TYPE OF VACCINE		
Coast	84.02	54.29	52.24	67.08	46.43
Urban	87.40	58.07	56.01	70.05	50.14
Lima	90.31	62.49	60.22	73.96	53.88
Slums	91.24	58.35	55.50	74.42	50.02
Rural	62.44	30.14	28.13	48.10	22.71
Mountains	49.99	18.31	17.94	39.31	12.99
Urban	77.16	41.56	41.86	59.70	30.29
Rural	39.42	10.11	9.51	32.13	6.89
Jungle	57.06	32.42	31.23	50.44	27.63
Urban	84.20	61.46	60.01	74.02	55.82
Rural	43.16	17.48	16.42	38.30	13.13
National total	67.62	37.81	36.51	54.40	31.31
Urban	85.36	55.47	53.87	68.56	47.14
Rural	44.34	14.66	13.75	35.82	10.57

	NONE	SOME PRIMARY	COMPLETE PRIMARY	SECONDARY	HIGHER
		BY MOTHER'S EDUCATION			
Coast	31.59	41.97	50.60	60.23	69.66
Urban	37.19	46.70	53.29	61.28	69.56
Lima	37.37	59.16	55.10	62.67	69.45
Slums	38.29	66.99	59.30	65.23	62.01
Rural	23.47	27.76	32.70	42.38	81.09
Mountains	10.778	14.18	25.68	35.81	51.39
Urban	27.02	30.51	30.57	39.30	50.37
Rural	9.32	10.70	23.05	27.88	58.50
Jungle	16.42	23.94	40.18	60.52	79.70
Urban	36.08	44.58	56.08	66.74	83.43
Rural	15.04	17.33	29.29	43.85	50.00
National total	16.17	26.62	42.23	55.73	65.28
Urban	34.36	43.46	50.23	58.49	65.47
Rural	11.82	15.05	26.79	36.02	61.01

Source: National health and nutrition survey. Peru, 1984 (unpublished).

A somewhat similar pattern emerges when vaccination coverage is compared across educational levels. As the educational level rises, so does vaccination coverage, and the geographical inequality diminishes. It is also true that the lower the coverage in a given geographical area, the greater is the inequality across educational groups. Thus the most marked socioeconomic inequity occurs in the rural mountainous areas, where overall protection is extremely low, and the least inequity is found in Lima. Children of less educated mothers, presumably in poor families, are the last to be reached, except for urban slums. This pattern probably reflects demand for vaccination on the part of parents, and not simply differences in availability: better educated mothers are more likely to bring their children to be vaccinated, without requiring a public campaign to persuade them to do so, and are better able to pay a private physician for service if necessary. While the inhabitants of the slums of Lima may be very poor, Tables 4.2 and 4.4 also show that they are not a particularly underprivileged group in access to health care.

Summary measures of inequality

The emphasis in Tables 4.1, 4.2 and 4.4 is on all the differences among geographical regions or socioeconomic groups, since any of these differences may be particularly important for the interpretation of how equitable or inequitable a health care system is, and where its inequities are concentrated. It is also possible to calculate summary measures of inequality, and to use them to form overall judgments about whether one distribution represents a more or less equitable situation than another (3). All such measures, however, discard information, and the way a particular statistic summarizes a distribution corresponds to assumptions that may or may not be appropriate when judging equity. Because it has an easy geometric interpretation, the Gini coefficient is often used for this purpose; it is applied, for example, in the Central Reserve Bank's analysis for Peru. The coefficient is calculated by first drawing the Lorenz curve, which relates the cumulated population across groups to the cumulated resource or utilization measure studied, ranking the groups from lowest to highest values of resources per capita. The Lorenz curve corresponding to the departmental distribution of physicians in Peru, calculated from Table 4.1, is shown in Fig. 4.2 It indicates, for example, that the departments where physicians are most scarce have 70% of the country's population but only about 28% of its physicians. The diagonal line corresponds to perfect equality in the ratio of physicians to population. The Gini coefficient is the ratio of the area between the diagonal and the Lorenz curve, to the total area under the diagonal, a measure which increases from 0 to 1 as inequality increases. As Table 4.1 shows, this measure is higher for physicians than for any of the other health-related resources considered. The Lorenz curve can also be used to represent inequality or inequity without calculating the Gini coefficient or any other summary statistic.

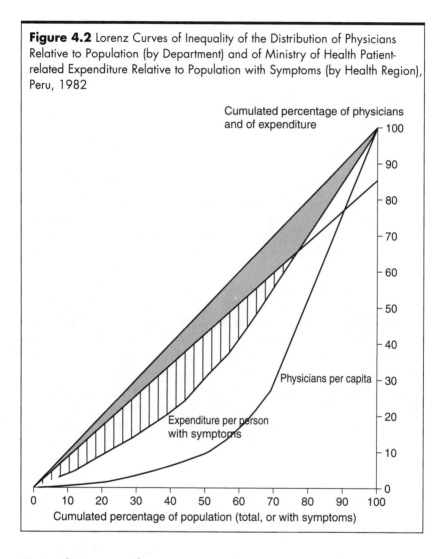

Figure 4.2 Lorenz Curves of Inequality of the Distribution of Physicians Relative to Population (by Department) and of Ministry of Health Patient-related Expenditure Relative to Population with Symptoms (by Health Region), Peru, 1982

Cumulated percentage of physicians and of expenditure

Physicians per capita

Expenditure per person with symptoms

Cumulated percentage of population (total, or with symptoms)

Financial Measures of Equity

Physicians, nurses, drugs, vaccines and other resources and supplies are used to produce health services, but none alone is an adequate measure of resources used in health care. The best overall measure of the resources dedicated to health services is the cost of producing those services. This raises two equity-related questions. The first concerns the equality of expenditure across population groups; the second concerns the relation between the cost of providing health services and the contributions different groups make to that cost, either by direct payment (fees for service) or by taxation. Both questions are particularly important for the equity of ministry of health services, which are typically financed largely from general government revenues and which are usually intended to cover the population groups too poor to pay for private medical care, and unlikely to be protected by the medical services of the social security system.

Equity in the distribution of expenditure

Variations in expenditure per capita on health care can be separated into differences in the likelihood of being sick or needing care, in the likelihood of receiving care, and in the cost per patient of the care given. Estimates of total cost by health region in Peru have been made for the years 1982–1984; these can be separated into costs related to individual patients, and those attributable to preventive and maintenance activities. Costs for the former can then be compared to total population, to the population presenting illness or symptoms and needing care, or to the population which actually receives care. Some of these estimates for 1984 appear in Table 4.3, classified by health region. The first of these measures—cost per capita—is often used as an indicator of equity, but like the indicators in Table 4.1, it suffers from the untested assumption that needs are everywhere proportional to population. At the other extreme, cost per consultation leaves out much that is important for equity; the cost per consultation could be uniform, yet the health system would not be equitable if the chance of getting attention varied widely among population groups. Thus the best measure of equity in spending on health care seems to be expenditure per person needing assistance—ideally this indicator would not include persons with symptoms too minor to require medical attention.

Expenditure and morbidity. It appears from Table 4.3, that patient-related expenditures are distributed more equitably in Peru than are some of the resources which help account for those costs. The Lima health region, for example, has about one-third of the country's population, a slightly larger share of those with illness or symptoms, two-thirds of Peru's physicians, but less than half of spending attributable to individual treatment. This perception is confirmed by Fig. 4.2, which compares the Lorenz curve for expenditure per sick person to that for physicians per capita. The former distribution is systematically much more equitable: the very unequal distribution of physicians undoubtedly overstates the inequity of the Peruvian health care system. Differences in unit costs contribute to total inequality, but their impact is *small* compared to the effect of differences in the likelihood of receiving treatment: costs per consultation, for example, vary over a range of only 2:1 in most of the health regions, and even those differences may depend on regional variations in the incidence of particular diseases or conditions, some of which in fact cost more to treat than others. These results only reinforce the conclusion that the chief source of health care inequity in Peru is variation in the probability of getting medical attention when sick.

Inequality without inequity. Equity is related to, but not identical with equality: thus, as remarked earlier, there can be inequality which is not necessarily inequitable. Suppose, for example, that while the cost per consultation in 1984 ranged from 8,845 to 23,843 *soles* among Peruvian health regions, adequate care could be given for a unit cost of 15,000 *soles*. That is, higher unit costs represent inefficiency, use of overqualified personnel, etc. Then, adequate medical care could have been given to all those patients attended, for only 85% of what was spent. This situation is shown in Fig. 4.2, where the hatched area represents real inequity, and the dotted area represents inequality. The former is due mostly to differences in the probability of receiving care, plus some inequality in unit costs below 15,000 *soles*, suggesting inadequate care, on average, in some regions. The latter is due entirely to average expenditures exceeding that level in some health regions. While the choice of a unit cost of 15,000 *soles is* arbitrary and used here only for illustration, the argument that not all inequality represents real inequity in health care is quite general. The logic of this comparison is similar to that involved in drawing a "poverty line" in the distribution of income, and regarding as inequitable the fact that some incomes are below that line, without being concerned with differences in income among those above the poverty line.

Equity as getting what you pay for

The comparison of costs or expenditure to population or to medical needs still does not ask how those expenditures are paid for. To medical professionals, equity is usually interpreted in terms of the satisfaction of needs, and questions of payment arise only as possible obstacles to obtaining medical care. This is a somewhat different matter from the satisfaction felt by the patient or consumer, because his demand for health care may not coincide with his need as determined by a physician. Equity could also be considered to require the satisfaction of wants or demands. To economists, however, equity has another meaning: that the distribution of health care expenditure should be less unequal than the distribution of income, or that there should be a net subsidy (expenditure minus tax contributions) to population groups with low incomes, and a net contribution by groups with high incomes. Equity then becomes a question of the amount and direction of net subsidies. Studies with this orientation commonly find that public health care spending is progressive when compared to the distribution of income, and also that it is more equitable than some other kinds of public social expenditure such as spending on education (4). That is, compared to what they pay in taxes, the poor usually get a net benefit from public health care, whereas they may suffer a net loss in certain other categories of government expenditure. This kind of analysis has not yet been conducted for Peru, although studies have been completed in several other Latin American countries. The first of these recent studies to be published concerns Chile[3].

It is important to note that these two concepts of financial equity in health care—expenditure relative to need, and expenditure relative to payment—may, but will not necessarily, coincide. If a particular population group contributes nothing and receives little or nothing, that will be equitable according to one criterion but not the other. This question becomes particularly important if the object is to judge the equity of a public health service system, when there is also private fee-for-service medical care available. Is the public system equitable if it provides access to those who cannot afford private care, ignoring those who can and do buy medical attention from private providers? Or does equity require the public system to reach, and subsidize, those poor consumers who now pay for private services because they are more accessible, or believed to be of better quality, than public services? The answers to these questions determine which indicators to construct, and how to interpret the available information.

Concluding Reflections

Equity is too complex a concept to be reduced to a single indicator; to analyze it necessarily requires a great deal of information and some subjective judgment as to what kinds of inequality in fact constitute inequity. However, many indicators can be constructed which are related to equity, or which help to measure it. The empirical discussion of the Peruvian case illustrates both the difficulties of analyzing equity in health care and the possible uses of administrative, financial and household data to form some overall judgment and to identify where inequity is concentrated, or with what factors it is associated. This is much more valuable than arriving at some single over-all measure of how equitable a particular health care system is.

The need to compare medical consultations and expenditures not just to population but to morbidity and perceived needs for assistance, indicates that relatively full assessments of equity must draw on population-based data and cannot be constructed only from the kind of information normally available to a ministry of health. The infrequent collection and high cost of such population data mean that equity is more easily studied in the cross section than in year-to-year changes. However, given a baseline assessment of how equitable a system is and where its principal problems are, changes over time in the distribution of resources and effort can give a good idea of whether the system is becoming more or less equitable. It is less important to calculate elaborate statistical measures such as summary coefficients of inequality, than to have a clear view of the range or variation in the proba-bilities chosen for study. All such efforts, to be useful, must take account of the diversity of health conditions and of responses to them, and of the dif-ferent dimensions of the population according to which equity can be evaluated.

Notes

[1] Central Reserve Bank of Peru. *Mapa de Salud en el Perú.* Lima, 1984.
[2] Chirinos, 0. et al. [*Health sector financing and expenditure.* Study 6.2, Financing and costs sector, ANSSA-Peru, Taller seminar III]. Lima, 1986 (in Spanish).
[3] Rodriguez Grossi, J. [*The distribution of revenue and social expenditure in Chile, 1983].* Santiago, Latin American Institute of Social Sciences and Studies (ILADES), 1985. (In Spanish).

References

[1]   PAN AMERICAN HEALTH ORGANIZATION. *Health for all by the year 2000: plan of action for the implementation of regional strategies.* Washington D.C., PAHO, 1982. (Official document no. 179).
[2]   PRESIDENT'S COMMISSION FOR THE STUDY OF ETHICAL PROBLEMS IN MEDICINE AND BIOMEDICAL AND BEHAVIORAL RESEARCH. *Securing access to health care: the ethical implications of differences in the availability of health services. Volume* 1: report. Washington D.C., US Department of Health and Human Services, 1983.

[3] MUSGROVE, P. Equity in health system services—concepts, indicators and interpretation (summary in English). *Boletin de la Oficina Sanitaria Panamericana,* 95 (6): 525-546, 1983.

[4] JIMENEZ, E. The public subsidization of education and health in developing countries: a review of equity and efficiency. *The World Bank Research Observer,* I (1): 111-129, 1986.

CHAPTER 5

What Should Consumers in Poor Countries Pay for Publicly-Provided Health Services?

Acknowledgments

An earlier version of this paper was presented at the National Council on International Health Conference, Washington, D.C., June 1982. Nothing said here represents the position of the Pan American Health Organization or its Member Governments. I am grateful to Robert Robertson, Dayl Donaldson, David Dunlop and anonymous reviewers for a large number of helpful comments, some but not all of which have been taken into account in the revised version; responsibility for errors of fact or interpretation is mine alone.

Definition of the Problem

The question to which this paper is addressed was defined for me by the Coordinator of Health Services of the Ministry of Health and Education of one of the smaller Caribbean countries. Publicly-provided health care in that country is free, in accord with the government's ideological commitment that no one should be denied medical attention for economic reasons. However, it is extremely difficult to raise the revenue required to operate the existing health care system, especially in the current economic situation, and the difficulty will only be compounded if coverage is expanded. Under

Reprinted from *Social Science and Medicine* 22 (3), 1986, with permission from Elsevier Science.

these circumstances, the government would like to recover some part of the cost from the consumers or beneficiaries, while doing the least violence to its principles; the question is, what prices or fees for service should they adopt?

Thus expressed, the question is not the same as, What should the price(s) of health service(s) be? In particular, prices are not assumed to determine supply; the government decides on the number and type of facilities to build and staff and the services to offer, on other grounds. Prices are not even assumed to determine resource allocation within the existing or planned level of supply, in the short run. Consumers will have to respond to prices, but suppliers in the public sector will not. This does not mean that it is of no interest to operate the public health system more efficiently, only that prices to patients are not to play a role in that effort.

In these circumstances, what is sought is clearly a second-best solution. It is irrelevant to a ministry of health—and most if not all ministries of health in Latin America and the Caribbean find themselves in this same situation—that a first-best solution might involve restructuring the entire tax system, or changing a great many other prices in the economy. The ministry of health does not control taxes: it simply faces pressure both from within the government and from international donor agencies and from the International Monetary Fund, to recover some part of its costs, either so as to permit expansion of its services or so as to make smaller demands on the budget. When allotments to all ministries are cut as part of an austerity program, imposing fees may be the only way to avoid reducing services. In any case, the question of what, if any, fees to charge would still be present even if the tax system were modified and the economy otherwise made to operate more efficiently.

Given the restricted role of prices in this view of the problem, and the short-run pressures on the public health system, two other limitations of the question are important. The first is that there is no requirement that fees cover any particular fraction of total cost or bear any particular relation to marginal costs. The second is that equity considerations are vital: the government does not want to purchase efficiency at the expense of its view of equity. Its goal is essentially that espoused by the U.S. Presidential Commission, which studied the issue of securing access to health care [1, pp. 20, 111], that of an adequate level of health care for everyone, without economic difficulties causing people who need care to forego it or to postpone it until their medical problems are much worse. I have argued elsewhere that medical equity should be interpreted as an equal probability of receiving care when it is needed [2], and it is this probability which the government wants to reduce as little as possible as a consequence of charging fees. This is distinct from concepts of equity which consider how health care is to be financed, but the government is also interested in financial equity. This issue is addressed later. The question of what the government wants is taken up in more detail in the next section.

Given some strong assumptions about the welfare function implicit in the ministry of health's actions—a welfare or objective function which I assume is characteristic at least of most governments in Latin America and Caribbean countries and perhaps in poor countries generally—it is possible to derive conditions for the optimum level of prices or fees to charge. Because this level depends on the demands of consumers for health care, the following section considers what assumptions are reasonable to make about those demands. Given the emphasis on equity, the relation of health care demands to income may be particularly important. Other determinants of demand are considered more briefly.

Although it is convenient to speak of 'the' price for medical attention, in fact medical care consists of a great variety of goods and services. Moreover, these are not independently produced and consumed; one level of utilization (consultation) may be a prerequisite to another (treatment). Even for a particular element of care, the price may vary among consumers, geographic areas or other dimensions; the next section therefore considers price discrimination, particularly with respect to income and to the other (non-fee) costs which consumers must meet in order to obtain medical attention.

Conditions for an Optimal (Single) Price

Under the assumption that the price charged for medical care is not to determine the supply, the optimum price is to be determined taking account not of the cost of production but only of the government's welfare function, i.e. its objectives in providing care. Governments do not usually specify welfare or objective functions in such terms as to permit the derivation of optimum policies, for prices or for anything else. The member governments of the Pan American Health Organization, for example, have subscribed to a mixture of objectives [3, p. 15], some of which specify measurable results in terms of death rates, immunization coverage, etc., while others refer to general goals of "reorganization", "improvement", etc. to achieve higher levels of (undefined) "equity, efficiency and effectiveness".

I will assume as a first approximation that for the purpose of deciding what fees to charge, the government's welfare function may be regarded as having just two components, which do not interact with one another. These are $N(p)$, the number of consultations or utilizations by patients, expressed as a function of price; and $pN(p)$, the total revenue obtained from these consultations.

The first element is a reason for wanting fees to be low, while the second may justify high fees, depending on the elasticity of demand for medical care. In order to form a welfare function, $W(p)$, from these two elements, a parameter is required for comparing the volume of service to the monetary value of revenue. If this parameter is called λ, and is assumed to be constant—each consultation is treated as of equal monetary value, although its value may not be the same as its price—then

$$W(p) = \lambda N(p) + pN(p).$$

It is assumed that for a given need, all consumers benefit equally from treatment; there is no discrimination either according to individuals' subjective valuation of how much they benefit from care, nor according to any more objective criteria such as the effect on earning power.

Note that the same formulation would result if the ministry were assumed to try to maximize $N(p)$ subject to a budget constraint in which total expenditure were equal to resources from the treasury plus the revenue generated by fees. Differentiating $W(p)$ with respect to p yields, after some manipulation,

$$0 > \varepsilon_N = -1/(1 + \lambda/p) > -1$$

where ε_N is the price-elasticity of demand.

If demand is elastic (falling more than proportionally as the price is raised) at a zero price, then the price should be raised until demand becomes inelastic. Just how inelastic it should be depends on the relative sizes of λ and p. If the ministry cared only about revenue ($\lambda = 0$), the elasticity should be exactly -1; whereas a high value on attending to patients (λ large compared to the price p) means a low elasticity. At the extreme of caring only about consultations, price should be zero.

This very simple form of the objective function requires only that the ministry decide for itself how much a consultation is worth, compared to the revenue obtained from it—i.e., establish a value for λ—and then learn enough about how demand depends on price to adjust price and therefore $N(p)$ to the optimum level. The analysis can be complicated in a number of ways, such as by introducing other elements into the objective function or by distinguishing different types of demand. Two of these possibilities are considered next.

The government's concern with equity, for example, might be explicitly incorporated into its objective function by including a third term,

$$\mu \sum_{i \varepsilon C} U_i(Y_i, p)$$

where U_i is the utility of the ith consumer, expressed as a function of his income Y_i and the price p. Charging that price will reduce the utility of any patient who actually is attended, compared to treating him for free; the sum is therefore taken only over the set C of patients who are seen when the price is p. The parameter μ compares the value (to the ministry) of these utility losses, to the revenue obtained: the loss for any customer is greater as p is higher or as Y_i is lower, so if a concave utility function is assumed, the total loss of utility will be greater as the distribution of income is more unequal, leading to a lower price. It is assumed here that interpersonal comparison of utilities is appropriate, and that income, properly defined, is a reasonable basis for such comparisons. This assumption is necessary to the 'ability-to-pay' approach to price setting [4, Chap. 5], however dubious the idea is; and more generally, it is the 'old welfare economics' assumption for necessities such as food, shelter and health care [5], for which everyone's needs can be assumed to be very similar if not identical, in the same physiological circumstances.

Prices usually are not given the role of protecting equity in the economy, and for the producer of a typical good or service the distribution of income matters only as it affects sales and therefore revenues and profits. Ministries of health do not appear to think this way, however; and as they have some control over prices but no control over their clients' incomes, they may try to use prices to affect welfare apart from the effect on the number of patients cared for. If this term is included, and $W(p)$ is differentiated, then so long as the same set C of customers is considered, the condition for the optimum price becomes

$$\varepsilon_N = \frac{-1 - \mu E(dU/dp)}{1 + \lambda/p}$$

where E refers to the average or expected value of the change in utility, dU/dp, when the price is increased. Since this is negative, the effect is to bring the optimum elasticity closer to zero and to lower the optimum price. Changing the price will have the further effect of shrinking or expanding the set C of clients who use the medical service, so that some people's utility losses due to the price will cease to be, or will become, of interest to the ministry. Formulating the objective this way means representing the ministry as caring both about the total number of consultations $N(p)$ and about the group of patients who account for those consultations, whereas the previous formulation is concerned only with utilization and does not distinguish one patient from another. It may seem like double-counting to consider both the utilization $N(p)$ and the welfare loss that results from paying the price p for that utilization, but public health officials do express both objectives, at least rhetorically. This formulation of their objectives attempts to reflect the cost associated with a highly inelastic demand, so that a high price can be considered undesirable even if it does not reduce utilization.

In fact, not all consultations are equally necessary or desirable on medical grounds. Some can be considered frivolous, so that while they are welcome for the revenue they generate they should not be considered to contribute to welfare, and they still represent a cost to patients. The ministry's objective function can be rewritten to separate necessary (N) and frivolous (F) demand, both as functions of price, as

$$W(p) = \lambda N(p) + p\{N(p) + F(p)\};$$

Differentiating yields, after some manipulation, the condition

$$N(1 + \varepsilon_N) + F(1 + \varepsilon_F) + \lambda dN/dp = 0$$

where ε_N and ε_F are respectively the price elasticities of N and F, which may be different.

Whether N and F will be different functions of price will depend on whether consumers' views of the necessity for care coincide with doctors' opinions. The formulation shown allows for different elasticities with respect to p, but—since patients may be poor judges of how much they need medical care—does not require it.

In order for the maximum condition to be satisfied at a positive price, $1 + \varepsilon_N$ or $1 + \varepsilon_F$ or both must be positive; otherwise all three terms in the expression are negative. This means that if demand is elastic (falling more than proportionally as price is raised) at zero price, the price should be raised until at least one of the demands becomes inelastic. If necessary demand is inelastic to start with, as is likely if patients correctly recognize the more serious needs, then any increase in price will have little effect on medically needed utilization, but may still reduce less-needed demand F. Whether in that case price should be raised above zero will depend on the levels of both kinds of demand; it is not necessarily the case that price should increase until ε_F also becomes inelastic. Rewriting the optimum condition to separate ε_N, as in the previous analysis, yields

$$\varepsilon_N = \frac{-1 - (F/N)(1 + \varepsilon_F)}{1 + \lambda/p}$$

which depends on the relative amounts of frivolous and necessary demand and on the elasticity of the former. Since ε_F can be more or less than one in absolute value, the optimum price to charge can go either up or down compared to the case where all demand is necessary. If both kinds of demand exist but react the same way to price, then

$$\varepsilon_N = \varepsilon_F = \frac{-(1 + F/N)}{1 + \lambda/p + F/N}$$

reflecting the fact that a higher price has the good effect of reducing frivolous demand but the disadvantage of also reducing needed consultations, and the balance of these two effects depends on F/N. Introducing patients' utilities explicitly affects the optimum levels of elasticity and price, but not the need for at least one of the demands to be inelastic.

Consumer Demand and its Determinants

The demand for health care, whether or not it is separated into necessary and frivolous components, can be presumed to depend on the price charged for care; on the costs in time of reaching a medical facility and waiting for attention; on the income foregone by seeking care; on income; on one's general condition of health; on the specific conditions or symptom(s) of illness or accident; on the consumer's ability to diagnose and treat himself, which depends among other things on education; and on his opinion of the quality of care he is likely to receive [6]. With respect to price and income, I am assuming that the consumer's demand function has the shape shown in Fig. 5.1. Two consumers are represented, with incomes OY_1 (poor) and OY_2 (rich). Facing a relatively high commercial price P_C such as a private doctor would charge, the amount of care demanded by the richer consumer, C_2, is much larger than that demanded by the poorer one, C_1. This corresponds

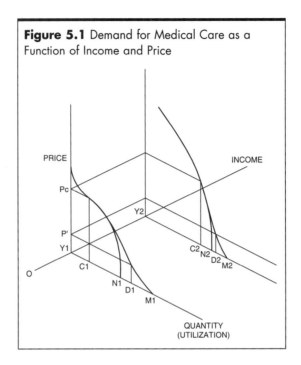

Figure 5.1 Demand for Medical Care as a Function of Income and Price

to the empirical finding that total private spending on medical care in Latin American countries typically shows an elasticity with respect to income of slightly more than 1.0 [7]. (For specific components of spending the elasticity may be quite different: for drugs, for example, it starts high but quickly declines as demand approaches saturation.)

At a zero price, the poor consumer's demand M_1 may actually exceed that of the richer consumer, M_2, because the former is less healthy or less well able to treat himself, or because his time is less valuable. It is not obvious which consumer will exhibit the greater necessary demand (N_1 and N_2) when the price is zero, but it is to be expected that except at low prices, raising the price will reduce the necessary demand more for the poorer consumer. For both consumers, the horizontal distance between M and N represents frivolous demand; this is presumed to be more sensitive to price than necessary demand, and is likely to be greater for poorer consumers, at least if the non-fee costs of seeking medical care (travel and lost income) are low.

Under these conditions, the optimum price discussed above is something like p^*, established at a level where the demand curve has become inelastic; compared to a zero price, necessary demand is reduced only slightly and frivolous demand considerably more. Exactly where the optimum is depends also on the importance (if any) of consumers' disutility from having to pay the fee, and on the weight (λ) assigned to consultations in the government's objective function; these are not shown in the figure. The demands resulting from p^* are D_1 and D_2.

Two further observations concerning the assumed demand function and the consequent optimum price are in order. The first is that the suggested rule for determining price is in one sense the opposite of what a private monopolist would follow. Here the price is set in relation to where the originally elastic demand becomes inelastic, as price rises; a monopolist would set price at the other end of the inelastic range, where the price has become so high that raising it more begins to reduce even necessary demand sharply and so revenue falls. The second observation is that if the optimum price were determined separately for each consumer, it is conceivable that it would be lower for the richer one, despite his greater ability to pay. This is because of his presumed more inelastic demand. Setting the optimum relative to all consumers together takes account of the distribution of income among them and also of the possibility of extracting more revenue from those with higher incomes.

Finally, it should be noted that both the government's supposed welfare function and the consumer's demand refer to instances of medical care, not to health in general or to other kinds of behavior which influence health. Medical care is undoubtedly sought to maintain or improve one's (perceived) health, and the government's ultimate objective is a healthy population, but models of the 'demand for health' [8, 9] are too general and too long-term in focus to help determine what fees should be charged. Both consumers and the government take actions designed to promote health by other means than the provision of medical services; these actions can best be thought of as shifting the demand curve through better self care, more prevention and less cure, and otherwise reducing the number of instances in which medical care is necessary.

Optimum Price Discrimination

The argument thus far has assumed that all consumers will pay the same price, but it is probably preferable to discriminate in price-setting. The most obvious reason is the disparity of incomes: richer patients can afford to pay more, without significantly reducing their necessary demand. Calculating the optimum price separately by income level will lead directly to prices being higher for the rich, provided the utility-loss term reflects decreasing marginal utility of income at a rapid enough rate. If no account is taken of utility loss as a function of income, the elasticity analysis alone could lead, as indicated above, to the poor being charged more. (Alternatively, λ can be considered to depend on income, but then all patients are not considered equally valuable in medical terms, which seems unethical.) Introducing price discrimination among consumers of course raises two problems: patients have to be classified by some sort of means test, which creates some administrative expense, and it has to be decided for which services to charge differentiated prices. Governments do often recognize the greater ability of some patients to pay than others, and introduce higher fees for the former, but even then the price may remain very low, hardly justifying the administrative burden and bearing little relation to incomes. This is perhaps especially likely to occur with hospital charges [10]. At the other extreme, discrimination may mean treating indigent patients completely free of charge.

Discrimination among consumers by income level may be of limited potential in many countries, simply because the better-off are unlikely to be clients of the ministry of health in the first place; if there is medical coverage under social security, it is the better-paid workers who are most likely to benefit from it. Of course, the arguments in favor of fees to reduce frivolous demand apply equally well in a social security medical care system, but the revenue argument is unimportant if the system is already financed by payroll taxes which the beneficiaries regard as their contribution to paying for the service.

As for where to apply price discrimination, the simplest procedure is probably to set fees for particular services and then to apply uniformly a scale of adjustments based on income. However, the administrative burden would be reduced, and a considerable revenue could still be collected, if a uniform fee were charged for consultation (set low enough not to have much effect on necessary consultations by poorer consumers), and price discrimination were introduced only at the stage of treatment. In particular, hospitalization seems an appropriate stage at which to set differential fees, both because of the large share of hospital costs in total government health budgets, and because higher-income consumers sometimes use private doctors for consultations, but go to public hospitals for treatment.

One of the arguments for setting fees at all is that this will reduce unnecessary demand, ideally with minimal effect on necessary utilization. It is more correct to say that the total cost of obtaining medical care will reduce frivolous demand; and if the cost of travel, waiting time and income lost are high enough, most or all unnecessary utilization will already have been eliminated. In that case there will be no role for fees except to raise revenue, and so the optimum fee will in general be lower. (This argument is offset, to the extent that a given fee represents a lower share of total cost when other costs are high, so that the price-elasticity of necessary demand, ε_N, is reduced, permitting the optimum fee to be somewhat *higher*.) This suggests a second form of price discrimination may be desirable: fees should be lower for consumers for whom the *other* costs of obtaining care are higher. In particular, fees should perhaps be lower in rural areas of dispersed population and difficulty of access than in urban areas with good transportation and relatively easy access. This kind of geographic basis for discrimination has the advantage that it does not require classifying individual patients. Moreover, since the population of thinly-settled rural areas is typically poor, the lower fees would not usually benefit high-income consumers.

The argument is sometimes made that introducing fees is a way to make the revenue of a particular health facility reflect the quality of service it offers its clientele, and therefore to stimulate managers of hospitals and clinics to operate more efficiently and to satisfy their patients better; it not only permits but rewards decentralization. Among facilities serving the same class of consumers, this is a reasonable defense of fees, but it ceases to be valid once the non-fee costs of obtaining care differ. Applied to the sort of urban/easy-access and rural/difficult-access facilities just described, it would mean either that the urban facility would have extra funds with which to expand service where it is already better than average while the rural facility would not, or else that necessary demand would be reduced more in the already-under-served rural area. Equity in the raising and use of revenue from patients' charges probably requires either that fees raised in one place be (partly) transferred to less-favored facilities and populations, or that regular (tax-financed) budgets go preferentially to those locations where the optimum fee is lower.

References

[1] President's Commission for the Study of Ethical Problems in Medicine and Biomedical and Behavioral Research. *Securing Access to Health Care: the Ethical Implications of Differences in the Availability of Health Services, Vol.* I (Report): 20, 111. Washington, 1983.

[2] Musgrove P. La equidad del sistema de servicios de salud. Conceptos, indicadores e interpretación. *Boletín de la Oficina Sanitaria Pan-Americana.* 95, 525, 1983.

[3] Pan American Health Organization. *Plan of Action for the Implementation of Regional Strategies: 15.* Official Document 179, 1982.

[4] Musgrave R. *The Theory of Public Finance.* McGraw-Hill, New York, 1959.

[5] Cooter R. and Rappoport P. Were the ordinalists wrong about welfare economics? *Journal of Economic Literature* 22, 507, 1984.

[6] Newhouse J. P. The demand for medical care services: a retrospect and prospect. *Health, Economics and Health Economics* (Edited by Van der Gaag J. and Perlman M.). North-Holland, New York, 1981.

[7] Musgrove P. Family health care spending in Latin America. *Journal of Health Economics.* 2, 245, 1983.

[8] Grossman M. The demand for health: a theoretical and empirical investigation. NBER Occasional Papers 119, 1972.

[9] Muurinen J. M. Demand for health: a generalized Grossman model. *Journal of Health Economics* 1, 1, 1982.

[10] Pan American Health Organization and Agency for International Development. *Belize Health Sector Assessment,* 1982.

CHAPTER 6

Compensatory Finance in Health: Geographic Equity in a Federal System

Acknowledgments

I am indebted to Rena Eichler for much useful information about the United States Medicaid Program; to colleagues from the World Bank, the Inter-American Bank and the Brazilian Ministry of Health for the discussions which eventuated in the formula for assignment of federal funds to states in the two Banks' REFORSUS project; and to Barjas Negri of the Ministry for his urging to put these comparisons together and draw conclusions from them. Atilio Alsogaray of the University of La Plata provided the stimulus to write this paper.

Introduction: Relations Between Nations and Localities

The health of the population is often considered a responsibility of the national government, whether specified by law or constitution or through political consensus. At the same time, it is common for sub-national governments to control the public provision of health services, and even to assume the responsibility of financing private providers. This situation creates the need to determine the relation between one and another level of government, particularly with respect to financing. Two characteristics are relevant: the differences among parts of the country, and the specific capacities of the national government.

Translated and revised version of a paper in Spanish presented to the Third International Seminar on Fiscal Federalism, La Plata, Argentina, 24 April 1998.

Local inequalities and inequity

In general, a federal country is characterized by differences among regions, states or provinces, and municipalities. Relative to health, these may be differences in:

The degree of poverty, which limits private spending on health;
Local fiscal capacity for public spending on health;
Total health expenditure;
Needs for health care (the epidemiological situation); and finally,
The overall state of health.

These differences, especially in health status and access to services, are often considered unjust or inequitable, requiring compensatory or redistributive interventions.

The role of the national government

At least in comparison to the poorest states or provinces in the country, the national government generally has a greater capacity to generate tax revenues. The tendency—more marked, the more public functions are decentralized—is for the federal government to raise resources and transfer them to sub-national governments. In addition to the purely fiscal responsibility, the nation also is expected to assure equity or even equality among its citizens. This implies, among other things, reducing geographic differences. This function can be exercised either for universal programs, to which everyone has a right, or for targeted programs.

An Example: The Medicaid Program of the United States

The United States depends, more than is typical for a rich country, on private financing of health care, largely through employment-related insurance. Nonetheless, there are two large federal health programs: Medicare for the elderly, which is financed by a specific tax, and Medicaid for the poor. Both are shared between the federal government, which legislates the rules under which they operate and contributes to financing them, and the state governments, which administer the programs and also spend on them. (In contrast to what happens in some other countries such as Brazil and Chile, municipalities do not figure in the definition, financing or operation of these programs.)

Logic and objectives of the program

The poor, by definition, can hardly pay for health care out of pocket. On the other hand, they seldom have jobs that allow access to adequate insurance at reasonable cost. The chief objective of Medicaid is to provide subsidized insurance coverage for poor people. Another goal is to allow considerable freedom to state governments, not only to administer the program but to define the beneficiaries, the benefits to which they are entitled, and the corresponding cost. In contrast to some other programs, such as those described below, Medicaid does not operate by distributing a fixed federal budget.

Determining expenditures and their distribution

The state government (**s**) defines the beneficiary population (**Bs**) to be eligible for the program, subject to the regulations in the national legislation. Similarly, and also subject to federal rules, it determines the set of health services to be covered by the insurance. The combination of beneficiary characteristics and the list of services determines the quantity of care (**Qs**) to be utilized.

On the other hand, and also subject to federal approval, the state government determines, or negotiates with providers (mostly private), the prices (πs) it will pay. These prices should be the lowest necessary to guarantee a supply of services of adequate quality. A provider who agrees to serve Medicaid beneficiaries promises not to require co-payments or additional fees from patients. Together, the prices and quantities determine the total cost of the program in the state, $Cs = Qs^*\pi s$.

What the federal government determines is the fraction (ϕs) of that cost that it will contribute in that state. This depends on state per capita income; at incomes above about \$ 22,000 (in 1995), the share ϕs reaches its minimum value of 50 percent. That is, in the richer states the federal government finances half the cost of the program. In the poorer states the federal share is larger, reaching a maximum of 83 percent.

Federal or national expenditure in the state is therefore $CNs = \phi s^*Qs^*\pi s$, while the state government's expenditure is $CSs = (1 - \phi s)^*Qs^*\pi s$. The relation of federal to state spending is then $CNs = [\phi s/(1 - \phi s)]CSs$, with a minimum of equal expenditure at the two levels and a maximum of federal spending being five times that of the state government.

Observations: who decides what

The federal government influences the determination of the beneficiaries, the services to be subsidized, and the prices to pay for them. However, the only parameter it directly determines is the share it contributes to financing—on the basis of income per person, which neither the national nor the state government can influence appreciably. The other decisions are taken by the states. This has an important consequence for equity: two equally poor people in two different states can be treated differently. This can happen because of inclusion among the beneficiaries in one state and not the other, or because more services are covered in one state than in the other.

To put it another way: the federal Medicaid program is redistributive—it contributes much more to paying for health in poor states than in rich ones—and thereby compensates for differences in the number of poor people as well as in the capacities of states to assure them adequate health care. But the program does not impose equality of treatment, leaving it to state governments to decide how "generous" to be in applying the rules. This represents a relatively high degree of decentralization of decisions. It also has the consequence that the decisions by the states influence the total expenditure to which the federal government is committed. Finally, as occurs with some other programs, especially that of Aid to Families with Dependent Children, differences from one state to another may motivate migration from a less-generous to a more-generous state. There are no estimates of whether this happens on a significant scale.

A General Example: Explicit Redistribution

Another way to define a redistributive health financing scheme is to begin with a uniform level of expenditure per capita, or a uniform set of services, for the entire beneficiary population of a public insurance. Then one determines how the cost is divided between different levels of government. This logic corresponds more to the Canadian health system than to that of the United States, particularly as the former operated in Canada a decade or more ago, when there were specific federal transfers to the provinces to finance health. (Nowadays the transfers also pay for education and other programs, and it is left to the provinces to decide how to distribute the funds among different uses.) In general, such a system can be universal, as in Canada, or it can exclude part of the population because it is rich, or has private health insurance, or for some other reason (as occurs in the Netherlands). The definition of a public system which takes into account the coverage of private insurance, avoiding subsidy to those who do not need it, while assuring equity among the whole population, is of particular interest for countries with mixed health systems such as the majority of countries in Latin America.

The logic of a national health insurance

What follows describes a system for defining compensatory transfers from the national government to sub-national governments, which allows the latter some liberty in spending their own resources but imposes common national norms for the beneficiary population, the services covered, and their costs. Another difference from the Medicaid program is that the sharing of costs depends not on per capita income but on the revenues of the states—including any non-tied transfers which the state or province receives from the federal government for spending as it chooses. This leaves more control to the state for determining its own taxes and consequent revenues, but simplifies the determination of how much the state will have to spend on health. Revenues are known more quickly and more precisely than incomes, especially in countries with less-developed information systems. The central objective is to guarantee a uniform minimum coverage: to impose a floor but not a ceiling. The other objective is to control federal spending, although not rigidly—that expenditure is still influenced by the decisions of sub-national governments.

A redistributive formula

The national government defines (perhaps through negotiation with the states or provinces, as in Canada) the population which, because it is already privately insured (**A**), is not eligible for the full benefits of the public insurance. If private insurers cover fewer services than the public program, that insured population can participate as partial beneficiaries and still receive transfers. If **Ps** is the population of a state, the fully-covered beneficiary population is **Bs** = **Ps** − **As**.

The national government also determines the minimum level of per capita expenditure (**C**), or alternatively the minimum set of services (**Q**) to be financed. (Trying to specify both quantities and expenditures leads to rationing, if the spending is insufficient, or to expenditure which can buy more services than the minimum defined.) This determines the committed level of spending by each state, which can be expressed as **Cs** = **C*Bs**, or **Cs** = **Q*π*Bs**, where π are the prices, specified nationally. (This ignores the potential complexity of allowing different federal prices in different states, because providers' costs differ. However, that complication is often relevant for hard-to-reach rural areas or dispersed populations.) The state, for its part, retains the right to offer more services than are negotiated with the federal government, **Qs** > **Q**, or to pay higher prices for them, πs > π. In either of these cases, it has to spend its own resources: the federal commitment is limited to financing only **Q*π**.

If the privately insured population receives a more limited set of services than the national minimum, **Qas** < **Q**, the formula for the total expenditure committed has to be modified to include the services not guaranteed by private insurance. The result is

$$\mathbf{Cs = C*Bs + (Q - Qas)*\pi*As},\ \text{or}$$
$$\mathbf{Cs = Q*\pi*Bs + (Q - Qas)*\pi*As},$$

which can be expressed as **Cs = Q*π*Ps − Qas*π*As**. The program pays the cost of the minimum set of services for the whole population of the state, less the cost represented by the services provided by private insurers to their clients.

The last element of the system is the determination of how this total cost is shared between the federal and sub-national governments. There can be many different formulas, the simplest being that the state or province is required to spend on health, a fraction β of its revenues **Rs** (own tax revenues plus non-tied federal transfers). This way the state contribution becomes **CSs** = β***Rs**, and that of the federal government is **CNs** = **Cs** − **CSs**. Federal expenditure is purely compensatory, guaranteeing the minimum stipulated spending or services for the whole population, including any shortfall of private insurance coverage relative to the public insurance.

Observations on political decisions

In a system like that just described, the states or provinces can participate in two types of decisions. If the parameters **C** or **Q**, π and β are not fixed by law or the constitution, but negotiated (for example, annually), the sub-national governments share in determining them. The best way to fix the parameter values depends on the country's political situation, and in particular on the relative power of different states or provinces to benefit from these decisions. In the case of Brazil, the constitution was amended, first for education and later for health, to specify the responsibilities of the different levels of government (federal, state and also municipal). This was done to prevent the states with greater wealth and political power from continuing to obtain inequitably large federal transfers because the ceilings on federal resources were determined more on the basis of the distribution of providers than in relation to needs for health or financing.

In the second place, each state determines its own taxes, which affects the revenues **Rs** of which a share β must be spent on health. There is some risk of moral hazard, in that a state can pass more of health costs on to the federal government by reducing its tax rates. This danger is not entirely imaginary: it happened with a corrupt and irresponsible government in the state of Alagoas, in Brazil, which went effectively bankrupt by reducing taxes on the sugar industry and waiting for the federal government to pay for public services such as health. However, in general there are two strong protections against such moral hazard. One is that reducing taxes so as to pay less for health means losing larger revenues for other uses, especially if β is low, say 10 or 15 percent. The other protection is relevant if besides its own taxes, state revenues **Rs** include non-tied or general transfers from the federal government. In a poor state, these transfers can be a large share of total revenue, which effectively assures that the federal government will finance much of health expenditure and thereby protect the neediest. However, this requires that the non-tied transfers themselves not be very inequitable, to the point of annulling the equity due to the tied transfers for health.

Equity in Investment: The REFORSUS Project in Brazil

The two examples just discussed refer to *recurrent* spending in health, that is for the purchase of services. The problems of geographic inequality or inequity and the need for compensatory actions also can arise for *investment* spending, that is for the creation of capacity to produce services. The REFORSUS investment project in Brazil, begun in 1996 and financed partly by the World Bank and the Inter-American Development Bank, was designed to complete, equip or remodel hospitals and other health facilities. It required some arrangement to distribute the resources of US$590 million among the states of the country in an equitable and politically acceptable way. It therefore offers an illustration of how the ideas discussed here can also be applied to investments.

Background and objectives

Federal health expenditures in Brazil at the outset of the project (before the constitutional amendment mentioned above, which specifies values of β for states and municipalities) were distributed very unequally among states—largely because the public system (*Sistema Único de Saúde*) paid according to the production of services, and capacity for provision was very unequal and concentrated in the richest states. The resulting inequity was limited, at that time, by federal spending ceilings established for each state, besides a general ban on paying for the hospitalization of more than eight percent of a state's population in any one year. The ceilings were negotiated annually, but because of the unequal political power of the state governments, did not succeed in equalizing expenditure per capita, much less to adjust it according the fiscal capacities of the states for financing health from their own revenues.

The goal in the REFORSUS project was to establish ceilings for investment in each state, which would correct part of the existing inequity. They would also have to respect three important limitations:

according to budgetary law, at least 50 percent of the funds would have to be assigned on the basis of population;
no state should receive more funds than could be absorbed in justified investments; and
the criteria had to be transparent and the formula simple.

Determination of state-by-state ceilings

Many criteria were proposed for distributing the total investment fund **F** among the states or determining the values **Fs**. Among these were the level of income, the prevalence of poverty, age-standardized mortality, and many other indicators. In principle all were relevant, but they would have yielded a formula too complex to be understood and accepted. In consequence, and after much discussion, it was decided to base the allocation of funds solely on the state's population, **Ps**, and recurrent federal health spending per capita in the state, **Cs**. In addition, it was evident that the formula should be linear in these two variables, so as not to give very high or low allocations to states with extremely high or low population or per capita expenditures much above or below the mean. (Note that according to the rules for the Medicaid program, the fraction φs is linear in per capita income, up to the maximum income; and in the second example above, the state's contribution is linear in its revenues since β is constant.)

A "gap" was defined between federal expenditure per person in a state, **Cs**, and the maximum per capita spending among all the states, **Cm** (in the state of Paraná). The total gap or deficit of federal spending for any other state is calculated as **Ds = (Cm − Cs)*Ps**. This is the additional spending the state would need to receive in order to reach the same per capita level as the most-favored state **m**. The sum of these deficits is the total additional spending needed in Brazil to bring per capita federal expenditure in all states up to the level in Paraná: that is, $\mathbf{D = Cm*P - \Sigma s(Cs*Ps)}$, where **P** is total population.

To complete the allocation formula, one arbitrary parameter α was needed, which represents the relative weight of population. The fraction $\mathbf{1 - \alpha}$ is then the relative weight of the state's deficit in recurrent spending. This parameter is arbitrary in the same sense as φs or β in the previous examples; it must be decided politically. The difference is that instead of determining federal and state contributions, it fixes the assignment among states of a purely federal fund.

Incorporating α, the formula becomes $\mathbf{Fs/F = \alpha*(Ps/P) + (1 - \alpha)*(Ds/D)}$. The fraction of the total fund assigned as a ceiling to a state, **Fs/F**, depends on the state's share of the country's population and on its share of the total deficit or gap in recurrent federal health expenditure. Only the second term is explicitly redistributive, but in the circumstances of Brazil, even proportionality to population improves equity for various states. In the end, a value of 0.70 was chosen for α, so the redistributive adjustment has a relative weight of 30 percent.

Potential long-term adjustments

Obviously, if a formula such as this were applied during a long interval of investment, eventually the value of federally-financed installed capacity per person in health would become equal among all the states. If payment continued to be based on production of services, this would also tend to equalize recurrent spending among states. Eventually this might not be desirable, because differences in the epidemiological pattern among regions and states would justify unequal expenditures. Moreover, this adjustment toward greater equity says nothing by itself about the distribution of spending between the federal government and the states (not to mention the municipalities, which in Brazil operate much of the network of health facilities and sometimes contribute substantially to financing it). The subsequent constitutional amendment is aimed at equity in this larger sense. Not only should federal investment resources be directed more toward those states where spending has been lower in the past, but states should, by assuming responsibility for spending according to their own resources, liberate federal recurrent expenditure for a more equitable distribution.

Concluding Reflections

These three cases have several features in common which are worth empha-sizing. First, they deal only with geographic equity, leaving for lower levels of decision the allocation of funds among particular interventions, health conditions, or population groups. Geographic equity is at least partly a necessary condition for more detailed distributional justice according to needs, but not a sufficient condition. Second, the variables which go into the formulas for distribution—per capita income, revenues, population, or expenditure—are relatively easy to observe, more so in the case of revenue and spending, and do not require additional efforts to gather information. Third, these variables are subject very little or not at all to manipulation by either federal or sub-national governments. (Fraud may be possible, and estimates of population or income can always be controversial, but moral hazard is essentially nonexistent.) No government at either level can obtain more funds for itself, or reduce its financial contribution, by playing with variables under its control. Fourth, each formula contains one and only one arbitrary parameter: ϕs, β and α, respectively. As a result, the unavoidable political negotiation can focus on a single number rather than dealing with a multitude of effects or relative weights of several different variables. The resulting formula is transparent and politically comprehensible. It seems reasonable to suggest that these four characteristics are valuable for any allocation formula in pursuit of equity. The case for such simple formulas with a minimum of arbitrary parameters is strengthened when information is limited or of doubtful accuracy, or when relations between national and sub-national governments are characterized by mistrust or incomprehension.

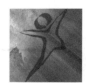

CHAPTER 7

An Ounce of Prevention Is Worth How Much Cure?

The conventional wisdom in health care is that an ounce of prevention is worth a pound of cure: preventing illness or injury not only avoids pain and suffering, it is also cheaper than treating those ill or hurt. Sometimes this is clearly true, but in other cases it is questionable. At the least, the right balance of prevention and cure in health care spending must depend on the costs of the two approaches, and those costs in turn may depend on the numbers of preventive and curative actions taken. Unless these costs are properly taken into account there is no way to tell how far to emphasize prevention, and at what point to give up and treat the cases that were not prevented. Still less is it possible to judge *a priori* how expenditure on health care ought to be divided between prevention and cure—and yet it is common to hear the complaint that 80 percent of a government's health budget goes for curative care and only 20 percent for prevention. If prevention really *is* so much cheaper than treatment, that may even be the right outcome: many cheap preventive actions and fewer, but more expensive, curative treatments. The fact that rice is much cheaper than meat does not by itself imply that rice will, or should, take up more of a family's food budget.

In order to minimize the combined costs of prevention and cure—the total cost of keeping people in good health or restoring them to it, supposing that such restoration is possible—the latter should take over from the former at the point where their marginal costs are equal. Here marginal cost means the cost of providing for the next *person*, whether what is provided is preventive or curative. So long as prevention costs less than cure, everything should be spent on prevention; but if at some point curing

Reprinted, with permission, from "An Ounce of Prevention Is Worth How Much Cure? Thinking about the Allocation of Health Care Spending". *A View from LATHR.* Latin America and the Caribbean Technical Department, the World Bank, 1990.

people becomes cheaper, spending from that point on should go for cura-tive care. What matters is not average but marginal cost, and these will not be equal if the cost per patient is not constant but depends on the number of patients for whom service is provided.

Figure 7.1 illustrates this argument, for the simple case in which preven-tion is always cheaper than cure. The population at risk is N, of whom some number NV receive preventive care: V is the marginal cost of prevention, shown by the curve from V_0 out to V. The symbol V is chosen to suggest vaccination, which is close to the ideal of prevention in both effectiveness and cost. This cost may initially decline as more people receive preventive care, reflecting the fixed costs and consequent economies of scale as coverage starts to expand. Before the whole population can be covered, however, the marginal cost is likely to rise again, surpassing its initial level. This reflects the increasing difficulty of reaching people as they are geographically scattered, resist being treated, or respond poorly to the

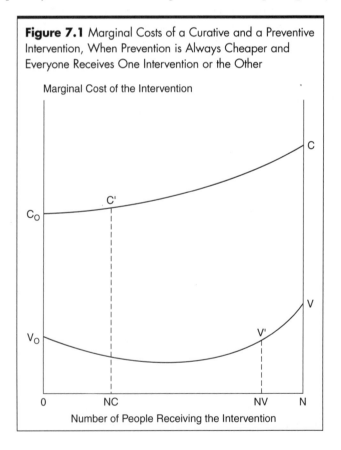

Figure 7.1 Marginal Costs of a Curative and a Preventive Intervention, When Prevention is Always Cheaper and Everyone Receives One Intervention or the Other

Marginal Cost of the Intervention

Number of People Receiving the Intervention

measure. The total cost of reaching NV people is the area under the V curve, from zero out to NV, and the marginal cost at that point is V'.

The other, higher curve in Figure 7.1 shows the marginal cost of curative treatment for the same health problem, C. If NC patients are treated the total cost is the area under the curve out to NC, and marginal cost at that point is C'. This cost curve may also show an initial decline and a subsequent rise, but it need not be shaped anything like the preventive-cost curve. The analysis is unchanged if the marginal cost C includes the non-medical cost of being sick or hurt, such as loss of income, or even an allowance for pain and suffering.

In this example, the cost of prevention never becomes as high as the cost of treatment, even if the whole population is covered. The right policy is therefore to reach everyone possible with preventive care even though this will raise the marginal (and average) cost of prevention above what it would be with lower coverage, since the last people reached are relatively expensive to provide for. The share of preventive spending is 100 percent, whether coverage is provided to the whole population or only to a small fraction of it. This probably is the model most people have in mind when they argue that (almost) everything should be spent on prevention. And there are doubtless cases where it applies: measles is easier to prevent than treat, and in an unvaccinated population, essentially every child runs a high risk of getting measles.

This example is far from universal, though. It contains two features which make prevention very attractive. First, the cost of prevention stays low even when everyone is covered: there is no technological barrier to reaching the whole population and the expense of doing so is bearable. Second, it is assumed that everyone who does not receive preventive care will, in consequence, require treatment—every individual gets one or the other. Even for measles, this is not strictly true. As more children are vaccinated the likelihood that an unvaccinated child will get sick is reduced, because transmission of the disease may be interrupted with less than full coverage by the mechanism of herd immunity. And for most diseases and injuries the probability of requiring treatment is well below 100 percent, even in the absence of any preventive action. Not everyone got polio before a vaccine was found.

If the probability of needing curative treatment when one has not received any preventive care is P, then the right comparison to make is not between V and C, the marginal costs per *patient*, but between V and PC. The latter is the *expected* expenditure on an individual who gets no preventive care, allowing for the possibility that he may or may not get sick or hurt; put another way, it is the cost per *person* of treatment when only a fraction of persons become patients. (If only a fraction of the entire population are candidates for the preventive measure—are at risk for the disease or injury it is desired to prevent—there is no need for a second concept of probability to apply to V; instead, N is simply defined as the population at risk, so that the probability for V continues to be unity.) Now when P is very low, cure must be much more expensive than prevention in order to justify preventive action, $1/P$ times as high, in fact. This will sometimes be the case— the cost of treating polio, for example, appears to be high enough to offset the low probability of paralysis among untreated children—but not always.

Figure 7.2 illustrates the two complications just discussed. First, the preventive cost curve V_O-V starts out low, just as in Figure 7.1, but then begins to rise so steeply that it becomes essentially impossible to cover the whole population at risk. Second, the curative cost curve is shifted down by the fraction P, to the position PC_O-PC. The result is that the two curves now

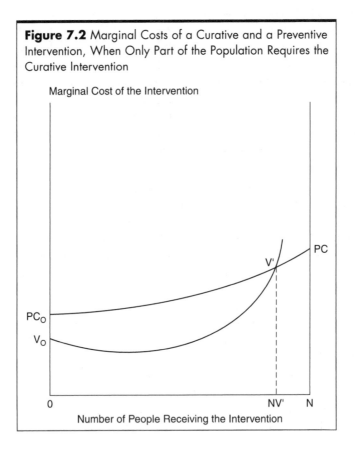

Figure 7.2 Marginal Costs of a Curative and a Preventive Intervention, When Only Part of the Population Requires the Curative Intervention

cross: beyond the point NV' it would be cheaper to start curing patients than continue to work at prevention, even though it is much cheaper to prevent NV' cases than to give curative care to the same number of people. For simplicity, the Figure is drawn supposing that P does not itself depend on the number of preventive actions. (Allowing for that possibility would generate a whole family of curative cost curves, each corresponding to one level of preventive coverage, which could cross the preventive cost curve at different places. Alternatively, the diagram would need to be three-dimensional, with the third dimension showing how P is related to preventive coverage.)

Figure 7.2 may seem to show that NV' is the correct level of preventive care, but of course that is not the case: costs are compared as though all individuals received both preventive and curative measures with the latter becoming cheaper for the next person after NV'. In fact, the expected cost of treating the first person who is not covered by prevention is shown by the height of the PC curve at PC_O at the left margin of the Figure. This will be equal to the marginal cost V' at NV' only if the cost curve is flat, with marginal and average costs equal. To find the correct (cost-minimizing) level of preventive action when the curative curve is not flat, the curve PC_O-PC is shifted (added) horizontally to the right until its starting-point meets the preventive cost curve. This is done in Figure 7.3, which shows the correct level of prevention to be NV^*. To the left of V^* the curve V_O-V^* shows preventive costs and to the right the curve V^*-PC shows curative costs. The first person for whom curative care is expected to be needed will cost exactly as much to take care of as the last person covered by preventive measures. In this example, prevention turns out to be the cheaper approach for much more than half the population at risk, but the total cost of curative care may still exceed total expenditure on prevention: the area NV^*-V^*-PC-N may be greater than the area O-V_O-V^*-NV^*. This distribution of resources is not evidence of inefficiency; it simply reflects the low probability of needing cure, and the sharply rising marginal cost of prevention. (The shaded, almost triangular area between the curve V^*-V' and the curve from V^* toward PC shows the additional cost that would be incurred by carrying preventive action too far, to the intersection of costs shown in Figure 7.2. A similar triangle to the left of V^* would show the extra cost associated with stopping the preventive measure too soon.)

Figure 7.3 shows how both total expenditure and its allocation between prevention and cure vary, as the total number of people reached by one measure or the other increases. It is important to note that so far as cost minimization is concerned, *every* point on the curve V_O-V^*-PC is an optimum,

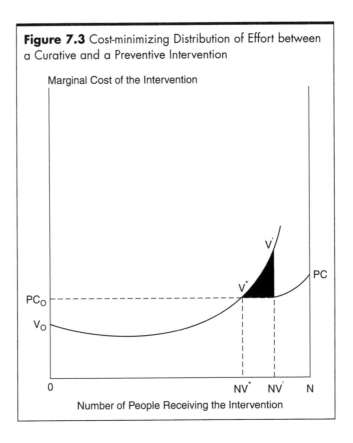

Figure 7.3 Cost-minimizing Distribution of Effort between a Curative and a Preventive Intervention

Marginal Cost of the Intervention

Number of People Receiving the Intervention

representing the cheapest way of reaching a given number of people. It is only in terms of health benefits, that one point can be said to be better than another—benefits increase steadily as one moves from V_0 toward PC. Whether those benefits are sufficient to justify the costs incurred is a larger question, which is considered briefly below. At this point, what matters is that the right balance of spending between preventing a health problem and curing it, depends on how much in total is spent on that problem. At low levels of total expenditure, the correct allocation may be 100 percent for prevention, but when enough is spent to do something for everyone at risk, the optimum share for prevention may be much lower, as in the Figure. The argument that too much is being spent on curative care, particularly in poor countries, is often implicitly an argument either that the situation in Figure 7.1 prevails, and nothing should or need be spent to cure people; or, that in the situation depicted in Figure 7.3, the country cannot afford to help everybody, that budgetary constraints impose an optimum close to—perhaps a little to the right of—V^*, and far from PC.

Does the real world ever look like what Figure 7.3 shows? In at least two important instances it does. One case is exemplified by diseases like malaria, where the preventive measures available work imperfectly—eradication of vectors is possible only in unusual circumstances, and is becoming more difficult, it is hard to avoid the vectors, and there is as yet no effective, cheap vaccine—and costs can become exorbitantly high as coverage is expanded. These problems do not mean that prevention should be abandoned, only that curative care is also part of a cost minimizing solution, and may have to absorb a large share of total costs. (Just how large depends also on the definition of the population at risk, N.)

The other typical case is exemplified by vehicular accidents. It is known how to reduce death and injury drastically by very inexpensive means such as always wearing seat belts and never driving while intoxicated. But these measures require repeated individual compliance: there is no vaccine yet against pigheadedness or drunk driving. Some people comply readily with the required preventive actions, producing a very low initial cost V, while others are impervious to safety propaganda and can be reached only by much more expensive measures such as air-bags or saturating the roads with police who will enforce the (appropriate) laws. It is these drivers who make the preventive cost curve rise so steeply. So do other elements outside the control of individual motorists, such as the high cost of making roads safer and cars more crashworthy. Nobody even knows what the cost curve looks like with any certainty: giving more money to the Ministry of Health (or anyone else) to reduce vehicular accidents does not translate into fewer victims as readily as more money for polio immunization translates into fewer paralyzed children. Hence the high, and growing, share of expenditure to treat accident victims.

Both these examples suggest that what is needed is not just more expenditure on existing preventive measures—and certainly not just less expenditure to treat victims—but the discovery of better prevention, cheaper and/or surer to work. That is why so much effort goes into developing new vaccines, and why governments experiment with laws, regulations and educational campaigns to reduce drunk driving, smoking, and other risks for which the curative costs can be very high, even, as in the case of AIDS, infinitely high. New preventive measures may eventually transform the optimum balance between prevention and cure, just as vaccines have done for measles and polio; and that in turn can be expected to redistribute spending between the two types of care. But at least when total expenditure is high enough, the outcome may be that curative care will properly get a larger, not a smaller, share of total health care resources. That will be the right solution, if effective prevention becomes very cheap for almost everyone, but still cannot reach some people—while curative treatment remains costly. Meanwhile, the relative spending on prevention and cure by itself says nothing about whether preventive efforts are inadequate, excessive, or about right: one must get beyond budget shares to relative marginal costs.

Strictly speaking, this analysis is valid only for a given health problem, which can be prevented (with more or less success) and for which some effective treatment exists (with greater or lesser probability of restoring full health). For that particular problem marginal cost analysis can in principle help determine the balance of preventive versus curative spending, to minimize the total cost of a given health outcome or to maximize the number of cases prevented or cured, for a given expenditure. Under these conditions, costs do not have to be compared to any measure of benefits, if one takes as given the budget for total spending on that problem. The preventive/curative distribution of total health care expenditure, however, depends also on the distribution of health problems on which money is spent. It is not possible to determine how much to spend in total on each kind of care without comparing the seriousness of different problems or, equivalently, the benefits of preventing them or curing them. If vehicular accidents are more of a problem than measles, there will be more spent on curative care, *in the optimum situation*, than if measles were the more serious problem.

Judging how serious a problem is means explicitly considering some measure such as loss of life, of years of life, or of quality-adjusted life years (which can also take account of non-fatal morbidity). The combination of such a criterion for comparison among *different* health problems and the marginal-cost criterion for allocation for each *particular* health problem, is in principle sufficient for specifying the optimum allocation of total health care spending between prevention and cure—again, for a given total expenditure on all types of health care. Arguments that too much is spent on curative care are often, implicitly or explicitly, arguments that too much is spent on certain problems, for which effective preventive measures do not exist or for which the known curative treatments are very costly. Such judgments can only be based on some comparison of benefits.

For a given health problem, prevention which is cheap and effective but cannot—for whatever reason—reach everyone in the population is likely to lead to an optimum in which curative care for a small number of people requires spending more than preventive measures for a much larger number. "Success" does not necessarily raise the preventive share in total spending, unless the prevention covers everyone at risk. The same phenomenon probably operates even more powerfully between health problems: successful prevention of one problem, such as measles, means that some other problem, such as vehicular accidents, becomes more important, with the consequence that the curative share of total spending *should* go up—at least until vehicular injury becomes as easy and cheap to prevent as measles is. At each moment, the correct balance of prevention and cure depends on total spending, on the epidemiologic situation and on the state of technical knowledge about how to prevent and how to cure health problems. The "epidemiologic transition" is largely just the product of successful prevention, whether by medical means (vaccination) or others (better diet, safer water), and it has cost consequences. How much should be spent in total on health care depends on comparing health benefits to the—incommensurable—benefits from spending on other things: there is no consensus on how to make that comparison.

It may be unwise to guess at a long-run equilibrium of health care cost levels and composition, since technical progress is rapid and there is little consensus on the seriousness of different health problems. But it is at least plausible that the correct distribution of spending in the long run will be even more weighted toward curative care than current spending is—because almost no one will die or get very sick at early ages, thanks to prevention, whereas the health problems people experience at later ages will not be amenable to prevention or even to cheap treatment. This might be the case even if society spent a smaller share of total product on health care—for example, if it stopped spending on "heroic" measures to prolong life by a few days or months, and spent nothing on people in comas or with Alzheimer's disease. A high proportion of spending on curative care may be the inevitable consequence of the fact that certain diseases and injuries can be prevented, but death can only be postponed.

CHAPTER 8

DALYs and Cost-Effectiveness Analysis

Acknowledgments

This note is the direct result of a request from Maria Paalman, the senior author-editor of the Review[1] {to which this article responded}, to read and comment on it. I am grateful to her for that impetus, and to Abdo Yazbeck, who worked on the 1993 *World Development Report*, for information and suggestions. Any misinterpretations are my sole responsibility, and in particular do not necessarily represent the views of the co-authors of the *WDR* nor of the World Bank.

Introduction

The article by Paalman et al. (1998) constitutes a fairly thorough and generally helpful guide to what is meant by the 'burden of disease' presented in the World Bank's 1993 *World Development Report, Investing in Health* (WDR), and how it is calculated. To a slightly lesser extent, the article is also useful for understanding how cost-effectiveness was estimated and used for setting disease control priorities,[2] and how these results were used in the WDR. As the title indicates, the piece is a critical review of these exercises and not simply an explanation of them. In this respect it is less acceptable, since some of the criticisms are misguided, a few are couched in somewhat irresponsible or evasive language, and some of them are plain wrong. This rejoinder proposes to sort out which criticisms are sound and which are not,

Reprinted from "A Critical Review of 'A Critical Review': The Methodology of the 1993 World Development Report, 'Investing in Health'." *Health Policy and Planning* 15(1), 2000, pp. 110–115, by permission of Oxford University Press.

or less sound, and thereby to clarify further what the WDR says and why it says it. I had the good fortune to be one of its authors, and so cannot claim neutrality in this discussion; but the experience of working on the Report and enduring much criticism of it even before it was published,[3] as well as in the 6 years since, may illuminate some of the issues raised. It is convenient to group the observations of the review by Paalman et al. (henceforth referred to as the Review) under four headings:

- the choice of cost-effectiveness, cost-utility or cost-benefit analysis;

- the various subjective parameters used to calculate Disability-Adjusted Life Years (DALYs);

- using the burden of disease and cost-effectiveness estimates (and other criteria) to set priorities; and

- things the WDR might have undertaken, but did not.

Choice and Appropriateness of Analysis

There are three distinct ways to compare the cost of some program or activity to its outcome: the analysis of cost-effectiveness (CEA), cost-utility (CUA) or cost-benefit (CBA) ratios or, in the case of CBA only, differences. The Review says that 'of the different economic evaluation techniques, the method used in the WDR is cost-utility analysis, a type of cost-effectiveness analysis used in the health sector' (p. 19). This is mostly right, although CUA need not be restricted to the health sector, and CUA is not so much a type of CEA as it is an extension of the latter that moves from purely objective measures of effects such as cases of disease, or lives, or people, to measures such as Potential Years of Life Lost (PYLL), Quality-Adjusted Life Years (QALYs) or DALYs, which explicitly introduce one or more subjective parameters in order to value the outcome. The distinction is clear and useful (Hurley et al. 1998), and it is perhaps regrettable that the WDR did not employ it; but there is a long tradition of using CEA to mean both things, and there is no convenient adjectival form of CUA comparable to 'cost-effective'.

The choice of CUA for the WDR meant that only *health* outcomes would be considered among the effects of an activity, precluding fuller evaluation of 'other sector interventions which are known to impact on health, such as girls' schooling, water supply and sanitation, and increased food consumption', as well as evaluation of the non-health effects of family planning (the Review, p. 14). The Review says of these interventions that 'in terms of total welfare they may be very cost effective', but this is a confusion of terms, just as it is to say that 'this has the effect of reducing the overall impact of an intervention, and thus reducing the resulting cost-effectiveness ratio' (p. 21). Such comparisons can be made only by assigning monetary values to the outcomes and applying CBA, as the Review recognizes elsewhere (p. 20). That raises problems of valuation far more vexing than those involved in CUA, such as whether to value results according to people's willingness to pay for them, which is dependent on the distribution of income and other factors that determine whether people act as though the intervention were worth its cost. Such comparisons are difficult enough within a single country, and would become almost meaningless across countries with very different incomes. The WDR authors chose to avoid these problems and accept the resulting limitations, and that choice cannot be criticized without implicitly favoring the monetization of benefits.

Subjective Parameters: Life Expectancy, Disability, Discounting and Age-weights

Even asking how much life is lost by a premature death, as in PYLL, requires choosing some life expectancy to define 'premature'. And any summing-up of mortality and morbidity, disability, or other notion of non-fatal health loss requires assigning weights to states between death and perfect health. Thus at least two of the four subjective parameters incorporated in the burden of disease calculations are inescapable in any such exercise, and the only question is what values they should take. There is a more subtle reason why the future should be discounted to some degree, which also makes a third parameter essential to avoid problems.

Life expectancies

The Review admits that it is 'ethically appealing' to assign potential lives of 80 or more years to everyone in the world (p. 16), but complains that 'the use of high standard life expectancies leads to very high burdens of disease in countries which presently have considerably lower life expectancies', so that 'it might be better to use realistic life expectancies when setting national priorities'. This is, regrettably, a common confusion: people dying young is clearly a 'burden of disease', or the phrase does not mean anything, and it is wrong to imply that the high burden of disease in poor, short-lived populations is somehow an overestimate. Probably what the authors meant, but did not distinguish, is that the amount of healthy life that could be gained by eliminating that disease alone might be relatively small, because in an unhealthy environment the people whose lives were saved would still die young from something else. That is, the effectiveness of interventions might be exaggerated, even if the burden were correctly estimated.

This is a plausible-sounding argument, and would imply the need for some adjustment when passing from the current burden to the potential gain from intervention. But it runs into a paradox which hardly any critics of the WDR have noticed: clearly if *all* the diseases contributing to the burden were controlled to the same extent that they are in Japan, life expectancy would rise to 80 or more years, just as in that country. (It does not matter that the cost of achieving such control, and the best choice of activities to bring it about, might differ from country to country.) Thus the gain from controlling all the diseases together would greatly exceed the sum of the gains from controlling each one separately, using the current short life expectancy. This adding-up paradox is a further reason, independent of the equity argument or the desirability of uniform international comparisons, for using the same long life expectancies everywhere when estimating the burden of disease.

Citing Anand and Hanson (1995), the critical review proceeds to another and much blunter confusion: the argument that if high life expectancies are used, 'the global burden of disease not only measures the burden of *disease*, but also indicates a burden of *'underdevelopment'*.' It should be superfluous to point out that by definition, every cause of death is classified as some sort of 'disease', taking the term to include perinatal conditions, malnutrition, and all forms of violence or external causes. Nobody dies directly of underdevelopment. The notion that there is a burden of disease up to a country's current life expectancy, and that the difference in years of life lost from there out to an expectancy of 80 years or more is due to something else, is simply wrong. The right way to think about underdevelopment is as a collection of risk factors, and it is true that disaggregating the burden of disease by risk factors is a much more complex undertaking than distinguishing the contributions of individual diseases. That is why the WDR attempted such an analysis for only a handful of risk factors: malnutrition (WDR Table 4.3), poor household environments (Table 4.5), and some other environmental threats (Table 4.6). These estimates are more preliminary and less thorough than those for particular diseases, and may be substantially revised when the World Health Organization finishes publishing the complete *Global Burden of Disease* series now in progress.

Disability weights

In contrast to the criticism of the other subjective parameters, the Review does not quarrel with the individual weights assigned to different disabilities—there are, after all, many of them, grouped into six classes—but focuses on how those weights were arrived at. In particular, the authors question the use of expert opinion, rather than that of patients or the general population, and complain that 'some of the criticisms might have been prevented if the process by which disability weights were established had been published and openly debated' (p. 18). It is certainly true that people with different relations to a disability—having suffered it, or treated it, or only thought about it—may evaluate it differently, but that does not establish whose view is more to be accepted; by definition, there are no right answers to these subjective elements, only answers that are reasonably consistent and defensible. And given the very tight deadline for producing the estimates that went into the WDR, there was no possibility of debate thorough enough to satisfy all the potential critics of the procedure. There was really no alternative to publishing the results and thereby opening them for discussion.

The Review points out that there is no allowance for conditions worse than death, but while one might admit there are such cases, they are surely rare enough, and often so short-lived as to make little contribution to the overall burden of disease. A more serious criticism is that severity and duration of disability are estimated separately, and the burden is simply the product of these two characteristics; there is no allowance for learning to live with a disability so as to suffer less from it, or for suffering more because there is no hope of cure or remission. This is an instance of a general issue that is confronted repeatedly in the definition of DALYs, which is that of *linearity*. The burden of disease adds linearly across individuals of the same age who suffer death or the same disability at the same time: this has the great computational advantage of permitting one to work with totals or averages. In contrast, DALYs are not linear with age, because of age weighting, nor through time, because of discounting; a year of disability differs in value according to when it occurs and the age of the person to whom it happens. Rather than imposing linearity everywhere, which would greatly simplify the calculations, or allowing everywhere for non-linear relations, the creators of the burden of disease estimates introduced nonlinearity wherever there seemed to be a strong specific justification for it, and not otherwise.

Finally, it is true that the assigned disability weights are uniform across cultures and circumstances, even though the ease with which someone can cope with a disability differs from place to place and person to person. Uniformity was imposed here partly for computational convenience, but also for equity reasons, so as to make no distinction among people according to where they happen to live and what resources they have for dealing with disabilities.

Discount rate

Since the burden of disease incident in any one year includes all the future effects of death and disability occurring in that year, it is necessary to decide how to value the future. The effects of choosing a high or low discount rate on the composition of the burden of disease are correctly described, as is the reason for not using short-term rates on risky investments. However, the discussion of this issue in the Review is unfortunately rather evasive. Thus, discounting 'purportedly' converts future lives to their present values, and 'is said to' avoid the time paradox (p. 18)—it is not recognized that it *does* avoid that paradox—and the paradox itself is consigned to a footnote. In a world where resources can be invested at a positive interest rate, if one does not discount future benefits, it will never pay to undertake an intervention because each year's delay means the benefit can be increased, for example by reaching more beneficiaries. The rhetorical question, 'Whose perspective and values should be considered?' ignores the fact that 'the long-term [average] yield on investments' is determined not by a cabal of experts but by all of society, which behaves as though it does discount the future at some rate not too different from 3%.

Age weights

These are easily the most controversial of the subjective parameters used in the calculation of DALYs, and as the Review says, 'neither universally accepted nor valued' (p. 17). This is partly because age weights are not intrinsically necessary for comparing mortality and disability, measuring years of life lost, or avoiding time paradox: this makes them the most optional of the subjective choices involved in going from CEA to CUA. However, a substantial part of the rejection they encounter is due to misunderstanding, in particular to supposing that the weights are determined by relative *economic* productivity. If they were, they would stay close to zero up to age 15 or so, reach their peak much later than age 25, and drop sharply at retirement age. They would also discriminate according to people's income-earning ability, so that their use to set priorities for health care would favour the rich—thus the 'obvious inequity' to which Murray (1994) refers. There is nothing inconsistent about rejecting such an economic measure and instead using age-weights that are designed to take account of the *emotional* loss to other people from an individual's death. The weights reach their peak at 25 years, because a person that age is likely to have a spouse and young children, and parents still living. They are low at very early ages because parents can often replace a lost infant, before they age much themselves, and low at high ages because one's parents are usually deceased and one's children grown by then. It *is* inconsistent to criticize parameters that try to incorporate the loss to those related individuals, and at the same time complain that DALYs do not include any of 'the burdens which fall on households' (p. 18).

More generally, treating all ages equally is also a subjective choice, and while it is simpler and more 'classical', it is not obviously better. Part of the sensitivity analysis conducted by Murray et al. (1994, p. 103) involves varying the age weights from the pattern used in the WDR, through three intermediate values with the same general shape but smaller age differences, to equal weight for all ages—not, as the Review says, 'shifting to more unequal age weights' (p. 19). Changing the age weights has complex effects on the composition of the burden of disease by age and by disease, effects partly compensated by the discount rate, but with essentially no effect on the composition by sex. There is no clear right answer to how to treat different ages, since it depends on how much one wishes to take into account emotional losses suffered by people close to the disease victim.

Actual Choices in Burden of Disease Estimates

As of mid-1998, there had been, in addition to the global estimates used in the WDR, 15 exercises in national priority setting in health in 17 countries and one large Indian state, which included estimates of burden of disease (Bobadilla 1998, pp. 12–15). Another such study was in preparation, and there had been another four efforts to determine priority interventions without estimating disease burden. These exercises covered as few as 10 major diseases and as many as 112. Several of them ignored morbidity and disability and estimated only the (much larger) health damage from premature mortality. 'Although the indicator to assess the burden of disease most commonly used was the DALY, half of the countries made significant modifications, and one (Russia) used a different indicator . . . Five countries did not discount future health losses, and . . . Five countries did not apply any age weights to health losses or used different weights from those proposed in the 1993 *World Development Report*. Finally, three of the countries that studied disability used a different disability scale to assess severity. In short, only seven of the 19 study results are comparable . . .' (Bobadilla 1998, pp. 17–18 and Table 3). This varied experience shows that what is proposed in the WDR is not universally imposed, for at least three reasons—a disease burden dominated by mortality from a small number of diseases, inadequate data (a problem on which the Review rightly insists) and subjective choices which depart from the logic outlined above. While this may be interpreted as a victory for local views and values, there is no reason to think it makes the different national studies any better than if they had all used the same methods and numerical values.

Priorities for Intervention

The Review summarizes well (p. 14) the idea that an intervention is a 'good buy' if it is cost-effective and also deals with a disease or risk factor that accounts for a sizeable burden of disease. In strict economic terms, the latter condition should be irrelevant: if at the margin, an intervention deals cost-effectively with a small disease problem, then it is worth buying. At least, this will be true so long as there are no large fixed costs to confronting small disease burdens, and the health care system can deal simultaneously with a large number of interventions. The reason for including the size of the burden as a criterion for priority setting is precisely that health systems in poor countries often cannot efficiently administer a large collection of programs, and dissipate their resources trying to do so. In consequence, it makes sense to maximize the health gains from a small number of interventions, economizing on scarce managerial and administrative capacity. There are, as the Review notes (p. 22), some very difficult issues of whether disease burden and cost-effectiveness criteria can be used for large-scale reallocations or only for marginal increments of resources, and of what the health system is currently doing or trying to do with its existing infrastructure, which cannot easily be re-directed. These difficulties mean that a simple ranking of cost-effectiveness cannot be treated as a list of priorities, even ignoring other considerations, unless the health system can—subject to overall resource limitations—actually offer any of the interventions on the list without interfering with the capacity to administer others.[4]

The Review observes, correctly, that when a disease is expanding rapidly, the current burden it causes is a poor guide to priority (p. 23, citing Bobadilla et al. 1994). But it does not recognize that the WDR applied this reasoning to argue 'Why AIDS is a special case', requiring urgent preventive measures to contain its spread (pp. 99–106). Nor do the authors of the Review take any account of the discussion in the WDR (pp. 54–59) of the rationales for government action in health other than that of obtaining value for money. Cost-effectiveness is, almost tautologically, the criterion for getting the most health gain out of a given quantity of resources, however the effect is measured. It is not necessarily the appropriate criterion for how *public* resources should be spent, except in the case of public goods for which markets do not exist, or services with such large externalities that markets will work quite imperfectly (Musgrove 1999). The emphasis in the WDR on disease burden and cost-effectiveness constitutes its principal novelty, and, not surprisingly, has drawn much more attention from the public health community than the more conventional discussion of public finance criteria and of equity.

Equity is a troublesome issue, because cost-effectiveness is concerned only with efficiency, and 'the fact that the most efficient interventions . . . tend to specifically benefit the poor is more a result of coincidence than of principle' (p. 24), a finding that has since been more fully substantiated (Gwatkin and Guillot 1998). And neither horizontal nor vertical equity is necessarily compatible with cost-effectiveness (Musgrove 1999); societies must choose how far to favor one or the other goal. Nonetheless, governments can do much to promote equity by how they *finance* health care, even if the interventions are chosen on the basis of value for money. And the essential package which the WDR recommends was designed specifically for very poor countries. At higher income levels, it becomes much harder to say what should go into a package, and cost-effectiveness becomes less relevant as a guide.

Giving some degree of priority to the poor, either because they are sicker than the non-poor or because they are less able to pay for health care, is ethically acceptable and is explicitly favored by the WDR. It does not follow that other distinctions among potential beneficiaries are equally justified. Thus giving 'greater weight to mothers and children than to adult males', as the Review says was done in the Oregon exercise to determine what interventions Medicaid would finance (p. 17), is *prima facie* inequitable, particularly since the greater life expectancy of children already gives them a measure of priority over adults, where death or long-term disability are concerned. And to judge that, *ceteris paribus*, a year of death or disability matters more for a woman than for a man is breathtakingly unfair. Priorities among population groups should not be imposed as part of the estimation of disease burden, but should emerge from the analysis of what health gains can be achieved, at what cost, given those groups' disease profile. That is the greatest conceptual advance in the WDR, the insistence that on grounds of both equity and efficiency 'it is appropriate to . . . prioritize health care interventions rather than population groups' (p. 23 of the Review). If this contradicts the common emphasis on 'vulnerable groups', so much the worse for that emphasis: everyone is vulnerable to some health problems, and not every vulnerability has a solution. The way to combine information on the main elements of the disease burden of particular age and sex groups, with information on the availability of cost-effective interventions that could significantly reduce that burden, is well illustrated in Appendix Tables B.6 and B.7 of the WDR. That exercise shows that children and women do indeed deserve priority *for certain health problems*, but not universally or independently of what diseases they suffer. Thus controlling childhood diarrhoea and respiratory infections should have priority, but dealing with congenital malformations probably should not.

The Review criticizes the idea of an essential package for poor countries, including a small number of interventions, on the grounds that it 'is not in line with the Alma Ata approach to comprehensive care, which has been pushed by WHO and donors for many years now', and that 'the call for specific packages could lead to vertical programs' (p. 24), as though it were demonstrated that vertical programs are a bad thing and that the Alma Ata approach has been shown to work adequately.[5] This sounds more like clinging to poorly justified positions than like real analysis. A more serious criticism is that 'the package arrived at by experts might not be acceptable to the public, and hence less cost-effective in the end' than if people's wishes were consulted in formulating priorities. This raises the general, and severe, problem of needs and wants not necessarily coinciding, and points to the urgency of finding out whether and why people may not use existing health services and reforming those services so as to attract the beneficiaries they are meant to help. The Review correctly emphasizes that the actual cost-effectiveness of an intervention depends on the scale of utilization and the degree of compliance by patients, which will vary with local cultural, economic and other conditions.

The Review is the result of conflating and editing separate papers by the four authors.[6] This may explain why it says in one place (p. 24) that 'Once the most cost-effective interventions are in place the burden of disease is expected to decrease', and then elsewhere (p. 25) claims that 'implementation of the advocated good buys will most likely not result in a reduction of the burden of disease, but in the transition of disease patterns and increased health care costs'. Certainly the former view is correct, or it makes no sense to do anything about health problems at all. The fact that the cost of gaining a DALY will rise if the cheapest DALYs are bought first is an indication of success, not of failure; it would still be true that the greatest number of DALYs could be bought for any given expenditure, or that for a given reduction in disease burden, the cost would be minimal. All that the WDR intended to do in this regard was to emphasize the huge differences in cost-effectiveness among known interventions—differences that are often much larger than the likely errors in estimation—and the large disease burdens that could be controlled at relatively low cost (although possibly requiring expenditures significantly larger than the poorest countries are now dedicating to health).

What the WDR Might Have Done, But Did Not

Unlike most publications from the World Bank or elsewhere, the annual *World Development Report* is produced on a timetable that does not allow even one day's deviation, and with a rigid ceiling on the number of pages. These constraints precluded doing a great many things that would have made for a more comprehensive volume.[7] A good deal of the criticism in the Review concerns such desirable but infeasible improvements as:

- generating more and better data on disease incidence, and especially on intervention costs and effectiveness, since the existing base of information is incomplete and includes many estimates and approximations;

- performing more extensive sensitivity analysis to see whether any of the conclusions or recommendations would be overturned by plausible changes in empirical data or in the values of the subjective parameters;

- incorporating more views into the estimation of disability weights and age weights, and forming a wider consensus on their values; and

- providing more help to countries wishing to use the recommendations of the WDR to restructure their health systems and reallocate resources, including 'practical advice for Ministries of Health on how to deal with political barriers' (p. 24).

The WDR was not intended as the last word on any of these issues; on the contrary, it was meant to stimulate more and better data and analysis, by showing what could be done even with the limited information available. And it could not, without becoming a multi-volume encyclopedia, deal with the specific economic, political and cultural circumstances of all the societies where its recommendations might be applicable. (A flood of country studies and project documents in the last six years have been dedicated partly to that end.) In particular, trying to give global political advice would be even more open to criticism than the global suggestions based on narrow economic criteria. Many of the recommendations in the Review for further research and refinement of recommendations are entirely compatible with the aims of the WDR and the views of its authors. However, no volume of data and no amount of analysis will do away with the need for subjective judgment about key parameters. More sensitivity analysis can at best show whether conclusions hold up under different numerical values—it cannot determine the right values. And wider debate about those values will not necessarily lead to agreement, as appears from the variety of assumptions adopted in the burden of disease exercises described above. More precision and clarity are possible, at a cost, and very desirable; certainty never will be. That is why the effort launched by the *World Development Report* is likely to continue for years and may gradually transform how people think about health sector priorities, without ever providing final answers.

Concluding Remarks

The authors of the Review are nothing if not critical; I hope that this reply will clarify where those criticisms are well-founded and where they are not, including the few instances of outright error. Still, the Review concludes that 'the World Bank is to be commended for this unique initiative, conducted in a self-critical spirit' (p. 25). In the same spirit, I believe the authors of the *World Development Report* can commend the thoroughness of the critical review which their work has received, and the obvious willingness of the reviewers to understand, explain, and improve on it.

Notes

1.   Maria Paalman, Henk Bekedam, Laura Hawken and David Nyheim. A critical review of priority setting in the health sector: the methodology of the 1993 World Development Report. *Health Policy and Planning*, 1998, 13(1): 13–31.
2.   In Jamison et al. 1993.
3.   It is probably safe to say that every single issue raised by Paalman et al. was debated extensively, and sometimes acrimoniously, within the Bank and WHO; arguments between orthodox economists and public health specialists were often particularly sharp.
4.   This is one of the crucial issues treated in *Better Health in Africa* (World Bank 1994), which is in many ways a companion volume to the 1993 *World Development Report*.
5.   Quite the opposite occurred in Bangladesh, where the development of an essential package of services led to the consolidation of more than 100 vertical programs, 66 of them supported by donors (Abdo Yazbeck, personal communication, June 1999; the details are in reference World Bank 1998).
6.   Maria Paalman, personal communication, June 1999.
7.   But as the author of Parkinson's Law (Parkinson 1957) says, referring to many things that were left out of his book, 'such a volume would take longer to read and cost more to buy', besides taking much longer to write.

References

Anand S, Hanson K. 1995. *Disability-Adjusted Life Years: a critical review*. Working paper series Number 95.06. Harvard Center for Population and Development Studies. Cambridge, USA: Harvard School of Public Health.

Bobadilla JL. 1998. *Searching for Essential Health Services in Low and Middle-Income Countries*. Policy Background Study Number Soc–106. Washington, DC: Inter-American Development Bank.

Bobadilla JL, Cowley P, Musgrove P, Saxenian H. 1994. Design, content and financing of an essential national package of health services. In: Murray CJL, Lopez AD (eds). *Global Comparative Assessments in the Health Sector: Disease Burden, Expenditures and Intervention Packages*. Geneva: World Health Organization.

Gwatkin D, Guillot M. 1998. *The Burden of Disease among the Global Poor: Current Situation, Trends, and Implications for Research and Policy*. Prepared for the Global Forum for Health Research. Washington, DC: World Bank.

Hurley J, Feeney D, Giacomini M, Grootendorst P, Lavis J, Stoddart G, Torrance G. 1998. *Introduction to the Concepts and Analytical Tools of Health Sector Reform and Sustainable Financing*. Centre for Health Economics and Policy Analysis,

McMaster University. Toronto, Canada. Written for the Economic Development Institute of the World Bank.

Murray CJL. 1994. Quantifying the burden of disease: the technical basis for disability-adjusted life years. In: Murray CJL, Lopez AD (eds). *Global Comparative Assessments in the Health Sector: Disease Burden, Expenditures and Intervention Packages*. Geneva: World Health Organization.

Murray CJL, Lopez AD, Jamison DT. 1994. The global burden of disease in 1990: summary results, sensitivity analysis and future directions. In: Murray CJL, Lopez AD (eds). *Global Comparative Assessments in the Health Sector: Disease Burden, Expenditures and Intervention Packages*. Geneva: World Health Organization.

Musgrove P. 1999. Public spending on health care: how are different criteria related? *Health Policy*, 47.

Parkinson CN. 1957. *Parkinson's Law*. Cambridge, UK: Houghton Mifflin.

World Bank. 1994. *Better Health in Africa: Experience and Lessons Learned*. Washington, DC: World Bank.

World Bank. 1998. Bangladesh Health and Population Program Project, Project Appraisal Document, Report No. 17684-BD, June 1. Washington, DC: World Bank.

CHAPTER 9

Criteria for Public Spending on Health Care

Acknowledgments

This note grew out of an impromptu lecture during Module 5 ('Designing a Cost-Effective Benefit Package') of the Flagship Course in Health Economics and Sustainable Financing, organized by the Economic Development Institute (now the World Bank Institute) of the World Bank in October-November 1997. I am grateful to Ricardo Bitrán, who developed Module 5, for the opportunity to participate in that part of the course and for his reactions to the ideas presented here; to my colleagues Paul Shaw, Anne Johansen and Hadia Samaha; and to the audiences for the Flagship Course in Washington and at seminars or courses in Moscow, Santiago, Bogotá, Brasília and Riyadh during the next several months, for opportunities to pursue these ideas and improve their logic and presentation. Julio Frenk, Lant Pritchett and an anonymous reviewer also provided helpful comments. Any remaining errors or confusions are no one's fault but the author's.

Introduction

It is standard practice in courses on health economics to explain each of the several justifications for the state to intervene in this sector. These include the different kinds of market failure that can occur in health care interventions and insurance, together with the equity reasons for intervention, such as to assure some minimum coverage of health insurance or access to health care for the poor or for some other group. What is almost always missing from such a course is any explanation of how these different criteria are related to one another. In particular, the participant seldom gets any help understanding two kinds of potentially very important relations between one criterion and another. One question is whether they are compatible with each other or are in conflict, requiring one to choose between them in deciding how to use public resources. The other question is whether they are connected sequentially or hierarchically, so that one should examine one criterion before asking if another one is applicable.

This note asks and answers these two questions—about compatibility and about hierarchy—for nine frequently used criteria. Working out the connections among these criteria leads to a partial decision tree concerning three possible outcomes: a particular service should be financed publicly (or subsidized in part), it should be left to private markets to provide or it should not be produced at all. Helping to reach such decisions is one of the main goals of public finance theory [1], and making the decisions is among the principal tasks of government.

Which Criteria Matter?

Fig. 9.1 displays the nine criteria, and classifies four of them as being primarily economic (about efficiency), four primarily about equity, and one as neither of these. To keep the analysis as simple as possible, each criterion is considered chiefly as a reason for spending public money on health care, or choosing how to spend it, rather than as a justification for other, non-financial kinds of government intervention.

The economic efficiency criteria start with cost-effectiveness, or the relation between the cost of an intervention and the resulting outcome or health gain. Two reasons for market failure which occur primarily in the market for health care are also included: health interventions which are public goods and therefore have no market or which produce such marked externalities that markets will not produce the efficient amount of the service. The fourth efficiency reason is the catastrophic cost of some health care, which is an argument for risk sharing via insurance.

The equity criteria include both horizontal and vertical equity. Both these concepts of fairness are considered only in relation to health care, not to how health services are financed, although the horizontal/vertical distinction also applies there. Poverty is another criterion in this group; that is, the emphasis

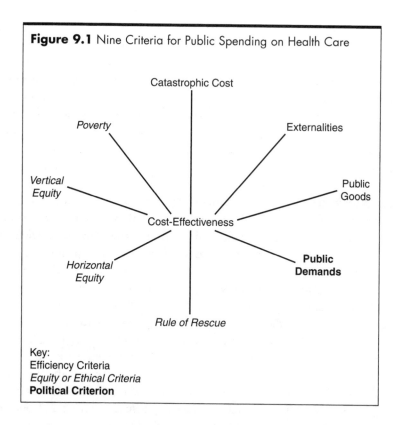

Figure 9.1 Nine Criteria for Public Spending on Health Care

Catastrophic Cost

Poverty

Externalities

Vertical
Equity

Public
Goods

Cost-Effectiveness

Horizontal
Equity

**Public
Demands**

Rule of Rescue

Key:
Efficiency Criteria
Equity or Ethical Criteria
Political Criterion

is on the equitable or moral aspects of providing preferential treatment to poor people, not on whether that would be efficient because it made them more productive, lifted them out of poverty, and so on. The fourth criterion of equity is the 'rule of rescue', the admonition to give priority to saving lives over interventions that do not make a life-or-death difference.

Finally, there is something rather lamely called 'public demands', which is meant to encompass an important political aspect missing from these more technical criteria: that is, what does the public think its money should be used for? Public beliefs and wishes may be many and contradictory, but probably include a mixture of equity and efficiency concerns, and it is worth asking how they also may be related to cost-effectiveness. (Other demands and pressures for public expenditure arise from providers of health care and from suppliers of equipment, drugs and other inputs; these are not considered here.)

The full set of possible binary relations among the nine criteria would require an unwieldy 36 comparisons. Only eight of these are considered, comparing every other criterion with that of cost-effectiveness. The reason is that this is arguably the most misunderstood criterion, partly because it is usually not treated in relation to other reasons for intervening in the health sector. In consequence, it is thought by some people to be the only test that matters, and by others to be irrelevant or nearly so. Concentrating on the relations between other criteria and cost-effectiveness helps to clarify the role of cost-effectiveness in making decisions about public intervention in health care.

Cost-Effectiveness and Public Goods

This is the simplest relation among those considered: cost-effectiveness is the criterion for choosing which of a number of public goods are worth financing. Simply being a public good is not reason enough for the government to finance a health care intervention, because the result in improved health might not be worth the cost—the same resources could be better used for another health service or for some non-health activity [2]. But if something is a public good, there is no private market for it, and so there is no risk that government finance will crowd out private purchases. In consequence, the output that is paid for publicly is all the output there is, and there is a direct relation between public finance and the gain in welfare. How large that gain is depends on the health improvement and on the welfare evaluation of the health gain. Maximization of welfare under these conditions leads to cost-effectiveness as the way to choose among different public goods [3]. All that is necessary is that total welfare be monotonically related to total health gain, so that obtaining the largest possible improvement in health—which is what cost-effectiveness does, for a given amount of resources—also yields the largest obtainable total welfare.

The relation between public goods and cost-effectiveness is not only straightforward, it is also hierarchical. That is, one asks first whether some health care service qualifies as a public good, and then whether it can be provided cost-effectively. It might seem just as well to select all the cost-effective health services first, and then to ask which ones of them are public goods, but there are two reasons not to proceed in this way. First, too little is known about the cost-effectiveness of hundreds of health services to draw up such a set and choose from among them [4]. It reduces the demands on information to ask about cost-effectiveness only after applying some other, more easily determined, criterion. Second, the sequence public good? cost-effective? is the only pair of questions that need to be asked where public goods are concerned. In contrast, the question of whether a particular health service is cost-effective also arises in relation to several other criteria, as indicated below, and it is easier to deal with each of them in turn.

Externalities, or Partly Public Goods

If an intervention does not qualify as a pure public good, because private purchasers are willing to pay for it, there may still be significant effects on non-purchasers: that is, externalities. Measures to treat communicable disease can fall into this category, because while a person with the disease may be willing to pay to be cured, treating him or her also reduces the risk of transmission and thereby protects others. (Chemotherapy for tuberculosis is an often-cited example.) The service is then partly private, because there is a private or individual gain that can be bought in the market, but is also partly public because of the externality. For this reason it seems intuitively clear that cost-effectiveness should also be used to choose which services with externalities deserve to be financed publicly. But there are two other issues to deal with before asking about cost-effectiveness.

The first is whether the externality is significant: that is, whether it really makes for a difference between the private benefits to purchasers and the total benefits, including those accruing to non-purchasers. If the difference is quite small, the service has only a little public character, and it can properly be treated as if it were a purely private good. If however there is a large externality, it becomes appropriate to ask whether the private demand for the service is sufficient to assure realization of (nearly) all the potential social benefit. That is, will private individuals buy enough of the intervention that no public inducement or subsidy is needed? Or will they, for whatever reason (poverty, high cost, under-valuation of the benefits), fail to seek or to continue treatment, so that the preventive potential is not realized?

If the answer is that the private demand appears inadequate, then cost-effectiveness becomes relevant. That is, one should ask whether the potential social gain from publicly subsidizing the service with the externality is large enough to justify the cost. Since there is some private demand, the subsidy may be only partial, rather than total as in the case of pure public goods. The chain of questions becomes longer: significant externalities? adequate private demand? cost-effective?

For both public goods and services with externalities, the hierarchical relation to cost-effectiveness means that the question of whether the different criteria are consistent does not arise. One does not get into hypothetical problems such as, that a particular intervention ought to be financed publicly because it is a public good, but should not have public money spent on it because of low cost-effectiveness. The second decision dominates the first, and the service is not worth buying.

What If the Cost is Catastrophic?

Two health care interventions may look equally justified because they have the same ratio of cost to effectiveness—the same cost per life saved, per year of healthy life gained, or some other measure of results—but one may be an order of magnitude more expensive than the other ([5] Figure 3.2). People paying out of pocket will afford the cheaper service, but the catastrophically costly service will be available only if the financial risk is shared. The fact that some services cost too much for individuals to buy is often regarded as a reason for public finance, but it is really a reason for insurance. Whether that insurance should be public or private or a mixture of the two is a complex question, involving the risks of failure in the private insurance market and the costs of limiting those risks or eliminating them by public regulation, finance or other measures. If the cost of a service is not catastrophic, however—that is, if most people can pay for it out of pocket without being impoverished—then there is generally no argument for it to be financed publicly. (The exceptions are services which people could buy, but do not, because of incomplete information, such as preventive screening that would allow early treatment and avoid later catastrophic expenses. Subsidizing such services is one way of overcoming this market failure.)

This leaves two conclusions. One is that costs matter by themselves, and not only in relation to results. The other is that if the cost is low enough, individuals who contemplate buying the service can make their own decisions about cost-effectiveness. The two criteria, cost and cost-effectiveness, are independent, so they are compatible. Only when the cost is catastrophic, and there are good reasons for public finance of the service, does cost-effectiveness need to be separately taken into account. Then the two criteria may be in conflict, as will appear later.

There is one more question to ask about the criterion of catastrophic costs, and that is, catastrophic for whom? Some individuals, after all, can afford much more medical care than others. The easiest answer to this question seems to be to regard a cost as catastrophic if it cannot be paid by someone who is non-poor, without it making him or her poor. That is, the distinction between catastrophic and non-catastrophic depends on the distinction between being poor and non-poor, where poverty is defined by some criterion other than health, such as income, consumption of necessities such as food, etc. This leads directly to the next criterion: poverty as an ethical reason for public finance of health care.

Poverty and Cost-Effectiveness

Since poverty is defined independently of either the costs or the outcomes of health care, there would seem to be no obvious or necessary relation between these two criteria. The situation is not quite so simple, however, to the degree that the poor are not only sicker and die younger than the non-poor, but are afflicted by different diseases. Both the level and the composition of the burden of disease differ somewhat between poor and non-poor populations, with the poor suffering more from communicable diseases and from premature mortality, compared to non-communicable causes and disabilities ([1] Appendix B, Tables B.5 and B.8), [6].

It happens that some though not all of the diseases which differentially affect the poor are also diseases for which relatively cost-effective interventions exist. There is therefore a fairly marked relation between poverty and cost-effectiveness, but it is also an accidental and transitory association. It exists because the non-poor either do not need those interventions, or would benefit less from them, or have already benefited, while the poor still suffer a large reducible burden. Measles is a good example of this difference: the non-poor of the world are protected by immunization, but many of the poor still are not. And since the poor are more likely to be malnourished, and since malnutrition greatly increases the risk of death from measles [7], immunizing the poor prevents even more health loss than among the non-poor.

This suggests that poverty and cost-effectiveness are often compatible criteria: doing something to improve the health of the poor has a better than average chance of also being cost-effective—but not always. The poor also suffer from many health problems which do not now have cost-effective solutions, and it does not automatically follow that public money should be spent ineffectively, just because the intended beneficiaries are poor. The same question of value for money arises here as with the efficiency reasons for public expenditures. This is the basis for the idea of using public funds to guarantee access to a package of 'essential' or 'basic' services for the poor, and choosing those services partly on the basis of their cost-effectiveness ([51, Tables 3.2 and 3.3), [8]. Some of these services are public or partly public goods, so public spending on them is justified for the whole population at risk. The idea of a limited package of subsidized services for those in poverty is often attacked as being unethical, as representing 'poor health care for poor people', but that criticism is misguided on two grounds. First, the poor would, under such an arrangement, receive on average more cost-effective care than the non-poor. Second, there is nothing unethical about taking into account the wishes of those who pay the taxes to support the subsidy, for whom cost-effectiveness may be a reasonable criterion [9]. This issue is taken up again when considering what 'public demand' means.

To sum up: poverty and cost-effectiveness are somewhat related, but the association is partial and, historically, probably transitory. It did not exist a century or more ago, when the rich and the poor got sick and died of the same diseases and there was little effective health care, and it may not hold in the future, when the known cost-effective interventions will, one hopes, have been more fully applied to the benefit of the poor. Because the association is only partial, it is appropriate to ask first whether people are poor, and then whether a particular intervention justifies its costs.

Horizontal Equity in Health Care

This ethical principle implies giving equal treatment to people with equal health problems, that is, not discriminating among them as to how much or what kind of care to provide. If two people are really equal in the nature and severity of a disease or injury, and they get the identical treatment, then the results should also be the same. So horizontal equity implies equal effectiveness. In practice, outcomes often differ among patients who appear alike both in their problem and in their treatment, but the conclusion will still hold on average. The health gains will also differ if two people differ in age and therefore in life expectancy, with the younger beneficiary having more to gain from treatment. Similarly, there will be differences if one patient has an additional health problem (co-morbidity) which limits the effectiveness of care for their common problem. Other possible differences among people—in income, education, location, and so on—are irrelevant for this purpose unless they affect the outcome of all interventions.

All this implies that horizontal equity and cost-effectiveness are perfectly compatible, so long as the costs are equal, or nearly so, because then the cost-effectiveness of treatment will be the same for everyone with the same problem. But if the costs of treatment differ significantly between one patient and another, the two criteria are in conflict, and, as often happens [10], a difficult choice has to be made between equity and efficiency.

Fig. 9.2 illustrates this conflict: one population suffers from a problem treatable by Intervention 1, and another population from a problem for

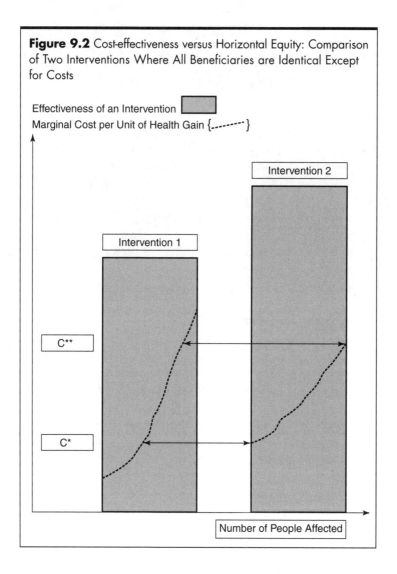

Figure 9.2 Cost-effectiveness versus Horizontal Equity: Comparison of Two Interventions Where All Beneficiaries are Identical Except for Costs

Effectiveness of an Intervention [ ]
Marginal Cost per Unit of Health Gain {--------}

Intervention 2

Intervention 1

C**

C*

Number of People Affected

which Intervention 2 is appropriate. The effectiveness of an intervention is the same for everyone who would benefit from it, but the cost of treatment is not the same. Some people live in remote areas, or are otherwise more difficult to reach or to treat, so that the marginal cost of an intervention, per unit of health gain, rises as more people are treated. Intervention 2 is uniformly more effective—yields more health gain—than Intervention 1, but even for the least costly patients, the cost is so much higher that the cost-effectiveness is initially lower than for Intervention 1. Horizontal equity says nothing about which intervention to finance first, and cost-effectiveness clearly gives priority to starting with Intervention 1. But before everyone in the first population is treated, the marginal cost rises to the level C^*, so high that Intervention 2 begins to give more value for money. Cost-effectiveness would require switching some expenditure to that intervention, slowing the rate at which Intervention 1 is extended. If C^{**} is the upper limit to cost per unit of health gain—any less cost-effective treatment is judged not worth buying—the result is to treat everyone with Intervention 2 but to leave part of the first population without treatment, in violation of horizontal equity. This kind of conflict can arise no matter which intervention is more effective; the problem is purely that costs differ among patients who are otherwise alike. Difficulties of this sort doubtless lie behind numerous conflicts between equity and efficiency in health care, such as those associated with urban/rural differences: it is usually easier and cheaper to treat urban residents than scattered rural populations, particularly if the intervention requires hospitalization.

Vertical Equity in Health Care

Horizontal equity presents a straightforward possibility of conflict with the criterion of cost-effectiveness, in which only one variable is involved—the cost of the intervention. The case of vertical equity and its relation to efficiency turns out to be much more complicated, because three variables are relevant. These are the cost and the effectiveness of different treatments, and the severity of different health problems. Since vertical equity concerns preferential treatment for people with worse problems, severity cannot be ignored the way it can be when dealing with horizontal equity. What particularly complicates vertical comparisons is that the effectiveness of a service need not bear any relation to the severity of the condition or disease it is meant to prevent or treat. Effectiveness, however it is measured, corresponds to the improvement in health from an intervention, which is the same thing as the reduction in the health damage caused by the disease. (The sum of this damage over a population is called *the burden of disease:* the same name is not commonly used, but the same concept applies, to the health damage for an individual.) One intervention may lead to a larger health gain than another, but cause a smaller proportional reduction in disease burden. For example, surgery following major trauma can be highly effective because it saves the patient's life, but still leaves him or her with severe disabilities, while surgery for some minor condition restores the patient to perfect health but causes less absolute improvement.

Fig. 9.3 illustrates some of these complexities. Four diseases or conditions are shown, affecting different populations. For each one, the figure also shows the size of the health loss (for an individual, this is the height above the horizontal axis); the effectiveness of treatment (the portion of health loss prevented or relieved by an intervention); and the cost of treatment (the length of the vertical bar below the horizontal axis). For each intervention, the cost is assumed to be uniform for all potential patients or beneficiaries, since the issue of costs differing among individuals has already been considered in discussing horizontal equity. Interventions 1 and 2 deal with the entire burden of the corresponding diseases, but Intervention 3 is effective for only some of the people with that health problem and will do no good at all for others, while Intervention 4 helps everyone, but only partly—the effectiveness falls far short of eliminating all the health damage.

Vertical equity requires giving preference to the sufferers from the second condition, since it causes the most health loss. Moreover, there is a fully effective intervention, which reinforces the choice. But the cost is much higher than for any other intervention, so that the cost-effectiveness of Intervention 2 is the worst of the four. Even Intervention 1, against the disease which does the least harm to people's health, looks better on the cost-effectiveness criterion. That relation can be changed only by changing how one measures the disease burden and the results of an intervention, so that for example Disease 2 looks not twice as awful as Disease 1, but several times worse. This issue is taken up again later.

Other kinds of conflict between equity and efficiency also arise in Fig. 9.3. Disease 4 causes an individual burden nearly as large as Disease 2, so equity according to severity would rank it second. And the treatment is no more costly than Intervention 1. The problem is that the service is, as indicated, not very effective, so that it is also not very cost-effective. Again,

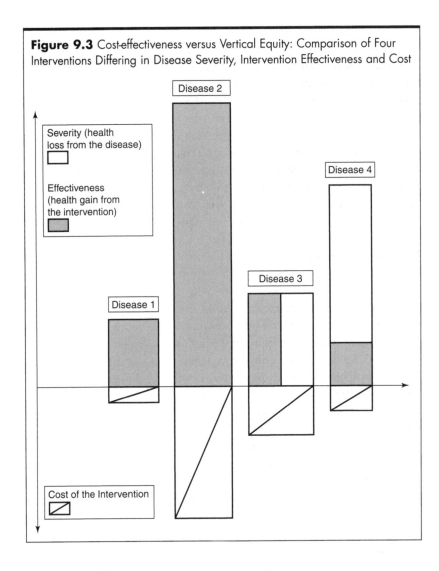

Figure 9.3 Cost-effectiveness versus Vertical Equity: Comparison of Four Interventions Differing in Disease Severity, Intervention Effectiveness and Cost

Disease 2

Severity (health loss from the disease)

Effectiveness (health gain from the intervention)

Disease 4

Disease 3

Disease 1

Cost of the Intervention

Disease 1 looks like the more efficient place to use resources. Disease 3 presents an even more complicated case, because the treatment is as cost-effective as Intervention 1 provided it is given only to those who will benefit from it, but yields much lower value for money if it is given to all sufferers, including those for whom it will do nothing. This discrimination of who should and who should not receive a treatment that will help some people but not others is one of the difficult choices medical professionals regularly make, usually without complete knowledge of the likely outcome. Erring on the side of equity then means wasting some resources.

It might seem that most or all of these problems could be resolved by redefining vertical equity, so that instead of "do more for those with worse problems", the principle were understood as "do more for those who can be helped more". That eliminates the severity of the condition as a relevant variable, leaving only the cost and effectiveness of treatment. But that does not solve the equity/efficiency conflict, because more effective treatments often cost proportionally more than less effective ones, which makes them less cost-effective. There is simply no systematic relation between cost and results, just as there is none between results and severity.

Is the Rule of Rescue Efficient?

This last ethical criterion is much simpler to deal with than those just discussed, because it does not involve comparisons among individuals, except of the simplest form—between those who will die without an intervention and those for whom the appropriate health care will not make such an all-or-nothing difference. This choice is the basis of triage, the custom of dividing patients into those whose lives can be saved by intervening, those who will die even if given treatment, and those in between because their lives are not immediately threatened. And that seems so obviously the rational thing to do that it appears there should be no conflict between efficiency and ethical considerations.

This conclusion is correct, with one important proviso: the rule of rescue and the criterion of cost-effectiveness are compatible, so long as 'saving a life' means keeping a person alive for long enough, and in good enough health, that the effect justifies the cost. This is what is usually meant by saving someone's life—rescuing him or her from drowning or some other accident, or curing a potentially fatal disease before it has done irreparable damage. The payoff can be decades of healthy life, so it does not matter that there may be a high cost. That is not the same thing as postponing death briefly, or keeping a person alive but terribly disabled. The effectiveness of any intervention depends on the instantaneous improvement in health, and also on how long that improvement lasts. Just as brief illness with full recovery contributes little to the burden of disease, no matter how severely one is sick, brief health gains, even if dramatic, do not yield much effectiveness. That is why, among other things, heroic measures to stave off death from chronic conditions are usually not cost-effective, and why the effectiveness of treatments for cancer is measured not by whether the patient leaves the hospital alive, but by the 5- or 10-year survival rate. This idea is explicitly recognized in any measure of health status that has a time dimension, such as potential years of life lost (PYLL) or more complex measures such as disability adjusted life years (DALYS) [11], or quality adjusted life years (QALYS) [12].

And What Do the People Want?

The rule of rescue is the last of the seven relatively technical, explicit criteria to be contrasted to cost-effectiveness. It remains to consider briefly how all this relates to what the public may think or want, and in particular to whether cost-effectiveness is likely to be compatible with those views and demands. This question cannot be answered conclusively, because what the public thinks varies from place to place and time to time, and is often either amorphous or polarized. There may be no such thing as a clear demand from people about which criteria should be used to determine how their money is spent. (In the case of public goods, there is no demand in the market sense, and there may or may not be one in the sense of public agreement as to what the government should do.) So it is possible only to speculate about how public wants fit in with the criteria under consideration: two hypotheses seem particularly relevant to this discussion.

First, the public is likely to mix up criteria or to misunderstand them. This is not surprising or reprehensible, in view of how complicated the relations can be between one criterion and another. To take one example, the decision of which health services to subsidize for the poor depends both on an assessment of who is poor and on a notion of how cost-effective something must be in order to justify public expenditure—and these are related to the distinction between costs that are catastrophic even for people who are not poor, and those that the non-poor can afford but the poor perhaps cannot. It is a combined technical and political task to decide on these matters clearly enough that a public subsidy for medical care for the poor can be put into operation at all, and its design is likely to involve many choices in both the medical and the financial spheres, as in the Medicaid program in the United States [13]. One of the reasons for separating a number of possible criteria and looking at their connections, as has been done here, is precisely to facilitate public discussion and understanding of the issues involved.

Second, most of the public would probably agree with the general proposition that one should get value for money when spending their taxes; but whether they would support a particular criterion of cost-effectiveness, and the allocations that result from it, might depend very much on how effectiveness is defined. And the relative weights to give to effectiveness and to costs might not be so simple as taking the ratio of the two measures and using it to rank different services. There is little explicit experience with the issue, but the development of the 'Oregon Plan', the list of health care procedures that the state of Oregon decided to include in its Medicaid plan, is instructive in this regard [14, 15].

The process began with an expert ranking according to perceived cost-effectiveness, using a measure that—as with PYLL, DALYs and QALYs— is linear across individuals. That is, 10 years of healthy life lost are valued the same whether they are all lost by 1 individual, or ten people each lose 1 year, or 1,000 people each lose 3 or 4 days. When this ranking was proposed to the voters of Oregon, they ended by modifying it in various ways, one of which was equivalent to regarding a concentrated loss for one person as worse than the same loss distributed among many [16]. This non-linearity of disease burden, and therefore of effectiveness of health care, makes calculation harder because one cannot simply use totals or averages when comparing different health problems. But it is perfectly defensible as an ethical view. And it affects some of the other criteria considered here. In particular, changing how one measures effectiveness must, at the least, affect the comparisons involved in trying to apply horizontal and vertical equity, although that will not change the possible conflicts between equity and efficiency discussed above. One conclusion from this experience seems to be that one cannot simply settle all the other connections among criteria and take up what the public wants at the end, because what the public thinks, or wants, or is prepared to support, can modify some of the other criteria and the way they are related.

Putting Everything Together: A Guide to Decision-Making

As promised in the Introduction, the object of this note is not only to examine the compatibility of different criteria, but to relate them sequentially or hierarchically when that is appropriate. If the different criteria can be taken up in some logical sequence, some of the problems of conflict among them are reduced, and it becomes easier to decide how to choose whether to finance a health care service out of public funds, leave it to the private market, do some of each, or conclude that the service will not and should not be paid for either publicly or privately.

Fig. 9.4 summarizes the results of the comparisons and connections studied here, in the form of a decision tree. Four conclusions deserve emphasis. First, it is possible to put together a clear sequence of questions, the answers to which ultimately determine in which of the three possible outcomes a given health care intervention falls. No single criterion ever suffices to justify public expenditure; however, depending on the character of an intervention,

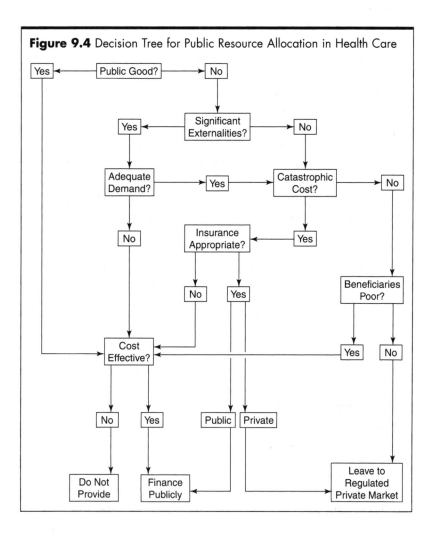

Figure 9.4 Decision Tree for Public Resource Allocation in Health Care

one or more criteria may be irrelevant, which greatly simplifies decision-making. Second, it is easier to arrange the efficiency criteria in this way, than those related to equity. Poverty is easy enough to locate in the decision tree, but horizontal and vertical equity are not, because they involve explicit comparisons among people and (in the case of vertical equity) among services. The question of how far to respect these two principles, in particular when they are in conflict with efficiency, probably has to be dealt with repeatedly rather than fitting neatly into one branch of the decision tree. The last ethical criterion, the rule of rescue, does not cause similar difficulties, since if 'rescue' is properly interpreted it is usually consistent with cost-effectiveness.

Third, there are some questions to ask about the use of public resources for health care that do not correspond precisely to any one of the criteria. This is most notably the case for interventions that are catastrophically costly, for which insurance is the appropriate mechanism for sharing risk and thus making the services available. The decision tree includes (but does not fully answer) two questions about insurance. One is whether a contributory insurance scheme is feasible—one in which there is explicit coverage of services in return for a premium that may be uniform, or related to capacity to pay. (The distinction whether one contributes or not is important, because public subsidy of health care for the poor is also a form of insurance, but one to which they do not contribute. If the poor are covered for catastrophically costly interventions, their premiums must in effect be subsidized.)

When insurance is feasible and appropriate, there is a further question whether it should be public or private or some of each. This is a complicated question not settled by appeal to any combination of these criteria—but it is evident that both horizontal and vertical equity are relevant to the decision. Private insurance is more likely than publicly financed care to violate one or both of these principles, by discriminating between people who have the same health problem but differ in their other health conditions, their age, capacity to pay, or other characteristics, or by making it more difficult to get coverage for more severe health problems, if the treatments for them are particularly expensive. These failings go far to explain why in most rich countries a large share of insurance is publicly financed, whether directly from the budget or through employment-related social security schemes [2].

Fourth, it turns out that the right way to use the criterion of cost-effectiveness is not once-and-for-all, as with some of the other criteria. Several different paths through the decision tree lead to the question whether a health care intervention's results are worth what it costs. One goes directly from the classification of a service as a public good, and is the only other criterion needed in that case. Another begins with the conclusion that a service has significant externalities, and that private demand for it is inadequate to secure all the potential social gains—the case of a partly public good. The question of cost-effectiveness arises again when considering what services to subsidize for the poor, although here the criterion is less clear-cut, as the experience of the Oregon Plan illustrates. It does not become irrelevant, though, because the people paying for the subsidy are almost certain to want some kind of value for money. And for similar reasons, if a service is catastrophically expensive, and it is not feasible to finance it through ordinary contributory insurance so that some separate and public funding must be found if it is to be provided, it is again relevant to ask whether the service is worth what it costs. This is the typical situation of a public program of re-insurance, superimposed on a large number of small private or semi-private insurance schemes which cannot afford the risks of a few extraordinarily costly interventions. Cost-effectiveness, in other words, is decisive in only one circumstance but important in several other situations.

To sum up: a fully thought-out decision of which health services to spend public money on and for whom, requires looking at all nine of the criteria considered, treating them in the proper sequence and taking account of whether they are consistent or in conflict. Public funds should be spent on public and semi-public goods when those are cost-effective and demand for them is inadequate, on cost-effective interventions which disproportionately benefit the poor, and on catastrophically costly care, when contributory insurance will not work effectively or there are good reasons to finance insurance publicly. Interventions which do not pass these tests either are not worth paying for at all, or they can be left to regulated private markets to finance because the costs are bearable without insurance, or private contributory insurance is feasible.

References

[1] Musgrave RA. The Theory of Public Finance, A Study in Public Economy. New York: McGraw-Hill, 1959.

[2] Musgrove P. Public and Private Roles in Health: Theory and Financing Patterns. World Bank Discussion Paper No. 339. Washington, DC: The World Bank, 1996.

[3] Hammer JS. Prices and protocols in public health care. World Bank Econ Rev 1997; 11.

[4] Jamison DT, Mosley WH, Measham AR, Bobadilla JL, editors. Disease Control Priorities in Developing Countries. Oxford: Oxford University Press, 1993.

[5] World Bank. World Development Report: Investing in Health: Figure 3.2. Washington, DC: The World Bank, 1993.

[6] Gwatkin DR, Guillot M. The burden of disease among the global poor: current situation, future trends and implications for research and policy. Washington, DC: The World Bank, 1998. Prepared for the Global Forum on Health Research.

[7] Beaton GH, Martorell R, L'Abbé KA, Edmonston B, McCabe G, Ross AC, Harvey B. Effectiveness of Vitamin A Supplementation in the Control of Young Child Morbidity and Mortality in Developing Countries: Summary Report. Toronto: University of Toronto, 1993.

[8] Bobadilla JL, Cowley P, Musgrove P, Saxenian H. Design, content and financing of an essential national package of health services. In: Murray CJL, Lopez A, editors. Global Comparative Assessments in the Health Sector: Disease Burden, Expenditures and Intervention Packages: 51, Tables 3.2 and 3.3. Geneva: World Health Organization, 1994.

[9] Musgrove P. Cost-effectiveness and the socialization of health care. Health Policy 1996:32:14.

[10] Okun AM. Equity and Efficiency: the Big Tradeoff. Washington, DC: The Brookings Institution, 1975.

[11] Murray CJL. Rethinking DALYs. In [16], 1.

[12] Goerdt A, Koplan JP, Robine JM, Thuriaux MC, Van Ginneken KK. Non-fatal health outcomes. In [16] 99.

[13] U.S. Social Security Administration. Annual Statistical Supplement, 1996, to the Social Security Bulletin. Washington, DC: Social Security Administration, 1996.

[14] Eddy DM. Oregon's methods: did cost-effectiveness fail? J Am Med Assoc 1996:266.

[15] Hadorn DC. Setting health care priorities in Oregon: cost-effectiveness meets the Rule of Rescue. J Am Med Assoc 1996:265.

[16] Murray CJL, Lopez AD, editors. The Global Burden of Disease, Vol. 1. Boston, MA: Harvard School of Public Health, 1996, on behalf of the World Health Organization and the World Bank.

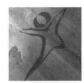

CHAPTER 10

Cost-Effectiveness and the Socialization of Health Care

Acknowledgments

In revising the paper I have benefited from extensive comments by Peter Berman and Howard Barnum.

Introduction: The Nature of the Problem

The World Bank's 1993 *World Development Report—Investing in Health* [1] treats cost-effectiveness as the principal criterion for choosing which health interventions governments should pay for. The *Report* recognizes the public-finance arguments that government must finance some interventions if they are to be provided adequately or at all, because private markets will under-provide public goods and goods with substantial positive externalities. However, even interventions which meet this requirement must still pass some test such as cost-effectiveness—a public good should not be financed simply because it is public. If it is accepted that the object of health expenditure is to improve health, rather than some more general concept such as welfare, and what is financed is a collection of interventions, then choosing to finance them in decreasing order of cost-effectiveness seems to be the way to maximize the health gain from any particular level of spending. "Value for money" implies cost-effectiveness, so long as "value" is measured in health gains.

There is an important technical objection to this simple view, which is that either the cost or the effectiveness of any one intervention may depend on what other interventions are offered at the same time. In that case the ranking by cost-effectiveness is not stable and one cannot just proceed down a list until the budget is exhausted or the next best intervention does not seem worthwhile. Taking account of interactions is difficult, but sometimes interventions can be "packaged" to exploit joint costs or synergies. Since a small number of interventions can deal with a large share of the disease burden, it is not necessary to consider all possible combinations: a cost-effective minimum package can be defined to absorb all health spending in poor countries and serve as the nucleus of a larger set of interventions in higher-income countries [2]. Less is known about cost-effectiveness, and it becomes harder to package interventions, as health expenditure rises, because the variety of interventions increases greatly.

A more serious difficulty is that while costs are, in principle, objective, the effectiveness of an intervention is always partly subjective. The quantification of Disability-Adjusted Life Years (DALYs), Quality-Adjusted Life Years (QALYs), Healthy Life Years or any other measurement of gains in health status depends on a long vector of elements. Some of these are objective, such as rates of mortality or incidence and prevalence of morbidity or disability, and the ages at which diseases strike.

Many other elements require subjective valuation. For example, the calculation used in the Bank's *Report* required choosing numbers for the discount rate; the relative value of life at different ages; life expectancy; and the relative disabilities associated with each of many non-fatal conditions [3]. If people differ in their evaluation of these numbers, each one may have his own ranking of cost-effectiveness, but the rankings will not agree enough for there to be a unique relation between cost and health improvement associated with any intervention, even for people of the same age and the same severity of health problems.

To say that people have different evaluations of effectiveness is equivalent to saving they derive different utilities from the same intervention because they differ in their views of the utilities associated with the prior state of ill health or health risk, the state of health after intervention, the disutility caused by the intervention itself, or some combination of these. If the objective is to maximize welfare rather than health, then the situation is still more complicated because people can also differ in their subjective evaluation of non-health benefits from consumption of other goods and services, in their aversion to risk, in income or in other factors.

This problem raises two related questions. First, should individual behavior in seeking and paying for health care be expected to be consistent with cost-effectiveness? Second, does socializing health care, whether through private insurance or through public financing, make collective behavior different in this respect from individual decisions? This paper argues that the more decisions about health interventions are socialized, the more appropriate it is to use cost-effectiveness as a criterion for health care spending. It does not presume to show that no other criterion does, or should, matter in making choices about health care, but only that the relative importance of cost-effectiveness increases with the degree of socialization. This tendency is reinforced when the socialization is compulsory, because people must contribute through taxes rather than voluntary insurance payments. That makes cost-effectiveness a particularly legitimate criterion for government decisions. The argument does not depend on the particular measure of health status, of which there are many [4, 5], which is used to derive the effectiveness of interventions.

Cost-Effectiveness and Individual Choice

In trying to answer the first question posed above, it is easy to invent examples in which people would not be expected to choose the more cost effective of two alternatives. Suppose, for example, that two drugs are available to treat a given health problem which poses a 30 percent chance of dying. One drug costs $2 and reduces the risk of death to 25 percent; the other costs $5 and reduces the risk to 20 percent. Each application of the first drug can be thought of as saving one-twentieth of a life, or one life for each 20 patients who receive it, while the other saves one-tenth of a life, or one life for every ten patients. The first drug is more cost-effective, because the cost is 40 percent as high while the health gain is half as large as with the second drug: the cost per life saved is $40 instead of $50 [6]. However, anyone who had $5 to spend would buy the second drug, unless the additional utility from spending $3 on something else outweighed the extra five percent reduction in the risk of dying. Choosing the more cost-effective drug can be interpreted to mean that the individual values his or her life at less than $60, or perhaps that unless the extra money is spent on food, he or she will die anyway.

In this example, the individual cannot spend $4 on two doses of the cheaper medication, and improve survival chances by the same amount as with one $5 dose of the costlier one. Spending $4 will, however, buy the same total survival gain for two patients, with $1 left over. The difference between the individual and the social decision turns on this possibility of treating more than one patient and on the indivisibility of individual benefits. The claim that the first drug is more cost-effective also depends on adding gains in survival probability linearly across individuals, or assuming that one-tenth of a life for one person is worth exactly the same as one-twentieth of a life for each of two people.

In a much more complex model [7], an individual with an additive, multiperiod utility function faces a health problem that reduces the probability of surviving into the next period and therefore the expected utility in that period, where utility depends on disposable income or income less medical expenditure. The utility-maximizing decision about how much to spend on health care this period is consistent with cost effectiveness, and does not depend on what will be spent in the next period if the consumer survives. The same conclusion holds when the model is complicated by discounting future periods, by allowing for nonfatal conditions and for expenditures which improve health status without affecting survival, and by admitting two or more possible interventions with different costs and different effects on survival and quality of life. Moreover, the optimal cost-effectiveness ratio is the same for both interventions, so that at the margin either of them buys the same amount of expected healthy life per dollar. This is possible only if—in contrast to the previous example—the patient can buy any amount of either intervention, up to the limit of income, with the prices of the interventions proportional to the marginal health gains.

The optimal relation between prices and health improvements suggests that the overall cost-effectiveness of health expenditure should depend on what interventions cost the consumer, from which it is commonly assumed that prices can be used to "rationalize" demand: raising the price of health care should increase value for money. This could happen because consumers were buying so much of all interventions that the marginal health gain was very small, and a uniform reduction in utilization would save money but have little effect on their health. Alternatively, consumers might preferentially reduce purchases of interventions yielding less health gain per unit expenditure. (If the prices in the two-drug example discussed previously were $200 and $500 instead of $2 and $5, the patient might choose the more cost-effective drug despite the lower health gain, because the $300 difference could buy much more compensating utility than $3 could.) However, if interventions do not produce steadily declining marginal health improvement but require some minimum expenditure in order to produce any gain at all, there is a risk that consumers would cut back or stop using more cost-effective services, causing substantial health losses.

What consumers will actually do depends not only on prices and on the true relation between utilization and health improvements but on their knowledge of that relation. In both the formal models just discussed, the consumer does not know for certain whether he or she will become sick or injured or die, but does know the survival probabilities, or the expected gains in health status, with and without each kind of health care. Real consumers are usually less well informed, because they do not try to find out, or because physicians mislead them, or simply because no one knows. Without that information it is impossible to buy care optimally, and so actual purchases cannot be expected to be consistent with cost effectiveness. Incomplete information is a pervasive reason why individuals' spending on health care might not be efficient even according to their own evaluations and preferences, leading them to prefer a collective solution in which lack of information is less damaging [8]. Add to this problem the variation in people's utilities, attitudes toward risk and other factors discussed above, and there is little reason to expect a collection of consumers to rank health care interventions by a single standard of value for money, and spend accordingly.

There are numerous empirical estimates of how utilization responds to price changes or differences [9], but very little evidence of how this affects cost-effectiveness. The RAND experiment of health insurance deductibles and co-payments in the United States found that for most consumers, higher prices reduced demand but did not much affect its composition, and had little effect on health status [10]. Thus there was no evidence of preferential reduction in the use of less cost-effective services— "cost sharing reduces appropriate and inappropriate care in about the same way"—but some evidence that average cost-effectiveness did increase. However, poor people, and especially poor people needing preventive care, tended to reduce utilization in ways that substantially threatened their health, so that their use of health services became less cost-effective. This result may be more relevant for poor countries than the average findings of slightly improved cost effectiveness.

One reason why individual consumers may not select health care according to cost-effectiveness is that they seldom choose between two interventions for entirely different health problems, although anyone financing health care for a large number of people must make such choices, if only implicitly. People typically suffer, and decide what to do about, one health problem at a time, and they have a clearer idea of the cost of doing nothing and the gains from health care for that problem than they have about other problems that might occur in the future. Ignorance about tomorrow's problems compared to today's makes it hard to make cost-effective multiperiod choices over different health care needs. Another source of difficulty is that *not* spending on care today may make only a small or uncertain contribution to one's ability to buy health care tomorrow. (The model described earlier assumes away such connections by supposing that future income and ability to pay for interventions is independent of today's health problems and expenditures [7].) The solution to the difficulty of paying for care needed in the future, of course, is insurance.

Socializing Decisions through Insurance

For any given health care intervention, insurance pools the financial risk across all the purchasers who are covered by insurance for that intervention. "Pure" insurance would eliminate out-of-pocket payments entirely by providing complete financial coverage. Most private insurance and some public insurance, in contrast, provides such zero-cost coverage only after the insured has spent a certain amount in the form of co-payments; thus it lowers the price for interventions up to some level of expenditure and lowers it all the way to zero only for expenditures beyond that limit. There may also be a floor up to which a deductible applies, with no effect on the price to the consumer. Thus the effect of insurance on consumption of health care depends in part on whether the insured are paying all, part or none of the cost of services. This in turn affects the administrative cost of providing the insurance.

Does socializing health care financing via insurance favor cost-effectiveness? The substantial literature on the effects of insurance on behavior and on welfare does not address this question but usually compares expenditure outcomes under insurance with the results of out-of-pocket purchases by individual consumers. It also concentrates on the subsidy to insurance which occurs when employers' contributions to buying insurance are excluded from corporate income and not taxed as income to workers; that issue is not considered here.

At first glance the answer to the question about cost-effectiveness and insurance would seem to be a simple no: insured individuals either face lower prices, or no longer have to consider costs at all, so they can consume health care without asking whether the health gain is worth the full cost. In fact, people may buy insurance partly to protect themselves from the need to consider cost, at a time of urgency and stress. Even if *all* the insured are spending in the range where prices (co-payments) are between zero and 100 percent of costs, and even if they continue to equate marginal costs to marginal benefits according to their individual utilities, they should be expected to buy services of lower marginal health gain and thus reduce cost-effectiveness on average.

The moral hazard intrinsic to insurance [12] is almost the antithesis of cost-effective behavior. To the extent that moral hazard leads people to take less good care of their health—particularly, to spend less on preventive measures not covered by insurance because they will not have to pay for curative treatment that is covered—insurance even appears to undermine cost-effectiveness in preventive and public health measures. More curative interventions may be required, at higher cost, to achieve the same health outcome [13].

The conclusion that insurance is inimical to cost-effectiveness because of moral hazard is modified when account is taken of adverse selection, the second kind of market failure characteristic of the health insurance market. Adverse selection arises because different people know they have different health status and anticipate different needs for health care, and this information is not available to insurers, who must charge the same premium to all. As a potential consumer of services, each insured person seeks to maximize the expected health gain from care for those problems he or she has or expects to suffer. As a purchaser, each one seeks to minimize costs. The insurance industry in effect allows buyers and users to bargain with one another so as to balance costs against health gains, with high-risk customers wanting to buy more insurance than low-risk customers. If low-risk consumers predominate in the market, they can force high-risk consumers to buy less insurance than they would like, offsetting some of the tendency of insurance to stimulate spending without regard for cost-effectiveness; the alternative for high-risk consumers is to pay the full cost of their anticipated health care instead of being subsidized by healthier and less costly customers [13].

Simulations based on the RAND experiment mentioned earlier show that more generous insurance plans with higher limits on out-of-pocket spending are squeezed out of the market, compared to plans which impose more cost on the insured [14]. Because it is difficult empirically to distinguish the effects of adverse selection from those of moral hazard, and because so much insurance is determined by employers (or by the state) and therefore limits adverse selection, it is not clear how much consumption is affected, and there is no specific evidence about cost-effectiveness.

These findings suggest that insurance is less inimical to cost-effectiveness than would follow from the reduction in out-of-pocket costs alone, but they do not indicate that purchases under insurance would be any more cost-effective than without it. The expectation of lower cost-effectiveness with insurance still follows if any consumer can buy any health service in any amount at reduced prices, with declining marginal health returns as more is spent, at all levels of consumption.

In fact, which services the insured person consumes depends on which services are covered, and insurance plans typically exclude certain services altogether or impose limitations on how often they can be used or how much can be spent on them. If everyone had the same evaluation of the relative cost-effectiveness of interventions, insurance plans would reflect that choice, and plans would be more cost-effective on average as they were cheaper and covered fewer services. It is only because potential customers differ in their utilities, risk aversion and incomes that insurance does not automatically favor cost-effectiveness. Even so, any insurance plan which is actually bought implicitly averages together the cost-effectiveness evaluations of all the people who freely buy that plan. This does not mean that every purchaser of insurance thinks about the cost-effectiveness of each intervention under the plan, because plans generally apply the same broad rules about deductibles, co-payments, ceilings and quantitative limits to a whole range of similar services. It does mean that the people who end up covered by a particular plan either have no choice, or are in rough agreement about the relation between the expected health effectiveness of the coverage and what it costs.

This implies that a competitive third-party insurance industry may lead to relatively cost-effective coverage *within* each of a number of policies or groups of insured, as people with the same tastes and desire for cost-effective coverage buy the same insurance. Similarly, when workers have a choice of employers but no choice about the insurance provided by each employer, each employer's workforce can be expected to be homogeneous with respect to the kind and amount of insurance wanted [15], also leading to local cost-effectiveness. Competition among insurers or employers will not, however, necessarily tend toward cost-effectiveness of interventions *across* all groups. Some groups will buy coverage for interventions of relatively low cost-effectiveness, while others will do without coverage for interventions that are more cost-effective. Limiting consumer choice, as by requiring everyone to have the same plan or at least the same minimum plan, can therefore improve overall cost-effectiveness.

The inclusion or exclusion of specific services is extremely important, because many health interventions are of an all-or-nothing character, or require a substantial minimum expenditure to yield any benefits at all. If there are eventual declining returns to further spending, these begin only at relatively high levels of expenditure. When people are relieved from worrying (so much) about the cost of care, they are free to concentrate on its effectiveness. Insurance can be expected to have little effect on the utilization of inexpensive services which people would buy anyway, but it stimulates the purchase of lumpy, expensive interventions, particularly if the need for these is hard to predict [16].

Since the cost and the cost-effectiveness of interventions are not highly correlated—there are more and less effective services at all cost levels [17]—stimulating utilization of expensive services does not necessarily reduce value for money. People who are still paying part of the cost should become more likely in particular to consume care which is both costly and cost-effective. This may offset much of the tendency to expand utilization of services which are inexpensive but not very effective. When expenditure reaches the out-of-pocket limit, cost-effectiveness might be expected to fall again, because all costly interventions become attractive if they provide any health improvement at all. This will be true unless the costs in pain, inconvenience or time lost—which, unlike financial costs, cannot be shifted to third parties—are too high. In summary, the expectation that insurance will undermine cost effectiveness by stimulating consumption of services seems to depend on two conditions. First, individuals react to lowered prices by expanding utilization at the margin, rather than by including expensive services which may provide large health gains but are too costly to buy out of pocket. Second, co-payments are so low that the tendency to equate marginal costs and benefits leads to over-utilization independently of price. By allowing purchases of costly but cost-effective services, and still providing an incentive to weigh marginal benefits against some cost to the consumer, insurance can promote cost-effectiveness even though it may raise total costs. This will be true even if the selection of which interventions to cover is independent of cost-effectiveness.

Of course, an insurance plan can be used to *impose* cost-effectiveness by covering services, or setting co-payments, in proportion to their health gains per dollar, but in a competitive environment such a plan will not be bought by all customers. In general, any uniform plan will not be Pareto optimal, in the sense of improving health or reducing costs for everyone compared to their individual choices [13]. Of all uniform plans, however, one based on cost-effectiveness appears to be the most efficient [7]. Cost-effectiveness is an appropriate criterion for designing insurance provisions, but its scope is limited by the heterogeneity of customers and the degree of competition among insurers.

More Complete Socialization: Second-Party Insurance

Under third-party insurance, physicians can provide, and possibly even create demand for, services of low cost-effectiveness because—like their patients—they are free to consider only the health gains and not the costs. This can happen even when medical professionals are scrupulous about not recommending or performing services with no expected health gain. However, if the physicians are also the insurers, they have to consider both the numerator and the denominator of the cost-effectiveness ratio.

Such second-party insurance is more fully socialized than third-party insurance because the patient and the doctor cannot pass any costs on to someone else. Insurance such as that provided through health maintenance organizations should therefore lead to a more cost-effective set of interventions than would occur with the same patients and the same doctors under third-party insurance. This may happen because coverage of less cost-effective services is explicitly restricted, or, when such services are covered because they are performed less often, at physicians' discretion, or the more cost-effective of two alternatives for treatment is used.

It is hard to estimate how much this occurs, because of differences in age, health status, education, attitudes toward medical interventions or other differences between those insured under second- and third-party coverage. The comparison is particularly difficult because of self-selection into one or the other kind of insurance: neither group is a random sample of the population [11]. And because outcomes are often uncertain, even health maintenance organizations sometimes spend heavily on procedures that turn out to be cost-ineffective. Nonetheless, the available evidence shows that second-party insurance controls cost better without sacrificing health gains [18], which suggests that it is more cost-effective. Certainly the criterion of cost-effectiveness is more clearly embodied in the way that care is paid for, than with third-party insurance.

Government Insurance and Taxpayer Support

If greater socialization of private health care expenditure favors cost-effectiveness, as argued above, then what happens under the most socialized way of paying for care, namely, public financing? It helps to split this question into three parts. The first concerns what governments can do, the second what they actually do, and the third the legitimacy of cost-effectiveness as a criterion for public spending.

Governments can make health spending more cost-effective, just by limiting public finance to the right interventions. The resulting cost effectiveness of what is paid for publicly will be partly offset by private purchases of less cost-effective interventions, but the effect of public finance can still be to improve the average value for money of health care. Any private insurance could, in principle, do the same thing—offer only services that are highly cost-effective—but it might lose customers as a result.

The advantage of government in this respect is that beneficiaries cannot choose a different insurer without paying twice, once in taxes and once in premiums. This kind of coercion, like that imposed by employer financed private insurance, may be unattractive to each consumer individually and yet acceptable when everyone knows that everyone else is subjected to the same control.

When publicly-financed services are universally available and sufficiently attractive that people actually use them, governments also can eliminate or reduce adverse selection—although, as indicated above, it is not clear how much that interferes with aggregate cost-effectiveness in private insurance. Of course, when only part of the population uses publicly-funded services, adverse selection can actually be increased, with the highest-risk population depending on public finance. This in turn may reinforce any tendency to limit services to those which are more cost-effective.

When governments fail to improve the cost-effectiveness of health care, it is because they do not know which interventions are cost-effective; or provide all services indiscriminately; or cover too few people; or waste resources in delivery; or provide such poor quality that people willingly spend their own money on care elsewhere. For all these reasons, governments in poor countries are often rightly accused of spending their health money badly compared to what could be achieved with an appropriate package of care. Nonetheless, they often do no worse than the private sector; and when they finance public health measures and interventions like immunizations which private markets cannot or do not provide adequately, governments are more cost-effective. This accounts for a large part of the extraordinary gains in life expectancy and in reduction of morbidity and disability in recent decades.

The share of public finance in health care spending generally rises as countries become richer, and a higher public share is somewhat associated with lower overall expenditure relative to national income, or with better health, or both. Even without examining the composition of spending by intervention, there is empirical evidence that greater public control of expenditure promotes value for money [8]. This presumably results from a concentration of public spending on some highly cost-effective interventions which private markets usually do not provide so thoroughly; it does not follow that public spending is intrinsically more efficient, only that it is better at covering some of the interventions that provide the most health gains per dollar. How far this interferes with Pareto optimality and consumers' freedom to follow their own notions of utility from health services depends on the range of services that are publicly financed and on whether there are differential subsidies according to the cost-effectiveness of the service. Finally, there is the question of whether it is *appropriate* for governments to base financing decisions on cost-effectiveness, or at least more appropriate than for individuals or private markets. Public insurance or direct public expenditure on health care typically differs from private insurance in providing subsidies not only from the healthy to the sick but also from the rich to the poor. The "purchasers" are taxpayers, who know that they are paying more than the average value of the services they can expect to receive. This makes them different from subscribers to an insurance plan, who know that the lucky will end up paying for the care of the unlucky, but who also know that *a priori* everyone is paying (approximately) a fair share.

Subsidizing health care is vastly more complicated than subsidizing food, but it still helps to compare the two cases. In both instances, taxpayers are willing to pay for what they think others need or deserve, but not for just anything they want. Thus food stamps cannot legally be used to buy alcohol or cigarettes; they can be spent on caviar, but then the buyer suffers for his choice in lower food intake. Cost-effectiveness offers a way to make a roughly parallel distinction in health care, with health gain corresponding to nutritional content in the case of food subsidies.

Governments cannot simply subsidize all demand for health care, because that leads to both inequity and runaway costs. They need criteria for what to finance, and cost-effectiveness is a relatively transparent basis for decision. The fact that any objective criterion is based partly on subjective evaluations of health burdens and gains does not invalidate that argument: what it means is that for cost-effectiveness to be understood and accepted as a basis for public finance, there has to be some consensus on those subjective choices. With private insurance, in contrast, it is only necessary to get agreement among all the people who buy a particular policy.

In fact, it may be that only government can promote the kind of public debate and understanding which can lead to consensus on those evaluations over the whole population, as the development of the "Oregon Plan" in the United States demonstrates [19]. However, this experience also illustrates that the public may not accept cost-effectiveness as the only or even the chief criterion for what services to finance. When the original list developed in Oregon turned out to give higher priority to some services with very small health gains but also very low costs than to some expensive but life-saving interventions, the cost criterion was dropped and the list restructured on the basis of effectiveness or health gains alone [20]. Even this contributes much more to health than a random choice with no regard for either outcomes or costs. Since cost-effectiveness is partly subjective, it is consistent with a greater priority for lifesaving interventions, if the disability weights for minor health losses are all revised downward so that death becomes more important relative to many diseases and injuries. The same ranking results if health losses are not added linearly across individuals, as cost-effectiveness implies, but priority is given to larger individual losses, ten healthy life years lost by one person being treated as worse than the loss of a year each by ten people.

Public finance of health care involves coercion, which means that it can enforce pooling solutions and eliminate the effects of adverse selection globally, whereas competitive private insurance can do so only over smaller and more homogeneous groups. This makes it easier to apply cost-effectiveness as the criterion of what to pay for. This tendency is reinforced by the explicit subsidy involved in having taxpayers finance care for poorer non-contributors: as with other subsidies in kind, individual preferences can be over-ridden in favor of what those paying think the beneficiaries need. Effectiveness certainly corresponds to that notion, and cost-effectiveness may also be both politically and ethically a reasonable criterion for public expenditure.

Much of the evidence used here comes from rich countries, and particularly from the United States. That country is an outlier even among OECD countries [8], in its reliance on employer-financed private insurance and its limitation of public expenditure to the poor, the elderly and a few other groups or types of spending. It is therefore legitimate to ask whether the argument developed here, that socialization of health care spending makes cost-effectiveness theoretically more appropriate as a criterion and easier to approximate in practice, is relevant to the issues of health care reform in poor countries.

There seem to be two strong reasons why it is. First, while there is undoubtedly scope for more socialization of health care spending in poor countries through private insurance, the danger from both moral hazard and adverse selection is arguably much greater than in richer countries. Such private insurance as exists or could easily be introduced is confined to the well-off minority, who are healthier on average than the poor majority, and who are particularly likely to obtain public subsidies enabling their insurance to provide costly, but not very cost-effective, services. These risks also exist for direct public financing, but can be attenuated if financing covers most of the population and therefore must be more limited as to the interventions it can cover. The argument that public financing offers potential efficiency gains over private insurance in such settings of poverty and inequality applies *a fortiori* to out-of-pocket expenditure, where the heterogeneity of people's conditions and utilities give no reason to think that spending will be particularly cost-effective.

Second, the poorer a country is, the sicker its population is likely to be and the smaller the range of interventions that can be financed for the bulk of the population. These circumstances make it easier to be sure what interventions are more cost-effective, and to compose an essential package of care which may be all that can be offered to the poor, but from which everyone can benefit [21]. Because many of these interventions are relatively cheap as well as quite cost-effective, people are not likely to buy private insurance for them—and such insurance is impossible for the public health measures with large externalities. People's information is also likely to be very incomplete, even regarding basic, life-protecting habits and procedures [1]. The welfare loss from not respecting individual preferences is therefore likely to be smaller, and the gains from socializing health care decisions larger, than in richer countries.

References

[1] World Bank, World Development Report 1993: Investing in Health. Oxford University Press, New York, NY, 1993.

[2] Bobadilla, J.L., Cowley, P., Musgrove, P., and Saxenian, H., "Methods and Data Used to Design the Minimum Package of Health Services." Background Paper to the World Development Report 1993: Investing in Health. World Bank, Washington, DC, 1994.

[3] Murray, C.J.L., "Quantifying the Burden of Disease: The Technical Basis for Disability Adjusted Life Years." *Bulletin of the World Health Organization*, 72 (1994) 429–445.

[4] Brooks, R.G, "The Development and Construction of Health Status. Measures: An Overview of the Literature." *The Swedish Institute for Health Economics, Report 1986.-4*, Lund, Sweden, 1986.

[5] Torrance, G.W., "Measurement of Health State Utilities for Economic Appraisal: A Review." *Journal of Health Economics*, 5 (1986) 1–30.

[6] Hammer, J.S., "The Economics of Malaria Control." *World Bank Research Observer*, 8 (1993) 1–22.

[7] Garber, A.M. and Phelps, C.E., "Economic Foundations of Cost-Effectiveness Analysis." NBER Working Paper No. 4164, National Bureau of Economic Research, Cambridge, MA, 1992.

[8] Barr, N., "Economic Theory and the Welfare State: A Survey and Interpretation." *Journal of Economic Literature*, 30 (1992) 741–803.

[9] Griffin, C.C., "User Charges for Health Care in Principle and Practice." Economic Development Institute Seminar Paper No. 37, World Bank, Washington, DC, 1988.

[10] Newhouse, J.P., and the Insurance Experiment Group, Free for All? Lessons from the RAND Health Insurance Experiment Harvard University Press, Cambridge, MA, 1993.

[11] Pauly, M. V., "Taxation, Health Insurance and Market Failure in the Medical Economy" *Journal of Economic Literature*, 24 (1986) 629–675.

[12] Arrow, K., "Uncertainty and the Welfare Economics of Medical Care." *American Economic Review*, 53 (1963) 941–973.

[13] Pauly, M. V., "Overinsurance and Public Provision of Insurance: The Roles of Moral Hazard and Adverse Selection." *Quarterly Journal of Economics*, 88 (1974) 44–62.

[14] Marquis, M.S., "Adverse Selection with a Multiple Choice Among Health Insurance Plans: A Simulation Analysis." *Journal of Health Economics*, 11(1992) 129–151.

[15] Goldstein, G.S. and Pauly, M.V., "Group Health Insurance as a Local Public Good." In R. Rosett (Ed.), The Role of Health Insurance in the Health Services Sector, National Bureau of Economic Research, New York, NY, 1976, pp. 73–110.

[16] Phelps, C.E., "Tax Policy, Health Insurance and Health Care." In J. Meyer (Ed.), Market Reforms in Health Care. American Enterprise Institute, Washington, DC, 1983, pp. 198–224.

[17] Jamison, D.T., Mosley, W.H., Measham, A.R. and Bobadilla, J.L., (Eds.), Disease Control Priorities in Developing Countries. Oxford University Press, New York, NY, 1993.

[18] Enthoven, A.C., Theory and Practice of Managed Competition in Health Care Finance. North Holland, New York, NY, 1988.

[19] Oregon Health Services Commission, "Prioritization of Health Services: A Report to the Governor and Legislature, State of Oregon." Portland, OR, 1991.

[20] Hadorn, D.C., "Setting Health Care Priorities in Oregon: Cost-Effectiveness Meets the Rule of Rescue." *Journal of the American Medical Association, 265* (1991) 2218–2225.

CHAPTER 11

Is the Eradication of Polio in the Western Hemisphere Economically Justified?

Acknowledgments

The central arguments in this article were developed in a previous draft (July 1986) that benefited from discussions with Ciro de Quadros, Marjorie Pollock, William P. McGreevey, Phillip Nieburg, T. Stephen Jones, and Alfred Thieme. None of them bears responsibility for the ideas presented here or even necessarily agrees with those ideas. I am further indebted to Luis Locay, Warren Sanderson, Dieter Zschock, and Dennis Young for helpful comments when the draft was presented (in May 1987) to a seminar at Averell Harriman College for Policy and Management at the State University of New York in Stony Brook, New York, USA.

Introduction

Since the eradication of smallpox in the 1970s, no other disease has been eliminated from the world by vaccination. Advances in mass immunization campaigns using oral vaccine have successfully interrupted the transmission of wild poliomyelitis virus in many countries, however, and have sharply reduced its incidence in many others (1,2). The benefits of polio immunization appear from some studies to outweigh its costs (3). And the

Reprinted, with permission, from *Bulletin of the Pan American Sanitary Bureau* 22(1), 1988.

cost-effectiveness of mass campaigns relative to other means of reaching the susceptible population has been established, at least in some circumstances (4). It therefore seems possible, by a suitable intensification of such efforts, to eradicate polio—if not all over the world, then at least in the Western Hemisphere—within the next few years.

In view of the success of the PAHO/WHO Expanded Program on Immunization (EPI) in the Americas since its inception in 1977, in April 1985 (5) PAHO recommended that its Member Governments support a five-year, US $46 million campaign to eliminate polio entirely from the Americas, after which it would be relatively easy to deal with whatever cases might be imported. The Member Governments ratified this proposal in September 1985 (6); and since then PAHO has been developing the campaign's detailed strategy and obtaining financial commitments from private, bilateral, and multilateral donor agencies.

To satisfy some of these agencies' requirements, a cost-benefit analysis was prepared. This article describes the assumptions and findings of that analysis, which indicate the eradication of polio is economically justified, and discusses some of their implications. Its concluding section considers the terms according to which the eradication of polio can be deemed an alternative to curative care.

Assumptions

The analysis that follows attempts to answer one specific question: Is the cost of eradicating polio, through the program adopted by PAHO, justified through the medical costs saved by not having to treat or rehabilitate polio victims? This estimate of the benefits from polio eradication takes no account of the gains from reduced pain and suffering, from the greater economic productivity of individuals who would otherwise be paralyzed and rendered unproductive, or from the reduction in other vaccine-preventable diseases that can be expected to result from a successful campaign against polio. If eradication is economically justified by reduced medical costs alone, then there is no doubt that it is still more justified when account is taken of other benefits.

The logic of the argument is as follows. For each of the five years of the eradication campaign, and then for each of 10 years thereafter, estimates are made of the following: the number of cases of paralytic polio that would be prevented; the cost of treating and rehabilitating that number of polio victims; the cost of the eradication effort; and the net benefit (in terms of reduced medical expenses minus the cost of eradication). These net benefits are then discounted at 12% per year, meaning that $1.00 saved next year is worth only $0.88 saved today, etc.[1] (This is the discount rate used by the Inter-American Development Bank for project evaluation, and is chosen because the Bank is helping to finance the eradication campaign.)

Because the campaign is superimposed upon continuing national efforts to control polio through the EPI, two cost-benefit calculations are made. One compares the total cost—US $74 million in national effort and $46 million from international donor agencies over the first five years, plus $10 million per year in national resources thereafter—with the total cases and costs that could be expected to occur in the absence of *any* substantial effort to control polio. The other calculation finds costs derived from the current estimated incidence of polio and compares these to the cost of the resources being sought from donors in order to ensure polio eradication by eliminating the relatively small numbers of cases that still persist after nearly a decade of the EPI. The first calculation compares total costs to total benefits (in terms of reduced medical expense), while the second compares marginal or incremental costs to the marginal benefits of going from the present case incidence to eradication. In both cases it is assumed that every polio victim would receive treatment, so that the comparison is really between the cost of preventing polio and the cost of treating all those who would otherwise get the disease. This assumption that all victims receive treatment is relaxed later, so that no benefit is attributed to cases not actually treated.

A number of additional assumptions underlying the calculations deserve further explanation. These assumptions are as follows:

1. The background or "natural" level of polio incidence is derived from the situation existing before the EPI began, when about 3,000 cases of paralysis and 350 deaths were reported annually in the Americas. It is recognized that before the EPI started, polio was greatly underreported (5), perhaps by a factor of five.[2] If this estimate is accurate, then the true pre-EPI incidence would have been about 15,000 cases per year. This should probably be regarded as an upper bound.

2. The EPI helped to reduce the hemispheric total of reported polio cases to about 500 a year in 1984 and 1985. Assuming no change in the degree of underreporting, this means the actual incidence would have been

about 2,500 cases annually. Of course, the improved surveillance that accompanied the EPI might also have reduced the underreporting significantly, so that the true incidence might have been lower, say on the order of 1,500 cases per year. It is also possible that expecting the level to remain at 2,500 cases per year for the near future without eradication is being over-optimistic. In the absence of an eradication campaign, national efforts might not be able to keep the incidence that low. For one thing, polio fluctuates cyclically, and the 1984–1985 level of cases appears to represent a cyclical trough from which a slight rebound could be expected. For another, vaccination coverage could actually decline because of financial difficulties and a false sense of confidence about the extent of control in the absence of a reliable surveillance system.

The example of Jamaica illustrates this latter risk. After over five years of reporting zero cases, levels of coverage declined; an outbreak then occurred in 1982 that produced over 50 cases. The cost of controlling the epidemic and treating the victims has been estimated at more than ten times the cost needed over the preceding five years to prevent the outbreak *(7)*.

There were substantial polio increases in Brazil and Colombia from 1985 to 1986 *(8)*, although these were partly offset by declines in Mexico, Haiti, and Peru. The buildup of a pool of susceptibles and any decline in vaccination coverage would have the same results in other countries. For this reason it is assumed that 3,000 cases a year remain to be eliminated, rather than the 2,500 figure that would result from 500 observed cases with 80% underreporting. This 3,000 figure should also probably be regarded as an upper bound, the lower bound being about half as high.

The external funds to be utilized in the eradication project will go to ensure that a surveillance system is built up and that supervisory systems are in place—so as to guarantee continued high levels of coverage and eventual eradication of the wild poliovirus. Without these additional resources, it may be very difficult for the countries involved to organize the needed surveillance systems, and it is to be feared that prevailing levels of coverage will decline for lack of supervisory systems.

3. The cost of treating a polio victim has been estimated from a 1982 study conducted in Brazil *(9)*. The expenses included were those of treatment during the acute phase of the disease (US $880 on the average, within a

range of US $350 to US $2,800 in different hospitals), together with those of surgery, rehabilitation, and subsequent therapy.

Rehabilitation sometimes extends over several years, so rehabilitation costs must be discounted. In the Brazilian study, discounting was done at 6% per year and was applied over 10 years; for purposes of the present calculations, the results reported have been adjusted to reflect the discount rate of 12% used here. With that adjustment, the average cost of the surgery, rehabilitation, and therapy phase is estimated at $4,949. Hence, the total estimated cost of treating a polio case is $5,829.

The combination of such a high individual treatment cost and a large number of unreported cases means, of course, that the estimated total cost of treating all polio victims would be quite high. In that sense, cost and case estimates could bias the results in favor of the eradication campaign. However, any such bias is offset by excluding from consideration all of the other costs associated with paralytic polio. Furthermore, the calculations based on these high estimates are modified later in the analysis in order to determine whether eradication would still be justified with fewer cases or lower treatment costs.

4. The five-year eradication campaign could not expect to bring the incidence of polio down to zero in the first year. Instead, as surveillance and coverage expand, the campaign is expected to achieve zero cases by the fifth year. It is assumed for purposes of simplicity that the decline in cases is linear over the five years of the campaign. This means that net benefits increase from the first to the fifth year, increase sharply in the sixth year (when spending drops back to the maintenance level of US $10 million per year), and thereafter remain constant, apart from discounting. At the end of the campaign, some 15,000 cases per year are being prevented. If there are currently about 3,000 cases annually, the difference of 12,000 cases that do not occur can be attributed to the current level of control exerted through the EPI. The eradication campaign is assumed to prevent another 1,000 cases in the first year (for a total of 13,000) and an additional 500 cases in each succeeding year.

5. Benefits and costs are calculated for 10 years beyond the end of the eradication campaign, which carries the calculation to the end of the century. Net benefits continue to accrue beyond that point if eradication is maintained, but discounting makes their present value quite small ($1.00 is worth only $0.18 fifteen years from now).

Costs and Benefits When All Polio Victims Are Treated

The foregoing assumptions lead to the costs and benefits shown in Table 11.1. When total costs (including national efforts as well as donor contributions to eradication) are compared to total savings (assuming all cases are treated), there is a net present benefit, after discounting, of US $217.2 million in the first five years, and the eradication campaign is economically justified in each of the first five years, well before full eradication is achieved. This simply reflects the fact that the current level of EPI coverage is economically justified by the potential savings in treatment costs on the basis of the assumptions made here.

During the 10 years following eradication, these calculations indicate a further discounted net saving of US $264.2 million. Because of discounting, this is much less than the estimated sum of undiscounted savings over 10 years, which is US $774.4 million. (Savings in each year of the decade would be US $77.4 million, but discounting would reduce their present value to only US $41.5 million in the first year and even smaller values in each subsequent year.) Discounting would also reduce the present value of anticipated savings during the five-year eradication effort from US $288.0 million to US $217.2 million.

During the whole fifteen-year interval, the present value of net savings is estimated at US $481.4 million. Whether the prevention of 220,000 cases of paralytic polio would be worth this much (or more, or less) to the potential victims and their families is not considered.

This estimate is so high because it is very expensive to treat even one polio victim. However, the conclusion that eradication is justified does not depend on this cost being as high as US $5,829. In fact, if the treatment cost were only US $1,728 the net total discounted savings over the five-year eradication campaign would be zero, and the effort would still pay for itself over the next 10 years. (Net savings in each year would be US $15.9 million, for a ten-year discounted total benefit of US $54.3 million.) If the campaign had the entire 15 years to pay for itself, the cost of treatment could be as low as US $1,207.

Alternatively, the incidence of polio could be much lower than is assumed in Table 11.1. That is, assuming treatment costs of US $5,829 per patient, the number of cases could be reduced to about 3,100 and eradication could still be justified.

Given that the current level of polio control by vaccination is much cheaper than treatment of all the cases that would otherwise occur, it may

Table 11.1 Costs and Benefits Associated with Polio Eradication During a Successful Five-Year Campaign and an Ensuing Ten-Year Maintenance Period, Assuming all Polio Victims are Treated

| | YEARS OF ERADICATION CAMPAIGN | | | | | CAMPAIGN YEARS, TOTAL | YEARS 6-15, PER ANNUM | YEARS 6-15, TOTAL | ALL 15 YEARS, TOTAL |
	1	2	3	4	5				
Discount factor[a]	0.945	0.844	0.753	0.673	0.601	—	—[b]	—	—
Total costs versus total benefits (in millions of US$):									
Number of cases prevented (thousands)	13.0	13.5	14.0	14.5	15.0	70.0	15.0	150.0	220.0
Savings in treatment expenses (millions of US$)	75.8	78.7	81.6	84.5	87.4	408.0	87.4	874.4	1,282.4
Cost of eradication or maintenance	24.0	24.0	24.0	24.0	24.0	120.0	10.0	100.0	220.0
Net Saving (net benefit)	51.8	54.7	57.6	60.5	63.4	288.0	77.4	774.4	1,062.4
Net present value of discounted savings	48.9	46.1	43.4	40.7	38.1	217.2	—[c]	264.2	481.4
Donor costs versus marginal benefits (in millions of US$):									
Number of cases prevented (thousands)	1.0	1.5	2.0	2.5	3.0	10.0	3.0	30.0	40.0
Savings in treatment expenses (millions of US$)	5.8	8.7	11.7	14.6	17.5	58.3	17.5	174.9	233.2
Cost of eradication or maintenance	9.2	9.2	9.2	9.2	9.2	46.0	0	0	46.0
Net saving (net benefit)	-3.4	-0.5	2.5	5.4	8.3	12.3	17.5	174.9	187.2
Net present value of discounted savings	-3.2	-0.4	1.9	3.6	5.0	6.9	—[c]	55.2	62.1

[a] Discount factors are calculated at mid-years, thus the factor for year one corresponds to discounting at 12% annually for six months.

[b] This discount factor varies from 0.536 in year six to 0.194 in year 15.

[c] Because of variations in the discount factor from year to year, only the ten-year totals are shown.

still be asked whether the donor contribution of US $46 million for the eradication campaign would pay for itself in terms of reduced incidence and associated lower treatment costs. The amount requested from donor agencies is 38% of the total cost of eradication, but it would be used to eliminate only 20% of the pre-EPI level of incidence (3,000 cases per year out of 15,000), the other 80% being controlled by national efforts costing US $74 million during the five years of the campaign.

Consequently, as the second part of Table 11.1 shows, the donor contribution exceeds the anticipated saving (again assuming treatment of all polio victims) during each of the campaign's first two years. This is followed by positive net benefits as eradication is achieved, for a total net benefit of US $6.9 million during the five years of the campaign. There would also be a positive net benefit of US $17.5 million in each subsequent year, while eradication would presumably be maintained by national efforts without further donor financial assistance. Even with discounting, over the next decade this latter benefit would amount to a further US $55.2 million. The result is an estimated net discounted positive benefit of US $62.1 million over the entire fifteen-year period.

This calculation naturally depends more for its positive value upon the assumed high cost of curative treatment. For the campaign to break even in five years (showing zero net discounted savings from the donors' contributions), treatment could not cost less than US $4,874. That would result in total discounted savings of US $46.1 million over the ensuing decade. These savings (over all 15 years) would still be positive at any treatment cost higher than US $2,106. Therefore, roughly speaking, the eradication of polio appears justified if treatment costs at least US $2,000, purely on the grounds of reducing the total discounted costs of treatment plus prevention over a fifteen-year period.

In other words, while the donor contribution directed at eradication pays off more slowly than the level of polio control already achieved, it is still an economically justified investment compared to the cost of treating everyone who would otherwise get polio. This remains true despite the need to devote resources to activities other than immunization (surveillance and laboratory work) that are necessary in order to ensure that eradication is achieved and maintained. Moreover, as in the previous calculation, no account is taken of other benefits anticipated from this investment—such as an increased capacity to control other diseases and consequent further medical savings.

In sum, there is no reason to suppose that the current level of polio control has already absorbed all the potential benefit, leaving nothing more to be gained from complete eradication of the disease. Rather, making an additional effort to eliminate polio entirely appears justified. This conclusion seems invalid only if the cost of treating a polio victim is much less than that assumed here, or if the number of victims treated is far smaller. The next section considers the second of these possibilities.

Costs and Benefits When Treatment is Incomplete

The apparent economic justification for eradicating polio contradicts the findings of a cost-benefit analysis of polio vaccination in Brazil covering the mass immunization campaigns begun in 1980 (10). On the assumption that such campaigns would end in 1983, and that thereafter the normal, pre-campaign rate of vaccination would be enough to keep polio from reappearing before 1990, it was concluded that the mass campaigns did not justify their costs (US $30 million), and that no more than US $43.4 million per year should be spent to maintain the pre-1980 level of vaccination coverage.

This study made several assumptions that differ from those reflected in Table 11.1. For one thing, the discount rate was taken to be 18% rather than 12%, which made future benefits less valuable. For another, the fixed costs of treating children in the acute stage of the disease were assumed to be zero, because of supposed excess facility and staff resources at pediatric hospitals. This amounts to supposing that any such resources would not be used for other medical care and would not be released—in other words, that ministries of health would maintain superfluous staff and facilities. (The costs of the subsequent rehabilitation and surgery, which were acknowledged to require specialized personnel and facilities, were not regarded as zero.) The most important difference, however, is that savings were calculated only for the estimated number of actual curative treatments, rather than for the number of victims who could benefit from such care but did not always receive it. Primarily for this reason, the mass vaccination campaign appeared to be justified in Northeast Brazil, where the incidence of polio was relatively high, but not in the rest of the country.

Relating the costs of immunization to actual rather than potential costs of treatment in this way raises two important issues. The first concerns the appropriate way to deal with those victims who get polio but receive no medical care. These people are entirely ignored if only actual spending is considered, but of course they account for much of the potential benefit of immunization if any kind of price is put on pain and suffering (*10*). The second issue concerns marginal costs and benefits. Once polio has been brought partly under control by immunization, the remaining gain from greater coverage may be small. However, the cost of obtaining greater coverage is likely to be high, since the current level has to be maintained while immunization is extended to the rest of the population. This makes polio very different from smallpox, which could be combated by concentrating only on those areas still reporting the disease (only surveillance activities, not vaccination, were needed in areas where smallpox had already been eradicated).

As a result of this problem of increasing marginal cost and decreasing marginal gain in the case of polio, it may never seem justified to finish the job. The calculations in Table 11.1 indicate, however, that complete eradication is justified for polio if the extra expense of donors' contributions is compared to the extra gain made possible thereby. Among the benefits from complete rather than almost-complete eradication are the prevention of later outbreaks like the previously mentioned one in Jamaica. These can be expensive to control, but because of their uncertain magnitude and frequency no attempt has been made to estimate the present discounted value of the costs they represent.

It should also be noted that because of uncertainty in the estimates of costs and incidences it is impossible to determine either the marginal point where preventive efforts cease to be justified or the maximum vaccination coverage that pays for itself.

Both calculations in Table 11.1 assume that treatment would be provided to everyone who actually contracted the disease. Most of the estimated benefits, however, are only potential savings that greatly exceed realizable savings attainable through actual reduction in treatment expenditures. Therefore, the next task is to see whether those realizable savings, by themselves, are enough to pay for the cost of eradication, without attributing any benefit to cases where people are affected by polio but receive no medical care.

This requires estimating the number of cases that are or would be treated. Before introduction of the EPI, the number of cases treated was roughly equal to the number reported, in part because some countries reported only those cases actually treated. (This accounts in large part for the very high level of underreporting.) In the absence of control measures, the number of cases treated would be at least as large as it was a decade ago. Allowing for some improvement in coverage or expansion of treatment, and recognizing that in many pre-EPI years there were more than 4,000 reported cases of polio, it seems reasonable to take 4,000 cases per year as the background or "normal" level of treatment that would occur in the absence of immunization. As in the calculations reported above, it cannot be supposed that the eradication campaign would immediately eliminate the need to treat those cases. Instead, it is supposed that in the first year of the campaign there would be savings from 2,000 fewer treatments, and that this number would rise to 4,000 cases over the five-year period. This estimate, which appears in the first line of Table 11.2, shows that over the entire fifteen-year period some 55,000 fewer treatments would be required.

Following this assumption, net savings are of course much smaller than they would be if all polio victims were treated. Savings remain negative throughout the five years of the campaign and turn positive thereafter. The result is a total net discounted benefit of –US $27.3 million during the eradication campaign, followed by a positive net benefit, after discounting, of US $45.4 million during the next decade. Total net benefits during the entire fifteen-year period are estimated at US $18.1 million.

This means that eradication of polio would pay for itself by reducing the medical costs of treating those victims who actually are or probably would be treated. Hence, in order to justify an eradication campaign, it is not necessary to attribute any benefits to people who probably would not receive treatment. The magnitude of the net discounted benefit is drastically reduced (from US $481.4 to US $18.1 million), but it continues to be positive. However, because the number of treatments is much reduced, the cost per treatment could not fall appreciably without turning savings negative; specifically, the minimum cost would be $5,097.

Assuming that some polio victims are not treated has exactly the same effect on estimated savings as assuming that fewer people get polio in the first place. Ethically, of course, the two situations are very different; and the total benefits are also different once pain and suffering are taken into account. Nevertheless, for the purpose of this analysis the two are identical. Thus, the calculations in Table 11.2 can be interpreted as meaning that polio eradication would be justified if there were only 4,000 cases annually in the absence of vaccination with all cases being treated—in which case only about 1,000 cases would remain to be prevented by the eradication campaign. This implies that the results do not depend critically on the assumed high incidence of unreported polio; and so, as noted earlier, the level could be as low as 3,100 cases per year.

The profile derived in Table 11.2 of immunization expenditures and savings ascribed to reduced treatment costs is displayed graphically in

Table 11.2 Costs and Benefits Associated with Polio Eradication During a Successful Five-Year Campaign and Ten-Year Maintenance Period, Assuming only a Fraction of all Polio Victims are Treated. The Discount Factor is the Same as Shown in Table 11.1

	YEARS OF ERADICATION CAMPAIGN					CAMPAIGN YEARS, TOTAL	YEARS 6-15, PER ANNUM	YEARS 6-15, TOTAL	ALL 15 YEARS, TOTAL
	1	2	3	4	5				
Total costs versus total benefits (in millions of US$):									
Number of treatments prevented (thousands)	2.0	2.5	3.0	3.5	4.0	15.0	4.0	40.0	55.0
Savings in treatment expenses (millions of US$)	11.7	14.6	17.5	20.4	23.3	87.5	23.3	233.2	320.7
Cost of eradication or maintenance	24.0	24.0	24.0	24.0	24.0	120.0	10.0	100.0	220.0
Net Saving (net benefit)	−12.3	−9.4	−6.5	−3.6	−0.7	−32.5	13.3	133.2	100.7
Net present value of discounted savings	−11.6	−7.9	−4.9	−2.5	−0.4	−27.3	—a	45.4	18.1
Donor costs versus marginal benefits (in millions of US$):									
Number of treatments prevented (thousands)	0.6	0.7	0.8	0.9	1.0	4.0	1.0	10.0	14.0
Savings in treatment expenses (millions of US$)	3.5	4.1	4.7	5.2	5.8	23.3	5.8	58.3	81.6
Cost of eradication or maintenance	9.2	9.2	9.2	9.2	9.2	46.0	0	0	46.0
Net saving (net benefit)	−5.7	−5.1	−4.5	−4.0	−3.4	−22.7	5.8	58.3	35.6
Net present value of discounted savings	−5.4	−4.3	−3.4	−2.6	−2.0	−17.8	—a	18.3	0.6

aBecause of variations in the discount factor from year to year, only the ten-year totals are shown.

Figure 11.1. The upper panel of that figure shows the un-discounted profile while the lower one includes the effect of discounting. As a result of discounting, the area of net gain is shrunken compared to the area of net loss.

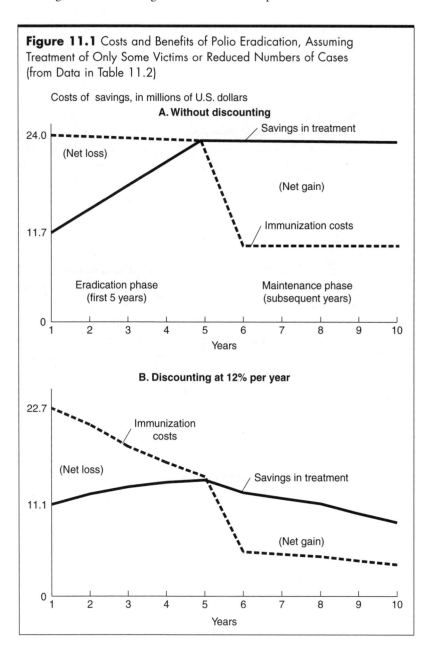

Figure 11.1 Costs and Benefits of Polio Eradication, Assuming Treatment of Only Some Victims or Reduced Numbers of Cases (from Data in Table 11.2)

Table 11.2 also compares marginal (donor) costs and marginal benefits in the manner of Table 11.1, assuming only a small number of cases treated. Here it is supposed that the reduction in treatments never exceeds 1,000 cases per year, starting from an approximate reduction of 600 cases the first year. This calculation shows a total discounted net benefit of only US $0.6 million over the entire 15-year period. Based on reduced medical costs alone, the donors' contribution almost exactly pays for itself, assuming treatment costs of US $5,829 per case.

In summary, these estimates indicate that the eradication of poliomyelitis is a justifiable investment, even without making any allowance for benefits other than those due to realizable reductions in expenditures to treat victims of the disease. Indeed, the cost of treating even a small fraction of those who need treatment is large enough to pay for the total prevention of polio. In other words, the eradication of polio would actually put money in the coffers of the Ministry of Health, or whoever now pays to treat polio victims.

It is important, however, to sound a note of caution. This projected result depends on there being enough current expenditure on treatment. It would no longer hold, for example, if the level of treatment were only one-fourth lower than that assumed in Table 11.2. This process of justifying an eradication campaign by its effect in reducing public expenditure depends on there being sufficiently high public expenditure to start with; and so the process can lead to effects that are clearly perverse. In our case, literally applied, and giving no allowance for non-monetary benefits in terms of reduced pain and suffering, it implies that the eradication of polio would be justified after spending millions of dollars over many years to treat polio victims, but would not be justified as an alternative to such a treatment expenditure. That is, eradication would be more justified the later it came, after increasingly large sums of money were spent for treatment.

Immediate Versus Delayed Eradication

To see how such justification of immunization, in terms of reduced costs alone, could lead to a delay in vaccination efforts, consider two hypothetical regions (A and B) with 15,000 cases of paralytic polio per year (the estimated pre-EPI level in Latin America and the Caribbean). Suppose that immunization has not begun in either region, and suppose further that in neither case are victims of the disease initially being treated. The costs of treating a case (US $5,829), conducting a five-year eradication campaign

(US $120 million), and maintaining eradication thereafter (US $10 million per year) are assumed to be the same as in the previous analysis.

In Region A, efforts are made to start treating victims for purely ethical reasons, treatment being extended to 1,000 patients the first year and 1,000 additional patients per year thereafter. At the end of five years, someone performs a cost-benefit estimate of the sort presented above and discovers that it would be cheaper to immunize people. Over the next five years, immunization is gradually extended to enough of the population to interrupt the transmission of wild poliovirus, and eradication is achieved. Thereafter, immunization of infants is maintained, and while treatment continues for the victims accumulated during the whole ten-year period (five without immunization and five after immunization began), no new patients are admitted for treatment in the eleventh and subsequent years. Assuming linear treatment and immunization trends, as shown in Table 11.3, 112,500 people get polio during the decade of whom 41,500 are treated and 71,000 receive no treatment.

In Region B, nobody worries about cost-benefit analysis of this sort. Immunization is begun immediately, rather than waiting for five years. Treatment of victims begins at the same time and is extended at the same rate as in Region A, except that because of immunization, treatment never rises beyond 4,000 cases per year and falls to zero in the sixth year. Over the ten-year period only 37,500 people get polio, of whom 11,500 receive treatment and 26,000 do not. This latter figure is only 37% of the number of untreated victims accumulated in Region A. From year 11 onward both regions are identical, in that they have no new polio cases and spend US $10 million each per year to maintain eradication. Any comparison of the two regions need therefore consider only the first 10 years.

What do costs look like in the two cases? Region A spends a total of US $241.9 million on treatment and US $120.0 million on immunization over the decade, for an undiscounted total cost of US $361.9 million. Region B spends only $67.0 million on treatment (just 28% of what Region A spends), but—since five years of maintenance are included after the five years of eradication—it spends US $170.0 million on immunization, US $50.0 million more than Region A. Region B's undiscounted total expenditure is therefore US $237.0 million, or 66% as much as Region A's.

Discounting expenditures at 12% per year has more effect on the costs in Region A, because spending there reaches its peak later, in year eight. This is due to initial postponement of the eradication campaign and also to the relatively slow expansion of treatment that is assumed; costs would

Table 11.3 A Comparison of Ten-Year Costs and Results of Two Hypothetical Polio Eradication Campaigns, One Immediate and One Delayed, Discounted at 12% per Year as in Tables 11.1 and 11.2

	YEARS 1	2	3	4	5	6	7	8	9	10	TEN-YEAR TOTAL
Region A (delayed campaign):											
Number of polio cases (thousands)	15.0	15.0	15.0	15.0	15.0	13.5	10.5	7.5	4.5	1.5	112.5
Number of cases treated (thousands)	1.0	2.0	3.0	4.0	5.0	6.0	7.0	7.5	4.5	1.5	41.5
Untreated Victims (thousands)	14.0	13.0	12.0	11.0	10.0	7.5	3.5	0	0	0	71.0
Cost of treatment (million US$)	5.8	11.7	17.5	23.3	29.1	35.0	40.9	43.7	26.2	8.7	241.9
Cost of immunization (million US$)	0	0	0	0	0	24.0	24.0	24.0	24.0	24.0	120.0
Total Cost	5.8	11.7	17.5	23.3	29.1	59.0	64.8	67.7	50.2	32.7	361.9
Discounted Total	5.5	9.9	13.2	15.7	17.5	31.6	31.0	28.9	19.2	11.1	183.6
Region B (immediate campaign):											
Number of polio cases (thousands)	13.5	10.5	7.5	4.5	1.5	0	0	0	0	0	37.5
Number of cases treated (thousands)	1.0	2.0	3.0	4.0	1.5	0	0	0	0	0	11.5
Untreated Victims (thousands)	12.5	8.5	4.5	0.5	0	0	0	0	0	0	26.0
Cost of treatment (million US$)	5.8	11.7	17.5	23.3	8.7	0	0	0	0	0	67.0
Cost of immunization (million US$)	24.0	24.0	24.0	24.0	24.0	10.0	10.0	10.0	10.0	10.0	170.0
Total Cost	29.8	35.7	41.5	47.3	32.7	10.0	10.0	10.0	10.0	10.0	237.0
Discounted Total	28.2	30.1	31.3	31.8	19.7	5.4	4.8	4.3	3.8	3.4	162.7

be shifted toward the early years if treatment were extended more rapidly. In Region B, total expenditure reaches its peak in year four, being higher than in Region A during each of the first five years. As a consequence, the discounted total costs are US $183.6 million in Region A and US $162.7 million in Region B, so that the Region B costs are 89% as high as those in Region A.

At the end of 10 years, neither region has any new polio cases. However, Region B is clearly better off. It has spent US $20.9 million less after discounting (US $124.9 million less without discounting); it has 30,000 fewer treated polio victims (who suffer some damage from the disease despite treatment); and it has 45,000 fewer untreated, paralyzed victims. Thus, making an immediate effort to eradicate the disease pays off both in reduced health damage and in lower total treatment and prevention costs. If either the cost of treating a polio victim or the number of victims were lower, the monetary saving in Region B compared to Region A would of course be smaller, but it would always be positive. If one assumed that eradication could only be justified by saving actual (not potential) expenditure on treatment, however, Region A pursued the right course by not starting immunization until the costs of treatment had become relatively high.

Concluding Remarks

What accounts for this perverse result? Part of it is due to discounting future costs and benefits. When the assumed number of treatments is reduced from 15,000 per year (Table 11.1) to 4,000 per year (Table 11.2), the un-discounted net savings fall from US $1,062.4 million to US $100.7 million. (This is much more than the approximately 15:4 reduction in treatment savings, because the costs of immunization are independent of treatment levels). Discounting means that net savings are reduced much more than ten-fold, because savings increase through time; thus, net savings of US $481.4 million become only US $18.1 million, a 24-fold reduction. What this means is that the higher the discount rate, the higher the number of current treatments necessary to justify the cost of eradication. If, as in Region A, immunization is delayed while treatment costs increase, the effect of discounting is to delay eradication still more.

It might seem that the answer to this problem is not to discount the future, but instead to base decisions on un-discounted costs and benefits. The logic of discounting, after all, supposes that a given individual, who is the same person today and tomorrow, values tomorrow less than today *(11)*. But the children who will suffer paralytic polio in the future, if the disease is not eradicated, have for the most part not been born yet. Discounting their future therefore means valuing them less than those are already here, which is very different from making inter-temporal choices for a given person.

However, to abandon discounting means being willing to wait forever, provided that eventually benefits outweigh costs. The resources required to eradicate polio could be applied to other uses, including medical uses, which might pay off more quickly. So even though discounting the future raises an awkward ethical question, there is no escaping the need to give priority to the present, at least so long as the benefits considered in the two periods can be compared.

The whole question of whether eradicating polio is worth the cost would not even arise if the private market for immunization worked properly. No parent wants to see his child paralyzed, and the cost of immunization is less than the expected cost of treatment per un-immunized child. Therefore, every parent should be more than willing to pay to have his child protected.[3] If this does not happen, the fault lies with some combination of poverty and ignorance. It is true that public expenditure to eradicate the disease takes resources away from competing private uses. But requiring that such expenditure "pay its way" amounts to supposing that the alternative private expenditures would be equally justified—which seems questionable in a world where private demand has not yet caused all susceptible children to be immunized. And if the rationality of private spending is to be doubted, then it is not clear why public spending must produce positive discounted net benefits.

But the most important reason why the eradication of polio may not appear to be economically justified (as in Region A) does not arise from distinctions between the present and the future or between public and private expenditure. It arises from the different way that curative treatment and preventive activities are judged. The "justification" for immunization is that it costs less than treating polio victims. If the aim is to minimize the expenditure required to avoid paralysis or death from polio, then eradicating the disease is clearly preferable to continued curative treatment. But if the aim is to reduce public expenditure on health, then immunization appears to be justified only if curative spending is high enough.

In general, the foregoing account assumes that some level of treatment will be provided, with or without economic justification, and then applies an economic test to see whether prevention should replace treatment as the way to deal with polio. Why should this be considered the right test of an eradication campaign's merit? After all, treating polio victims does not save money for the government; and if the aim were simply to reduce expenditure, then curative care could not be justified either. But if "it is unacceptable, given the technology presently available, that any child in this hemisphere should suffer paralytic poliomyelitis" (5, p. ii), then the eradication of polio is not only ethically justified but also economically sound.

Notes

1. If benefits in year t are designated B_t, while costs incurred in that year are C_t, $B_t - C_t$ is the net benefit. The corresponding discounted net benefit is $(B_t - C_t)/(1 + i)^t$, where i is the interest or discount rate used. The present value of this stream of net benefits (positive or negative) is the sum of these terms over all the years of a project, or in the present case through the first 15 years, after which net benefits are positive but, because of discounting, are quite small.

2. It is not easy to estimate polio underreporting, although surveys of residual lameness provide a basis (see 1, Session III, Section A). The assumption that before the EPI only about 20% of the polio cases were reported in Latin America and the Caribbean has been suggested by Ciro de Quadros and Marjorie Pollock as a reasonable estimate.

3. Once coverage by vaccination is almost complete a parent might consider that his unvaccinated child was adequately protected by the screen of vaccinated children, so that there would be no further gain from the child's immunization. This argument would apply, if ever, only when coverage was complete enough so that the risk of infection was essentially zero; it would not hold at the typically quite incomplete levels of coverage found in Latin America. Even at higher levels of coverage, this argument would make sense only if the cost of having the child vaccinated were high compared to the benefit, or the risk of paralysis from the vaccine itself were substantial.

References

[1] Horstmann, D.M., T.C. Quinn, and F.C. Robbins (eds.). International Symposium on Poliomyelitis Control. *Review of Infectious Disease 6* (Suppl 2), 1984.
[2] Sabin, A.B. Oral poliovirus vaccine: History of its development and use and the current challenge to eliminate poliomyelitis from the world. *Journal of Infectious Disease 151*:420–436, 1985.

[3] Willems, J.S., and C.R. Sanders. Cost-effectiveness and cost-benefit analysis of vaccines. *Journal of Infectious Disease 144*:486–493, 1981.

[4] Creese, A.L. Cost effectiveness of alternative strategies of poliomyelitis immunization in Brazil. *Review of Infectious Disease 6* (Suppl 2): S404–407, 1984.

[5] Pan American Health Organization, Expanded Program on Immunization in the Americas: Progress Report, PAHO document CE 95/15, 11 April 1985. Washington, D.C., 1985.

[6] Pan American Health Organization, PAHO member countries endorse polio eradication resolution. EPI Newsletter vol. 7. no. 5. October 1985.

[7] Ashley, D., and R. Bernal. Poliomyelitis in Jamaica: immunization policies and socioeconomic implications. *World Health Forum* 6:265-267, 1985.

[8] Pan American Health Organization. Polio in the Americas: Weeks 1–53, 1986. EPI Newsletter vol. 8. no. 6, 1986.

[9] Ministry of Health, Brazil, Memória sobre estimativa de custos dos casos de poliomielite no Brasil em 1982. Brasília. 1984.

[10] Garlow, D.C. Mass Vaccination to Combat Polio: A Cost-Benefit Analysis for Brazil. Mimeographed document. Instituto de Pesquisas e Estudos Econômicos. Universidade Federal de Rio Grande do Sul, 1983.

[11] Prest. A.R., and R. Turvey, Cost-Benefit Analysis: A Survey. In: American Economic Association and Royal Economic Society. *Surveys of Economic Theory* (vol. 3). St. Martin's Press. New York. 1967.

CHAPTER 12

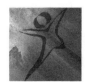

Cost-Benefit Analysis of a Regional Vaccination System

Acknowledgments

I am grateful to my former colleagues Robert Knouss, Francisco López Antuñano, Gabriel Schmuñís, Francisco Pinheiro, Ciro de Quadros, Alberto Pellegrini Filho, Victor Escutia, and Mario González Pacheco, as well as Drs. Guillermo Soberón, Akira Homma, and Armando Isibasi, for guidance and for the estimates on which this study is based. Any error, however, is the sole responsibility of the author.

Introduction

Although mass vaccination of vulnerable populations has been quite successful at reducing communicable disease morbidity and mortality, we still confront serious public health problems arising from diseases for which no adequate vaccines exist (1,2). Either a vaccine has not been developed, there having been only partial progress to date; or the existing vaccines are of limited effectiveness; or they are restricted to certain pathogenic serotypes and therefore would not protect the populations exposed to other serotypes; or they are too costly for mass application. In view of this situation, the governments participating in the World Children's Conference held in September 1990 proposed various measures including development of an "infant vaccine" for safe early protection against a variety of diseases (3).

Reprinted, with permission, from "Cost-Benefit Analysis of a Regional System for Vaccination Against Pneumonia, Meningitis Type B and Typhoid Fever" *Bulletin of the Pan American Health Organization* 26 (2), 1992.

Independently, in early 1989 the Pan American Health Organization began examining the prospects for undertaking a regional effort to perfect and disseminate certain vaccines. These vaccines would be directed against a limited number of diseases of particular interest to PAHO's Member Countries because of the high morbidity and mortality they caused or because of large expenditures needed to treat their victims. This initiative, named the Regional Vaccine System (Sistema Regional de Vacunas– SIREVA), was seen as including the phase of epidemiological research in the participating countries, basic research to develop the new vaccines, clinical and field trials, and construction and operation of a pilot production plant to support these other phases.

Once a vaccine had been found effective, safe, and affordable, production on a commercial scale would begin, possibly under arrangements with state or private laboratories; and mass vaccination of children would commence, perhaps through an extension of the Expanded Program on Immunization (EPI). The three diseases of bacterial origin considered targets of the effort are pneumococcal pneumonia, meningococcal meningitis caused by Group B *Neisseria meningitidis*, and typhoid fever.

SIREVA's original design included three options designated "A," "B," and "C." Option A dealt only with meningitis and typhoid fever, while options B and C included development of vaccines against all three target diseases. However, option B included only 10 participating countries with 10 collaborating national laboratories, while option C included 17 countries—thus envisioning vaccination of a larger population and implying greater development costs for SIREVA directed at identifying serotypes and testing vaccines in all 17 countries. All three options called for two principal laboratories or vaccine centers to be involved in the project, one associated with the National Institute of Public Health of Mexico and the other with the Oswaldo Cruz Foundation in Brazil, these being the centers with the greatest experience and technical sophistication in the Region.

On analyzing the costs and benefits the three options, it was concluded that the pneumonia vaccine should definitely be included in the system and that three vaccines could be applied in the countries of the Region where the selected diseases are now of major importance. However, it was also decided that the system would be developed in 11 countries, since a network of 10 national laboratories would be sufficient for the epidemiological work and the clinical and field trials. This option became the final version of the proposal (4).

The only variation still being considered deals with the number of people who would be vaccinated against meningitis, the cost-benefit calculations being repeated for two possible scales of operation that differ by a factor of two. It should be noted that the limit placed on the number of countries initially involved would not limit later administration of the vaccines in other countries of the Americas, or even in other regions, where the cost of vaccination might be justified by the benefits.

The purpose of the present analysis is to estimate and compare SIREVA's costs and benefits, and to establish under what circumstances the benefits would justify the costs, and thus justify establishment of the system.

With respect to costs, it is necessary to distinguish between two elements: expenditures for vaccine *development* (including field trials and adaptation to different epidemiological conditions) and expenditures for vaccine *administration* (that is, for vaccinating the population). Beyond that, however, it is not the purpose of this presentation to distinguish between different kinds of costs. Therefore, the account that follows makes no attempt to discuss the composition of the costs attributable to SIREVA (that is, their distribution among basic research, clinical trials, pilot production, etc.); only their distribution over time will be considered. Similarly, we will not consider the biologic, chemical, and epidemiological aspects of the target diseases and prospective vaccines. Rather, the information used in this analysis deals only with the number of people that would be vaccinated and the numbers that would become sick or die if unvaccinated; the costs of implementing SIREVA, vaccinating the population, and treating patients; and possible additional benefits attributable to vaccination. The last part of the analysis estimates the sensitivity of the results to changes in the parameters utilized, this type of estimate being especially crucial when neither the costs nor the benefits are known but must be estimated with varying degrees of precision.

The costs attributable to SIREVA as such (the vaccine development costs cited above) have been estimated for a period of 10 years under the assumption that, although the system could continue to function for many more years, the expenditures in the eleventh and following years would be dedicated to the development of new vaccines not contemplated in the initial plans. Therefore, it would not be correct to attribute or charge expenses of those future years to the first three diseases, and vaccination against them would have to justify only the expenses of SIREVA's first decade. These expenses, presented by year in Table 12.1, have been estimated at US $115.3 million in constant dollars.

Any cost-benefit analysis is based on what are called *present values* of cost and benefit flows over time, these flows being discounted according to how far in the future they occur. This procedure requires the selection of a discount rate (r), which is conceptually equivalent to an interest rate. A cost t years in the future is then estimated by dividing the present cost (C) by $(1 + r)$ for each of $t - 1$ years (5), the discounted cost being

$$C/(1 + r)(1 + r)(1 + r) \ldots = C/(1 + r)^{(t-1)} = C \times (1 + r)^{(-t+1)}$$

For example, if an item's present cost (C) were \$1,000 and the discount rate were 10% (0.10), then its discounted cost five years in the future (t = 5) would be \$683, calculated as follows:

Year 5 discounted cost

$$= C \times (1 + r)^{(-t+1)}$$
$$= \$1,000 \times (1 + 0.10)^{(-5+1)}$$
$$= \$1,000 \times (1.10)^{(-4)}$$
$$= \$1,000/1.1^{(4)}$$
$$= \$683$$

Of course, the total discounted cost (C*) over t years would be the sum of the costs in each of the years considered (from here on we shall use an asterisk [*] to designate a discounted sum). And so, if we let the letters CS stand for the SIREVA costs (for vaccine development), the total SIREVA costs appearing in Table 12.1, discounted over the decade, can be expressed by the formula

$$CS^* = SUM \; CS(t) \times (1 + r)^{(-t+1)},$$

Table 12.1 Cost of SIREVA, by Year, in Constant US\$[a]

YEAR	COST OF SIREVA (CS), IN MILLIONS OF US\$
1	5.41
2	26.36
3	11.23
4	10.33
5	10.53
6	10.48
7	10.43
8	10.43
9	10.06
10	10.06
Total (CS, not discounted)	115.32
Total (CS*, discounted)	80.31

[a]The analysis only attributes the costs of the first 10 years of SIREVA to the development of vaccines against meningitis, typhoid fever, and pneumonia because it is expected that initiation of vaccination with all three vaccines will occur in the first decade.

where CS(t) is the undiscounted cost in year t, $(1 + r)^{(-t+1)}$ is the discount factor, and SUM indicates the sum of the costs of all the years in question. The same method can be used to calculate discounted benefits.

Box 12.1 lists the multiplicative discount factors in the form $(1 + r)^{(-t+1)}$ for a discount rate of 10% per year (r = 0.10) from Year 1 of SIREVA (when the factor is equal to 1.0) to Year 30, which is the furthest horizon considered in this analysis and for which the factor decreases to only 0.063. This means that one dollar of costs or benefit that only occurs in Year 30 would have a present value of $0.063; and conversely, $0.063 invested today at a rate of interest of 10% per year would have a value of $1.00 after 30 years.

Box 12.1 Discount Factors, by Year, for a Rate (r) of 10% per Year

YEAR	FACTOR	COMMENTS
1	1.0000	Initiation of SIREVA
2	0.9091	
3	0.8264	
4	0.7513	
5	0.6830	
6	0.6209	
7	0.5645	Start of vaccination against typhoid fever
8	0.5132	
9	0.4665	Start of vaccination against meningitis
10	0.4241	Start of vaccination against pneumonia
11	0.3855	
12	0.3505	
13	0.3186	
14	0.2897	
15	0.2633	
16	0.2394	From year 16 on, the numbers of vaccinations do not vary.
17	0.2176	
18	0.1978	
19	0.1798	
20	0.1635	Sum for years 16 to 20 = 0.9981
		Sum for years 1 to 20 = 9.3647
21	0.1486	
22	0.1351	
23	0.1228	
24	0.1117	
25	0.1015	
26	0.0923	
27	0.0839	
28	0.0763	
29	0.0693	
30	0.0630	Sum for years 21 to 30 = 1.0045
		Sum for years 1 to 30 = 10.3692

The last line of Table 12.1 illustrates the effect of discounting the future costs of SIREVA at 10% per year over the course of a decade, which reduces the undiscounted figure (US$115.3 million) to a discounted cost of US $80.3 million.

The use of other discount rates would obviously give other totals. However, it has been judged that any reasonable rate would fall between 8% and 15% per year, and that changes introduced by using such rates as extreme values would be a good deal smaller than possible changes introduced by uncertainties regarding the value of other variables. For example, the cost of vaccinating one individual is not yet known, but it is conceivable that it could vary by a factor of 10, while a discount rate of 8% would not differ from one of 15% by as much a factor of two. Moreover, changes in the discount rate only affect the relative weights of costs and benefits occurring in the same year. Therefore, the question of whether the benefits justify the costs is not as sensitive to variations in the discount rate as it is to variations in the costs or benefits taken separately.

Anticipated Effects of SIREVA

According to the projections for SIREVA, it will be possible to begin vaccination against typhoid fever in Year 7 of the system's operation. Vaccination against meningitis would begin in Year 9, and vaccination against pneumonia in Year 10. In all three cases it is anticipated that vaccination will commence at a high rate, so as to reduce the number of susceptible individuals in the existing population. Later, the number of vaccinations carried out would be reduced to focus on newborns at relatively higher risk, though possible fluctuations could be occasioned by future outbreaks.

In the case of pneumonia, only one year of high coverage is foreseen. This high coverage phase would extend over five years for the other two diseases, and in the case of typhoid fever there would be a period of intermediate coverage followed by a second reduction in the coverage rate after another four years.

Table 12.2 shows estimates of the numbers of people who would be vaccinated against each of the three target diseases in any given year. However, the number of individuals vaccinated does not correspond to the number immunized, because development of vaccines that are 100% effective is not anticipated; rather, the estimates of disease cases and deaths prevented (see Table 12.3) are based on the assumption that the vaccines will be 90%

Table 12.2 The Projected Numbers of Individuals to be Vaccinated, by Target Disease and Year

| YEAR | NUMBER VACCINATED (NUM), IN MILLIONS, AGAINST: | | | TOTAL |
	MENINGITIS	TYPHOID FEVER	PNEUMONIA	
7		65		65.0
8		65		65.0
9	39.0–78	65		104.0–143.0
10	39.0–78	65	39.0	143.0–182.0
11	39.0–78	65	19.5	123.5–162.5
12	39.0–78	39	19.5	97.5–136.5
13	39.0–78	39	19.5	97.5–136.5
14	19.5–39	39	19.5	78.0–97.5
15	19.5–39	39	19.5	78.0–97.5
16	19.5–39	26	19.5	65.0–84.5
17	19.5–39	26	19.5	65.0–84.5
—	—	—	—	—
—	—	—	—	—
30	19.5–39	26	19.5	65.0–84.5
Discounted total number vaccinated (NUM*), in millions:				
20-year horizon	106–212	227	67	400–506
30- year horizon	126–251	253	87	466–561

Table 12.3 Total Discounted Numbers of Disease Cases Prevented, Deaths Prevented with Treatment of all Cases, and Deaths Prevented without Treatment of any Cases, over 20-Year and 30-Year Horizons

	20-YEAR HORIZON	30-YEAR HORIZON
Cases prevented (PREC*):		
Meningitis	9,547–19,094	11,313–22,626
Typhoid fever	305,897	341,075
Pneumonia	16,835	21,700
Deaths prevented, with treatment of all cases (PREDT*):		
Meningitis	477-955	565–1,130
Typhoid fever	3,059	4,411
Pneumonia	1,684	2,170
Total	5,220–5,698	7,146–7,711
Deaths prevented, without treatment of any cases (PRED*):		
Meningitis	4,774–9,547	5,657–11,314
Typhoid fever	30,590	34,108
Pneumonia	5,051	6,511
Total	40,415–45,188	46,276–51,933

effective. It should also be noted that the Table 12.2 data refer to individuals rather than to vaccine doses, since a series of two or more doses per person may be needed to complete the vaccination and achieve 90% immunization.

The cost-benefit analysis also assumes that the cost of vaccinating one individual will be independent of the number of people vaccinated. The latter number will always be large enough (at least 19.5 million per year) to benefit from possible economies of scale. Similarly, it is assumed the benefit obtained per individual vaccinated will be constant and independent of how many others receive the vaccine. Among other things, this implies that the chance of one unvaccinated individual becoming ill does not depend on the number of individuals immunized; that is, a possible "collective immunity" effect is not taken into account (6).

As a consequence of these assumptions, the total discounted costs and benefits can be found by totaling and discounting the number of people vaccinated and later applying to that discounted sum the costs and benefits per person. More explicitly, if the cost of vaccinating someone against disease 'i' is designated VAC(i), then by definition the total cost (CST) of vaccinating some number (NUM) of people against disease 'i' in some future year t is as follows:

$$CST\ (i,\ t) = VAC(i) \times NUM(i,\ t),$$

and discounting and totaling both sides of the equation yields

$$
\begin{aligned}
CST^*(i) &= SUM\ CST\ (i,\ t) \times (1 + r)^{(-t+1)} \\
&= SUM\ VAC(i) \times NUM\ (i,\ t) \times (1 + r)^{(-t+1)} \\
&= VAC(i) \times SUM\ NUM\ (i,\ t) \times (1 + r)^{(-t+1)} \\
&= VAC(i) \times NUM^*(i)
\end{aligned}
$$

The same type of calculation can be applied to the number of disease cases prevented (applying as a multiplicative factor the probability that a vaccinated individual would have acquired the disease if he or she had not been vaccinated); to the number of deaths prevented (successively applying the probability that an individual with the disease died of it, whether or not the effects of curative treatment on the probability of survival are considered); and to the total benefit obtained from vaccination (using the individual or unit benefit as the multiplicative factor).

In relating all these calculations to a discounted sum of individuals, one is not saying that an individual vaccinated 15 years from now is worth less than one vaccinated before that, but only that the economic value of the cost and the associated benefit are less today because they occur further in the future. This discounting and totaling of individuals instead of monetary sums is nothing more than a valuable mathematical simplification. Variables employed in making relevant calculations and the formulas used to discount and total them are summarized in Box 12.2, which also contains a glossary of all of the terms utilized in the analysis.

The discounted and totaled numbers of individuals vaccinated, designated NUM*, are shown at the bottom of Table 12.2 by disease for two different horizons −20 years and 30 years. In contrast to the SIREVA costs for vaccine development (CS), which end in 10 years, the costs of administering the vaccines (CST) never end, so long as the disease is controlled but the pathogens are not eradicated. Therefore, for the purpose of this analysis, it is necessary to choose a final year. It seems reasonable to think that if SIREVA could be justified, this justification would probably occur within 20 years, a period that would include more than a decade of application of each vaccine.

Beyond 20 years, any protection becomes very speculative; in particular, it is not known what might happen to the risks of acquiring a disease or the benefits of being protected. Solely to illustrate a longer horizon, the calculations have been repeated for a 30-year period. As will be seen, this extension of the period does not significantly affect the system's net estimated worth.

As the Table 12.2 projection shows, during the 20 years following SIREVA's initiation the equivalent, in terms of present value, of between 106 million and 212 million people would be vaccinated against pneumonia. Overall, in discounted terms, between 400 million and 506 million people would be vaccinated during the period, the actual figure depending on the extent of vaccination against meningitis. This total could refer to the discounted equivalent of 400–506 million individuals; or it could involve fewer individuals, some of them being vaccinated against two or even three of the target diseases.

On extending the horizon to 30 years these values increase, but much less than proportionately to the number of additional years of vaccination because the discount factors (see Annex 1) give little weight to the years furthest away. In terms of present values, the entire third decade has the same value as only the last five years of the second decade, which in turn are only worth the same as the first year by itself.

To go from the number of people vaccinated to the number of disease cases prevented it is necessary to multiply by the effectiveness of the vaccine

Box 12.2 Glossary of Symbols, Variables, and their Relationships—in their Approximate Order of Appearance in the Text

SYMBOL OR VARIABLE	DEFINITION
$t = 1,2,3 \ldots$	Years since initiation of SIREVA
$i = 1,2,$ or 3	Disease
NUM	Number of vaccinations administered; equal to the number of individuals vaccinated if every individual is vaccinated against only one disease. NUM refers to the number of complete vaccinations, not to the number of doses, if vaccination requires the application of two or more doses.
PREC	Number of cases of a disease prevented by the vaccination program
BEN	Total benefit obtained by prevention of disease cases
C	Total cost
CS	Cost of SIREVA (for vaccine development)
CST	Cost other than for SIREVA (vaccine manufacture, distribution, and administration)

Note: The variables C, CST, NUM, PREC, and BEN are classified by disease (i) and year (t). The variable CS is classified solely by year; CS(i) does not exist. By definition, $C(t) = CS(t) + CST(t)$.

SUM	Indicates the summation of a variable over a series of years t (up to 20 or 30 years in the calculations)
r	Discount rate for future years (0.1 or 10% in the calculations)
*	Indicates the discounted sum of a variable; for example, $C^* = SUM\ C(t) \times (1 + r)^{(-t + 1)}$ and $BEN^* = SUM\ BEN(t) \times (1 + r)^{(-t + 1)}$

Note: The variables C, CS, CST, NUM, PREC, and BEN are all transformed into $C^*, CS^*, \ldots$, by discounted summation. For all except CS, the sum can be obtained for a single disease (i) or for all three diseases taken together.

VAC(i)	Unit cost of vaccinating one individual against one disease (i). Thus $CST(i,t) = VAC(i) \times NUM\ (i,t)$, and $CST^*(i) = VAC(I) \times NUM^*(i)$.
VAC	Summing for all three diseases gives the average implied maximum cost of vaccination. It is calculated as follows: $VAC = (BENT^* - CS^*)/NUM^*$.
EFV(i)	Effectiveness of the vaccine (i). (In the calculations it is always assumed that EFV equals 0.9 or 90%.)
SUF(i)	The probability of a person not vaccinated against target disease (i) acquiring that disease. Thus $PREC(i,t) = SUF(i) \times EFV(i) \times NUM(i,t)$, which gives $PREC^*(i) = SUF(i) \times EFV(i) \times NUM^*(i)$.
MOR(i)	The probability that an individual with disease (i) will die if not treated.
MORT(i)	The probability that an individual with disease (i) will die iftreated.
PRED(i,t)	The number of deaths prevented by vaccination, assuming those ill would receive no treatment. $PRED(i,t) = MOR(i) \times PREC(i,t)$, and thus $PRED^*(i) = MOR(i) \times PREC^*(i)$. The corresponding totals for all of the target diseases taken together are PRED(t) and PRED*.

PREDT(i,t)	The number of deaths prevented by vaccination, assuming those ill would receive treatment. PREDT(i,t) = MORT(i) × PREC(i,t), and thus PREDT*(i) = MORT(i) × PREC*(i). The corresponding totals for all of the target diseases taken together are PREDT(t) and PREDT*.
UTU(i)	Unit benefit or utility of prevention—the benefit derived from preventing one case of disease (i). Thus the benefit of vaccinating one individual is UTU(i) × SUF(i) × EFV(i).
BEN(i,t)	The benefit derived from vaccinating NUM(I,t) individuals, so that BEN (i,t) = UTU(i) × SUF(i) × EFV(i) × NUM(i,t) = UTU(i) × PREC(i,t); and hence BEN*(i) = UTU(i) × PREC*(i). The corresponding totals for all of the target diseases taken together are BEN(t) and BEN*.

Note: The net unit benefit (benefit minus cost) of vaccinating one individual is UTU(i) × SUF(i) × EFV(i) – VAC(i), and the net total benefit is [UTU(i) × SUF(i) × EFV(i) – VAC(i)] × NUM(i,t) = BEN(i,t) - CST(i,t). The same relationship is valid for NUM*(i), BEN*(i), and CST*(i).

BTR(i)	Unit cost of treatment—the cost of adequately treating one case of disease (i).
BENT	The benefit derived solely from not having to treat disease cases. Note that BENT< BEN because the former does not include all of the benefits; hence BENT(i,t) = BTR(i) × PREC(i,t), and BENT*(i) = BTR(i) × PREC*(i). The corresponding totals for all of the target diseases taken together are BENT(t) and BENT*.
D	Delay (in years) between vaccination and the hypothetical onset of disease had the vaccinated individual not been vaccinated. The correct adjustment to the benefit derived from the prevention of one case can be calculated as follows: ADJD = $(I + r)^{-D}$

(which determines whether the person is really immunized) and then by the chance that the person would become sick if unimmunized. The effectiveness of all three vaccines is estimated at 90%, while the incidences of the three diseases (per 100,000 population at risk) are estimated at 10 (with a maximum of up to 50) for meningitis, 150 for typhoid fever, and 28 for pneumonia. These figures give the likelihood of preventing a disease case by vaccinating one person a probability of 9, 135, and 25 chances per 100,000 respectively. (Only the lower estimated incidence is used for meningitis, because this reduces the benefits without affecting the costs; and if SIREVA is justified under these circumstances, it would be even more justified if the disease incidence were higher.)

The probabilities of preventing a case are shown in Table 12.4, which will be discussed later, while Table 12.3 indicates the estimated numbers of cases that would be prevented, by disease, for horizons of 20 and 30 years. By far the greatest disease prevention occurs with regard to typhoid fever,

234 • Health Economics in Development

Table 12.4 The Estimated Cost of Treatment (in Constant US$), Probability of Preventing One Case, and Implied Maximum Cost of Vaccination,[a] by Disease, Independent of the Number of Vaccinations

	MENINGITIS	TYPHOID FEVER	PNEUMONIA
Probability of preventing one case, SUF(i) × EFV (i)	9.0×10^{-5}	1.35×10^{-3}	2.5×10^{-4}
Unit cost of treatment, BTR(i)	$3,000	$584	$6,306
Implied maximum cost of one vaccination, SUF(i) × EFV(i) × BTR(i)	$0.27	$0.79	$1.58

[a]The implied maximum cost of vaccination is the value such that the cost of vaccinating one person compensates exactly for the probable cost of having to treat that individual for the disease. It is calculated by multiplying the unit cost of treatment by the probability of preventing one case. For this calculation the fixed cost of developing vaccines against the target diseases is not considered.

because of its high incidence, the discounted number of cases to be prevented totaling over 300,000. For meningitis and pneumonia the estimated figures are lower by an order of magnitude, ranging from 10,000 to 23,000 for meningitis and from 17,000 to 22,000 for pneumonia.

In some cases a person who acquires the disease will die. The likelihood of this varies greatly, depending on the disease and whether the victim does or does not receive adequate and timely treatment. With such treatment almost no one dies of typhoid fever, since the death rate is estimated at no more than 1%; and even without treatment that rate rises to only 10%. Regarding pneumonia, it is estimated that the lethality is 3% with treatment and 10% without treatment, while for meningitis the corresponding rates are estimated at 5% and 50% (4). Therefore, the numbers of deaths prevented are not proportional to the numbers of cases prevented—the risk of death depending on the particular disease involved and also varying by a factor as great as 10, depending on whether one assumes that each patient does or does not receive appropriate treatment.

Table 12.3 shows the estimated numbers of deaths that vaccination would prevent, by type of disease, and also shows the total number of deaths preventable by SIREVA. Showing these latter totals is appropriate; for although it would be incorrect to total the numbers of cases of diseases that are very different with respect to severity and danger, it is legitimate to total the resulting deaths. Depending on the horizon selected, the totals range from 40,000 to 52,000 deaths prevented if no treatment is assumed, and from 5,000 to 8,000 if it is assumed that every victim receives appropriate care.

Economic Benefit: Treatment Cost Saved

The benefits obtained by preventing one case of a disease include some that are difficult to quantify or evaluate economically, such as reduction of the patient's pain and suffering. Other benefits, although possibly less important, are easier to evaluate in economic terms; among these is the treatment cost saved as a result of not having to care for the patient. Clearly, attributing this monetary benefit to vaccination depends on an assumption that the victim would receive the treatment if he were to contract the disease. This benefit is received by the person or institution that otherwise would have to pay the treatment cost, whether the paying party is the patient or not.

Thus, one way to compare costs with benefits is to relate the cost of vaccinating one person with the expected cost of treating that individual, considering these procedures as alternatives. Obviously, this last assumption is more reasonable when the treatment results in a complete cure, without permanent injury to the patient. When the patient dies despite the treatment (which is possible with all diseases and occurs in up to 10% of pneumonia cases) or is left with significant sequelae (as can easily occur with meningitis), treatment is a very incomplete substitute for prevention.

Of course, one must compare the cost of vaccination with the expected or probable cost of care, because not all vaccinated individuals would become sick if unvaccinated. The comparison depends, therefore, on the likelihood that the vaccine would prevent a case of the disease. This likelihood, as already noted, is shown on the first line of Table 12.4; it is calculated by multiplying the effectiveness of the vaccine (EFV) against disease (i) by the probability of suffering the disease, SUF(i). This is the same logic that has been used to justify eradication of poliomyelitis, through the savings in treatment costs that would result from vaccinating virtually the entire population at risk (7).

The second line in Table 12.4 shows the average cost of providing a patient with correct and timely care, designated BTR(i). This is estimated to range from less than $600 in the case of typhoid fever to more than $6,000 in the case of pneumonia. Taken together, the likelihood of preventing a case and the cost of treating that case determine a hypothetical cost of prevention where the prevention and treatment costs would equal one another, and so the net saving from vaccination would be zero. This cost can be viewed as *the implied maximum cost* of vaccination in the sense that at any lower cost the vaccination would be less costly than the treatment.

As can be seen on the third line of the table, this latter cost, $SUF(i) \times EFV(i) \times BTR(i)$, is calculated by multiplying the probability of preventing one case by the cost of treating one case. And the cost of preventing one case is the cost of one vaccination, $VAC(i)$, divided by the probability of preventing one case with one vaccination or

$$VAC(i)/[SUF(i) \times EFV(i)].$$

On relating this expression to the cost of treatment, $BTR(i)$, one sees that where

$$VAC(i) = SUF(i) \times EFV(i) \times BTR(i)$$

there is exact equality between vaccination and treatment costs; and likewise, where

$$VAC(i) < SUF(i) \times EFV(i) \times BTR(i)$$

vaccination offers a net economic benefit. In monetary terms (see Table 12.4), the corresponding values range from $0.27 per vaccination in the case of meningitis to $1.58 in the case of pneumonia. Regarding typhoid fever, it should be noted that the low cost of treating one case of this disease is partially balanced by its high incidence in the population, so that the implied maximum cost of vaccination against typhoid fever is $0.79, or almost three times the implied maximum cost in the case of meningitis.

As has been said, until the vaccines are developed and administered on a mass scale, there can be no exact picture of vaccination cost. The interpretation of the calculations in Table 12.4 is that vaccination will be justified—through savings in treatment costs, without considering other benefits—as long as it costs no more than $0.27 per vaccination against meningitis, etc. If, for example, it were feasible to vaccinate at a unit cost of $0.10—which would cover not only the cost of the vaccine but also the cost of distributing and administering it to the population, then clearly vaccination would be highly worthwhile. In contrast, if the unit cost were $1.00, only vaccination against pneumonia would appear to be justified, assuming no other benefits were considered.

Even if one compares only vaccination and treatment, however, the calculation presented in Table 12.4 is still incomplete because the vaccines involved do not yet exist and have to be developed. This implies that the benefits, in the form of saved medical costs, would have to cover not only the costs of vaccination (costs "outside SIREVA" or CST), but also the vaccine development costs "within SIREVA" (CS). In addition, SIREVA is attempting to develop three vaccines, without the total cost of the program being attributed to one or another of these products.

The first of these conditions implies that the maximum cost allowed for vaccination is going to be less than that shown in Table 12.4, since the benefits must also cover SIREVA's vaccine development costs. The second condition (of co-production or inseparability) implies that judging the worth of each vaccine individually makes no sense, because it will be necessary to judge the entire system with respect to the average cost of vaccination against the three target diseases.

This matter can be summarized as follows: For there to be a net benefit after considering both types of costs, it is necessary that

$$BENT^* > CS^* + CST^*,$$

where BENT is the total benefit in saved treatment costs—the cost of treating one individual times the number of cases prevented. (Table 12.3 indicates the number of cases prevented, and Table 12.4 shows the unit costs of treatment.) As noted above,

$$CST^* = VAC \times NUM^*,$$

where VAC denotes the average cost of vaccination within the time interval involved. Both $BENT^*$ and CST^* must be assumed for all the target diseases, and both must also be discounted and summed over time. Then, in order for the net benefit condition to be met, it is necessary that

$$BENT^* - CS^* > VAC \times NUM^*.$$

Table 12.5 presents the corresponding calculations. Starting with the values of CS^* and NUM^* from Tables 12.1 and 12.2, respectively, Table 12.5 proceeds to list values for the three ingredients of $BENT^*$, these being the saved costs of treating each disease, and the $BENT^*$ totals for 20-year and 30-year horizons. The last entries show the 20-year and 30-year values of $BENT^* - CS^*$ and of VAC.

The figures shown indicate that over a period of 20 years some US $80.3 million, at present value, would be spent developing the three vaccines, which would be administered to the discounted equivalent of 400–506 million individuals. The disease cases prevented would represent an estimated saving of $29-$57 million for meningitis, $179 million for typhoid fever, and $106 million for pneumonia. The total benefit would amount to $313-$342 million before subtracting the costs of SIREVA itself, yielding a net benefit of $233-$262 million. After dividing this amount by the total

Table 12.5 The Average Implied Maximum Cost of Vaccination (in Constant US$) Derived from the Number of Individuals Vaccinated, Treatment Costs, and the Cost of SIREVA, for 20-Year and 30-Year Horizons

	20-YEAR HORIZON	30-YEAR HORIZON
Costs of SIREVA (CS*), in US$ millions	80.3	80.3
Total number of vaccinations (NUM*), in millions	400–506	465–591
Saving on treatment costs (BENT*), by disease, in US$ millions:		
Meningitis	29–57	35–68
Typhoid Fever	179	199
Pneumonia	106	137
Total, three diseases	313–342	370–404
Net saving, after deducting SIREVA's cost (BENT* − CS*), in US$ millions	233–262	290–324
Average implied maximum cost of one vaccination–VAC (net savings divided by the number of vaccinations), in US$	0.52–0.58	0.55–0.62

number to be vaccinated, it can be concluded that SIREVA is justified with respect to the treatment costs saved as long as the population could be vaccinated for no more than $0.52–$0.58 each. If one individual were to receive all three vaccines, the permitted cost would rise to $1.56–$1.74. Applying these same calculations to the 30-year horizon yields an average permitted cost that is greater by a few cents because the costs of SIREVA would be distributed over more years of vaccination, and so their relative weight in the total costs would be less.

Overall Benefits from SIREVA and Vaccination Costs

The exercise in the previous section fixes a value on the benefit derived from SIREVA, equating it to saved medical treatment costs, and on this basis estimates the maximum cost of vaccination that would be compatible with a net positive benefit. This procedure can be reversed by first fixing a value on the cost of vaccination and then deriving from it an estimate of the *minimum* benefits could be of any type, without being limited to the treatment costs saved. The worth of preventing a death, the value of economic production saved by preventing death or illness, the reduction of physical and emotional suffering, and other benefits could be included. In this regard, since the disease cases and deaths prevented are the most quantifiable results of vaccinating the population, it seems natural to estimate minimum benefits in terms of these concepts.

The condition that must be satisfied is

$$BEN^* > CS^* + CST^* = C^*,$$

where C^* is the total costs and BEN^* is the discounted sum of *all* the benefits (including $BENT^*$, the benefit of not having to treat those who would become ill). If we then designate the benefit or "utility" per case prevented as UTU, and the number of cases prevented as $PREC^*$, we see that for case prevention alone to satisfy the condition it will be necessary for

$$UTU \times PREC^* > C^*,$$

or equivalently,

$$UTU > C^*/PREC^*.$$

Similarly, if we designate the benefit per death prevented as UTUD, we see that for mortality prevention alone to satisfy the condition it will be necessary for

$$UTUD > C^*/PRED^*,$$

where $PRED^*$ is the number of deaths that would occur in the absence of vaccination and treatment.

The corresponding calculations appear in Table 12.6. They are limited to the 20-year horizon, since it was determined (in Table 12.5) that extension of the horizon to 30 years does not significantly affect the results. Starting with the cost of SIREVA (CS^*), numbers of cases prevented ($PREC^*$), and numbers of deaths prevented ($PRED^*$) that appear in Tables 12.1 and 12.3, Table 12.6 derives the other component of the total cost—the cost of vaccination—from the total number vaccinated (see Table 12.2), using a unit cost (VAC) first of $1 and then of $10.

The resulting total cost (C^*) is then used to calculate the benefits per case prevented (UTU). It turns out that the first VAC cost ($1) yields values quite close to those that would permit justification of SIREVA solely on the basis of medical treatment costs saved, while the second VAC cost ($10) yields values so high that the benefits per case prevented would have to be substantially greater.

The results of attributing the entire benefit to the prevention of death (UTUD) are shown in the last line of the table. Naturally, the benefit

Table 12.6 Implied Minimum Benefit per Case Prevented and per Death Prevented as a Function of the Cost of Vaccination, without Considering Patient Treatment (20-Year Horizon)

	COST OF VACCINATION (VAC)	
	US $1.00	US$10.00
Total number of cases prevented (PREC*), in thousands	332–342	332–342
Total number of deaths prevented (PRED*), in thousands	40–45	40–45
Cost of SIREVA (CS*), in US$ millions	80.3	80.3
Cost of vaccination (CST*), in US$ millions	400–506	4,000–5,060
Total Cost (C*), in US$ millions	480–586	4,080–5,140
Minimum benefit per case prevented (C*/PREC*), in US$ thousands[a]	1.4–1.7	12.3–15.0
Minimum benefit per death prevented (C*/PRED*), in US$ thousands[b]	12.0–13.0	102.0–114.2

[a]The values for the minimum benefits do not change significantly on extending the horizon to 30 years.
[b]The minimum benefit per death prevented does not attribute any benefit to preventing nonfatal disease cases.

involved would have to be much greater. Given that, on the average, approximately 10% of the untreated cases would terminate in death, the minimum benefit per death prevented would have to be some 10 times greater than the minimum benefit per disease case prevented.

For example, at a cost of vaccinating one person for $1.00, SIREVA is justified so long as an average benefit per case prevented of between $1,400 and $1,700 is obtained. This is based on the estimate that a total of $480 to $586 million at present value will be spent in order to prevent a total of some 332,000–342,000 cases of the three diseases.

The minimum necessary benefit per case rises to $12,000 if the cost of vaccination is fixed at $10; it does not rise in the same proportion as the unit cost of vaccination because the actual expenditures of SIREVA are not affected. It should be noted, however, that when the cost per vaccination is $1.00 or greater, these fixed costs of developing the vaccines are of relatively little importance compared to what would have to be spent applying them. Therefore, justifying the vaccination is almost equivalent to justifying SIREVA, if there is no other way to develop the vaccines that is less costly than the system proposed.

The final calculations (on the last line of Table 12.6) are somewhat artificial, since they attribute benefits only to the prevention of death. This establishes a kind of "maximum of the minimum" for the necessary benefit justifying SIREVA—at levels on the order of $12,000 in the first instance and $100,000 in the second.

It should be noted, however, that benefits from cases prevented and deaths prevented can be combined. That is, it is appropriate to compensate for the costs of SIREVA through any combination of benefits per death prevented and benefits per non-mortal case prevented that satisfies the relationship

$$[UTU \times (PREC^* - PRED^*)] + (UTUD \times PRED^*) > C^*,$$

where UTU, the benefit per case prevented, would be substantially less than UTUD, the benefit per death prevented. The expression $(PREC^* - PRED^*)$ refers to the number of individuals who would become sick but not die if they were not vaccinated.

Both the calculations in Table 12.5 and those in Table 12.6 implicitly assume that the benefit associated with vaccination occurs immediately, simultaneously with vaccination. This assumption is justified if the target disease would probably attack an individual within a short time or never, as is typically true of the diseases targeted by the Expanded Program on Immunization, which affect primarily children (although those diseases can appear several years later than the normal age of immunization). If, on the other hand, a large proportion of those affected will typically become ill many years after vaccination—and if the vaccine retains its effectiveness for many years, so that it is not necessary to repeat the vaccination frequently— the calculations that were just presented can prove optimistic or overly favorable because they do not consider the interval between the moment of vaccination and the probable moment of becoming ill.

The greater this interval, the longer the benefits are delayed relative to the costs, and the greater they have to be to compensate for this delay. The way to adjust for the possible optimistic bias is to estimate the average interval between vaccination and illness in years (D) and then to discount the benefits with respect to the costs by the factor $(1 + r)^{-D}$, utilizing the same discount rate(r) applied elsewhere.

By way of example, Table 12.7 shows the sizes of adjustments associated with several different intervals of delay. Thus, if the benefits were delayed an average of 10 years, they would have only 38.55% of the value they would have if they appeared immediately. The rest of the table shows the impact of these adjustments on parameters calculated in Table 12.5 (the implied maximum cost of vaccination) and Table 12.6 (the implied

Table 12.7 The Effects of Adjusting for the Delay between Vaccination and Disease Onset upon the Implied Maximum Cost of Vaccination and upon the Implied Minimum Benefits of Preventing a Disease Case, in Constant US$

	DELAY (D), IN YEARS				
	0	5	7	10	15
Adjustment factor (AJUD)	1.000	0.7513	0.5132	0.3855	0.2394

Effects on the implied maximum cost of vaccination (original value multiplied by the adjustment factor), in US$:

	0	5	7	10	15
By disease, without counting the cost of SIREVA:					
Meningitis	0.27	0.20	0.14	0.10	0.06
Typhoid fever	0.79	0.59	0.41	0.30	0.19
Pneumonia	1.58	1.19	0.81	0.61	0.38
Average for SIREVA (all costs for three diseases):					
Minimum	0.52	0.39	0.27	0.20	0.12
Maximum	0.58	0.44	0.30	0.22	0.14

Effects on the implied minimum benefit per case or death prevented (original value divided by the adjustment factor) in US$ thousands:

	0	5	7	10	15
Per case prevented; vaccination cost = US$1.00:					
Minimum	1.4	1.9	2.7	3.6	5.8
Maximum	1.7	2.3	3.3	4.4	7.1
Per death prevented; vaccination cost = US$1.00					
Minimum	12.0	16.0	23.4	31.1	50.1
Maximum	13.0	17.3	25.8	33.7	54.3

minimum benefit per case prevented). As can be seen, a relatively short delay such as five years does not greatly affect the results; but longer delays such as 15 years produce much stronger effects—resulting in multiplication or division of the benefits or costs by a factor of four or more.

Conditions Justifying SIREVA and Sensitivity of the Results

It has not been possible to carry out a closed and precise cost-benefit analysis for the proposed system at this time because its exact costs are not known and there is no consensus on how to evaluate its benefits. Therefore, the analysis presented in the above sections is based on the relationships between these unknown elements, rather than upon definitive values assigned to them. For every level of benefit per disease case prevented, there is a corresponding maximum value for vaccination cost that still leaves a positive net benefit. And conversely, each unit cost of vaccination establishes a minimum for the total benefit of preventing one case (or one death) compatible with net benefit from the system. The corresponding calculation of these two ways of presenting the relationship, shown in Tables 12.5 and 12.6, can be considered the essence of the present analysis.

In general terms, the calculations allow one to conclude that SIREVA would be justified by its benefits if it were possible to develop the vaccines at the costs estimated for the different options and later to administer them to the population at a unit cost of half a dollar or less. At this level of expense, the system could generate sufficient treatment cost savings to compensate for the entire cost of developing and administering the vaccines. Even if it were assumed that in the absence of SIREVA not all the disease victims would receive adequate and timely treatment, the system would still be justified if benefits per disease case prevented were found to have a minimum average value between $1,000 and $2,000. Part of these benefits would derive from prevention of deaths; and if it were estimated that it would be worth spending somewhat more than $10,000 on the average to avoid one death, this benefit alone would justify the proposed expenditures.

How sensitive are these results to variations in the different parameters considered in the analysis? If a small change in one of them causes the system to stop appearing viable, then the proposal would be risky, given the great uncertainty in the estimated values. The analysis has taken into account all of the following factors: the cost of SIREVA itself (development of the vaccines), the cost of vaccinating one individual against one disease, the cost of treating one case of a disease, the number of individuals vaccinated, the effectiveness of the vaccine, the incidence of the target diseases, their lethality with and without treatment, the discount rate, and the possible delay between a person's age at vaccination and age at disease onset. For some of these factors, where less is known or it is possible to anticipate a large variation, an explicit sensitivity analysis has been made. For other elements the probable variation in the factor and the consequences for the results have been discussed briefly. To terminate this analysis, the sensitivity of the conclusions to the elements mentioned are discussed below. In general, there is no reason for hesitation in exploring the possibilities of changes on the order of 10% or 20%; the concern is whether one ought to anticipate variations of an order of magnitude or so in the system's estimated yield.

Actual cost of SIREVA. The importance of these costs depends on whether they are large or small relative to the total vaccination cost. If they are small, they can vary considerably without greatly affecting the total cost. For example, at the maximum cost calculated for which vaccination is justified in terms of medical costs saved, the costs of SIREVA itself are one-third or less of the total costs, so that they could be underestimated by 50% and still not have a great effect upon the system's yield.

Aside from an increase in SIREVA's cost, the relative importance of this element would be greater if the unit cost of vaccination were less than estimated. In that case, however, the reduced cost of administering the vaccines would compensate for a large increase in the cost of developing them. For example, consider the calculation in Table 12.5 and assume that the element CS* (the cost of SIREVA) were doubled. Then CS* would be $160.6 million, but the system would still be justified for any vaccination cost VAC less than $0.36.

Vaccination cost. As has been seen, this element is crucial; and if one calculates benefits only in terms of medical expense saved, this imposes a clear maximum value upon vaccination cost that is at the level of $0.50. Increasing the unit vaccination cost to $1.00 requires greater total benefits; and if the vaccination cost were as high as $10.00, the saving in treatment cost by itself would be far too small to justify the system. Hence, everything depends on whether vaccination is achieved at a reasonable cost, and the proposal assumes that result. To achieve such a result, it may be necessary to incorporate the new vaccines into the EPI; that way the logistic costs would be minimal, and little more would have to be spent beyond that needed to cover the costs of manufacturing the vaccines.

Treatment cost. It is assumed that this element is relatively well known, so that its possible variations need not be taken into account. In any case, if the scheme of analysis utilized in Table 12.6 is adopted to consider the *total* value of the benefits per case prevented, this treatment cost variable becomes less important—because it then constitutes only one component of the benefits, and perhaps not the greatest of them.

Number of individuals vaccinated. This factor is crucial for the simple reason that the costs of developing the vaccines must be offset by administering them to a large enough number of people. If it were not for this fixed development cost, the calculations in Table 12.4 could be applied directly; SIREVA's justification would be independent of the scale of operation; and the average cost of vaccination could be as high as $0.78. Comparing these calculations with the values listed in Table 12.5 shows how the need to compensate for the system's fixed costs affects the results. Both the maximum cost of vaccination and the implied minimum benefit vary directly with changes in the number of individuals covered by SIREVA. It is assumed, however, that the estimates of this latter number would not be in error by more than a small percentage.

Vaccine effectiveness. This factor cannot vary much because a vaccine would not be administered if it were not at least 70% or 80% effective. Therefore, vaccine effectiveness cannot affect the results very much. It would only be important if after expending millions of dollars on SIREVA, the effort failed and effective vaccines were not obtained; the entire proposal is based upon confidence that this will not occur.

Disease incidences. The estimates of these parameters are very low, the maximum value used being 150 cases per 100,000 inhabitants for typhoid fever. Any increase would only make the system more viable; and so the only consideration should be whether the incidences of the target diseases have been overestimated. Changes in the probability of getting sick affect the benefits the same way that changes in the number of people vaccinated do, but without affecting the cost—unless one could, at lower risk, vaccinate fewer people. The epidemiological studies constituting part of the system's development will help to define these risks better and so to adjust, if necessary, the projected extent of mass vaccination.

Disease lethality. This factor cannot vary much, even admitting that it is not known exactly. In any case, it is important only if one desires to attribute a specific benefit to the prevention of death, for there would clearly be great benefit in preventing each of the target diseases even if no one died of them.

Discount rate. As has already been discussed, this element cannot vary by more than a factor of two, and its influence affects the distribution of costs and benefits over time without affecting their comparison in a given year. Therefore, the results of the analysis are not considered very sensitive to the rate selected.

Delay between vaccination and prevented illness. As Table 12.7 shows, this factor becomes a matter of concern if it is necessary to assume a delay of more than about half a decade. If the disease presents risks over the entire human life-span, part of the benefit is left unperceived in terms of present value. Even though the probable impact of such a delay would only divide the benefits in half, this circumstance would require an average benefit twice as large, or a cost of vaccination half as large, as those projected.

It is clear that the justification, or lack thereof, of a project such as the one being analyzed depends upon how all of these elements are evaluated, and upon the values assigned to prevention of disease and death—values outside the purely economic realm. The present analysis only attempts to trace a dividing line between the possible combinations of factors, known or estimated, that show whether or not SIREVA would be viable in the sense of producing benefits that more than compensate for its costs of development and application, within a reasonable span of time.

References

1. Institute of Medicine, National Academy of Sciences. New vaccine development: establishing priorities (vols 1 and 2). Washington, DC: National Academy Press; 1986.
2. World Health Organization. Research and development in the field of vaccines; progress report by the Director General. Executive Board, 87th Session, Geneva: 21 November 1990. (Document EB87/6).
3. World Health Organization, UNICEF, and UNDP. Declaration of New York: the children's vaccine initiative. New York: 10 September 1990.
4. Organización Panamericana de la Salud. SIREVA: estudio de factibilidad, sistema regional de vacunas para los países de América Latina y el Caribe. Unpublished document. Washington, DC: 1990.
5. Drummond MF, Stoddard GL, Torrance GW. Methods for the economic evaluation of health care programs. Oxford: Oxford University Press; 1986.
6. May RM. Ecology and population biology. In: Warren KS, Mahmoud A, eds. Tropical and geographic medicine, 2nd ed. New York: McGraw-Hill; 1990. (Chapter 19).
7. Musgrove P. Is polio eradication in the Americas economically justified? Bull Pan Am Health Org. 1988; 22(1): 1–16.

CHAPTER 13

Cost-Effective Malaria Control in Brazil

Introduction

Although the Malaria Eradication Program of the Ministry of Health in Brazil had succeeded by the late 1970s in freeing the majority of the country from malaria transmission, it was unable to contain the rapid spread of the disease in the Amazon Basin. By June 1984, that region, including nine of the country's 26 states, accounted for 97% of all reported malaria cases, with high fatality rates. Between 1977 and 1988 the coefficient of mortality (deaths per 100,000 population) in the Amazon more than quadrupled. The enormous extent of the region, the substantial and hard-to-trace migration into and within it, and the existence of numerous transient and dispersed settlements, rendered ineffective the traditional eradication strategy based on active case detection for treatment and eliminating the vector through widespread use of insecticides. At the end of 1983, there were 280,000 reported cases of the disease, but with the number of people infected rising by 40,000 every year, incidence reached almost half a million four years later.

In 1986 the Government of Brazil requested World Bank technical and financial assistance to develop an Amazon Basin Malaria Control Project (known as PCMAM from its Portuguese title) to support the national program. The project was expected initially to be conducted over four years and cost US $200 million; it became effective in September 1989 and closed in June 1996, with a final cost of US $133.7 million, of which US $72.9 million was financed by a Bank loan (The World Bank, 1996). The project was originally aimed at getting the malaria outbreak in the Amazon Basin under

Co-authored with Dariush Akhavan, Alexandre Abrantes and Renato d'A. Gusmão. Reprinted from *Social Science and Medicine*, Vol. 49, No. 3, Copyright 1999, with permission from Elsevier Science.

control, preventing the spread into uninfected areas and strengthening institutional capacity. Like the program which it supported, the project consisted of vector control (application of insecticides in dwellings and fogging of high-risk communities), entomological surveillance, treatment, special efforts for disease control in indigenous areas and information, education and communication (IEC).

This paper provides an evaluation of the project during the interval of almost seven years corresponding to the World Bank loan. (There is no distinction between the Bank project and the pre-existing government program, so this is not an evaluation of the marginal contribution of the Bank-financed project.) A first estimate of the results of the project is provided by an extensive evaluation by one of the authors (Akhavan, 1996); some of these initial findings have been published in a World Bank evaluation (The World Bank, 1996) as well as in a government summary publicizing the results of this and a parallel project for the control of three other endemic diseases in northeastern Brazil (National Health Foundation, 1996). A more detailed state-by-state analysis was conducted later (Akhavan, 1997). The present study provides projections of three key variables in the absence of the project: the incidence, severity (proportion of *falciparum*) and lethality (case fatality rate) from malaria in the Amazon Basin during the period 1989–1996, and summarizes the estimated savings in lives, morbidity (cases) and disability-adjusted life years (DALYs) from malaria control.

Old and New Strategies for Fighting Malaria

Prior to 1991, malaria control was the responsibility of a semi-autonomous federal agency, the Superintendency for Public Health Campaigns (Superintendência para Campanhas de Saúde Pública, SUCAM), which carried out nation-wide malaria and endemic disease control campaigns through a workforce of 40,000. The agency was noted for its strong staff and line organization and had an excellent record in sustaining endemic disease control programs in remote areas, under very difficult conditions. Municipalities and States had no responsibility for endemic disease control. Hospitals and outpatient clinics affiliated with the National Health System (known from 1990 on as the Sistema Único de Saúde, SUS) did not treat malaria patients, who were routinely referred to SUCAM facilities or staff.

In 1991, SUCAM was extinguished and its functions transferred to a new agency, the National Health Foundation (Fundação Nacional de Saúde,

NHF), which went through a period of political and organizational turbulence, largely as the result of rapid decentralization (Brazilian Institute of Municipal Administration 1996a, b). This created something of a vacuum in the field, seriously undermined staff morale and jeopardized the operational capacity that had characterized SUCAM. These difficulties added to the natural complexity of controlling malaria by the traditional strategy of vector control everywhere that ecological conditions favored transmission and were only overcome starting in 1993.

Mortality from malaria had begun to fall in 1989, the year the project went into effect, and over the next three years fell to only half the peak level registered in 1988. Nonetheless, by 1992 it became apparent that this approach was inadequate, because the number of cases continued to grow. Beginning in late 1992, therefore, the Brazilian control program was reoriented in line with the new Global Malaria Control Strategy (World Health Organization, 1993a) emphasizing disease management, which replaced an earlier effort (World Health Organization, 1978) to define control strategies following the failure of eradication efforts. The Pan American Health Organization (PAHO) collaborated with the NHF in this first large-scale implementation of the new approach (World Health Organization, 1993b). A key element of the change was to stratify the population by risk and concentrate control activities accordingly (Pan American Health Organization, 1991). The project was refocused, with greater emphasis on early diagnosis and immediate and intensive treatment of patients, while the use of pesticides was more closely targeted to municipalities and communities with high malaria incidence.

The first of these changes aimed to prevent human deaths rather than kill mosquitoes, while the second emphasized killing those mosquitoes most likely to carry malaria, particularly the form, *P. falciparum*, which causes nearly all deaths (Miller and Warrell, 1990). This targeting drew on epidemiological studies in the 1980s (Sawyer and Sawyer, 1987; Cruz Marques, 1988), which had shown that malaria was concentrated in relatively few municipalities, often characterized by new and inaccessible agricultural settlements or wildcat gold mining areas (*garimpos*), where insecticide spraying or fogging is typically ineffective (Najera *et al.*, 1993, Table 13.2). In 1985, two states, Rondônia and Pará, accounted for over 73% of all cases in the region and were the source of infection of most cases identified in the rest of the country. In 1986, only 22 out of the 458 municipalities of the Amazon Basin accounted for 60% of reported cases of malaria. However, resources were not being allocated according to incidence: some 70% of the government program's resources were being used in areas with only 3% of cases. It is much easier to misallocate preventive efforts than treatment; in consequence, the cost-effectiveness of prevention is likely to vary much more, and may reflect more waste, than that of case treatment. This pattern shows up when cost-effectiveness is estimated separately for each of the nine Amazon Basin states (Akhavan, 1997).

The project developed new diagnosis and treatment protocols and carried out an extensive training program for health care professionals in SUS hospitals and ambulatory clinics, which also received supplies of antimalarials. As a result, parasitoscopic diagnosis efficiency improved by 20%; the number of hospital admissions for malaria, which had increased from about 10,000 in 1984 to 20,000 in 1988, rose to more than 50,000 in 1992 and 1994 before declining slightly; and the better care led to a 55% fall in the estimated overall case fatality rate.

One paradoxical effect of the changed strategy was initially to increase the apparent number of *municipalities* in every category of risk of infection, as Table 13.1 shows. In 1992, the Annual Parasitological Index (API), an indicator of the probability of contracting malaria, was available for only 80% of the 654 municipalities considered to have the ecological potential for transmission. Improvements in the NHF information system brought coverage up to 98% by 1993. To improve reporting and allow for greater focus on the highest-risk areas, the number of posts equipped for microscopic diagnosis of malaria was expanded from 405 in 1992 to 1,095 at the end of the project in 1996.

At the same time that more municipalities appeared to be at high risk, the concentration of disease control efforts greatly reduced the number of

Table 13.1 Population (Millions) and Number of Municipalities by Risk of Malaria Transmission, Based on API, 1988–1995

| | RISK CATEGORY | | | | | |
| | HIGH RISK (API≥50) | | MODERATE RISK (50≥API≥10) | | LOW RISK (10≥API≥1) | |
YEAR	POPULATION	MUNICIPALITIES	POPULATION	MUNICIPALITIES	POPULATION	MUNICIPALITIES
1988	21.78		26.41		16.82	
1989	22.79		25.19		17.26	
1990	23.85		25.79		17.70	
1991	21.66		24.75		16.56	
1992	22.09	63	25.24	103	16.88	188
1993	5.40	86	13.08	127	56.83	192
1994	5.86	105	4.41	113	10.33	174
1995	3.15	126	6.06	111	4.91	159

people at moderate or high risk (API > 10.0 positive blood slides per 1,000 population), by reducing the risk in the more populous municipalities. Focusing surveillance in those areas meant that between 1992 and 1995 coverage by prompt diagnosis expanded from 11 to 34% of the population at greatest risk, among whom the share of positive blood slides went from 24 to 42%. Increases in coverage and in positivity rates as a result of this concentration of effort were also observed for the populations at moderate, low and no risk of transmission. Collection of blood slides is more cost-effective when rates are high than when they are low and collection is maintained only to monitor eradication efforts (Najera *et al.*, 1993).

The change in treatment strategy meant giving each suspected malaria case presenting to any level of the program (any facility, from a health post to a hospital) a complete chloroquine treatment (25 mg/kg of body weight). This is still regarded as efficacious for *P. vivax* infections and partly effective in reducing the clinical symptoms of *P. falciparum* disease. Mefloquine, a synthetic antimalarial which allows effective early treatment of *P. falciparum* even in ambulatory settings, was also licensed and distributed widely in SUS. As a result of earlier and more aggressive treatment, 20% fewer *falciparum* cases required hospitalization in 1995 than in 1992. Mixed infections, patients who had both *falciparum* and *vivax*, were classified and treated as *falciparum* because of its greater severity.

Directly Observed Results: Malaria Cases, Severity and Program Expenditures

Figure 13.1 shows how the malaria epidemic began to come under control. The upper panel relates the total number of blood slides positive for malaria to the total expenditure on malaria control by SUCAM and subsequently by NHF; the lower panel shows the same information, but for *P. falciparum* only. These are all directly observed variables, involving no estimations or assumptions. The numbers in Figure 13.1 differ slightly from those used to estimate the total health benefits and the total costs of the program, which do involve assumptions. First, they refer to the entire country rather than just the Amazon Basin, but as indicated earlier, nearly all cases occur in that area, as do more than 90% of expenditures, so the difference is small. Second, the number of positive slides differs slightly from that of new cases, because two or more slides may be taken to confirm a diagnosis; the difference is small, probably of the order of 3%. Third, salaries of staff are not

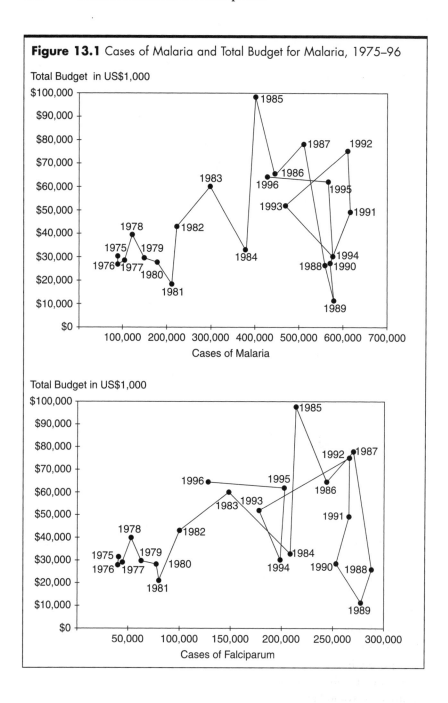

Figure 13.1 Cases of Malaria and Total Budget for Malaria, 1975–96

attributed to the malaria control program, so expenditures in Figure 13.1 reflect only other recurrent spending. However, salaries are small compared to those other costs, which do include the transportation and per diem expenses of field workers. Finally, expenditures are in current US dollars, without adjustment for US inflation or discounting to present value as is done when adding up total project costs. For year-by-year comparisons the second adjustment is irrelevant and that for price changes in the US is small.

What Figure 13.1 principally shows is that the epidemic expanded in every year from 1975 to 1989, irrespective of the level of SUCAM's expenditures on control and also of whether spending rose or fell from one year to another. Large annual increases in expenditure do seem to have slowed the expansion, but never enough to reverse the epidemic; in any case, the association is not robust. In 1987–1989, the program all but collapsed, with expenditure falling from US $78 million to just over US $10 million. With the implementation of PCMAM and the infusion of World Bank funds, the budget quickly returned to almost the 1987 level and the number of cases declined slightly in 1990 and then increased and stabilized in 1991–1992. There was a sharp reduction in cases in 1993, despite a decreased budget, and after a rebound in 1994, stabilization and further decline in 1995–1996, when the number of positive slides fell back to the level of a decade earlier at the same or lower expenditure. The pattern is very similar for cases of *P. falciparum* alone, through 1988; from 1989, the *falciparum* epidemic was better contained than that of malaria in general, with little or no rebound in 1991–1992 and then a return to the level of 1983. This appears to reflect the concentration of vector control in areas of high *falciparum* incidence and the consequent reduction of severity since the project adopted the revised control strategy.

Methods: Estimating Illness, Lives and Disability-Adjusted Life Years Saved

The malaria control program produced health gains partly by preventing cases, some of which would have ended in death while the rest produced only short-term morbidity, and partly by treating cases, particularly by preventing deaths from *P. falciparum* infection. The estimate of health benefits from vector control begins with the projected incidence of cases of malaria and proceeds through the expected severity (share of *falciparum* in total cases) and lethality (case fatality rate) to derive the losses in deaths and morbidity that would have occurred in the absence of the program.

To facilitate comparison with other diseases which also cause both death and disability, the savings in deaths and episodes of illness are then converted to estimates of DALYs saved, using the same disability weights for non-fatal conditions, the annual discount rate and the age weights as in the WHO-World Bank estimates of the global burden of disease (World Bank, 1993; Murray, 1994, 1996). On a scale in which perfect health is 1.0 and death is zero, the health loss due to *vivax* illness is assigned a weight of 0.22 and the disability from non-fatal *falciparum* is given a weight of 0.375, reflecting the greater severity of *falciparum* morbidity. The future is discounted at a constant annual rate of 3%, which matters greatly for death (the number of discounted years lost to premature mortality is much less than the number of calendar years or potential years of life lost) but has no effect on short-term morbidity. Finally, the value of life at each age, or the loss from illness or death at that age, follows an age-weighting function which starts at zero, rises rapidly to a maximum of 1.525 at age 25, and then declines slowly and almost exponentially toward zero. An extensive explanation of these subject parameter values (Murray, 1996) and a sensitivity analysis of the effects of variation in the discount rate and the age weights (Murray *et al.*, 1994) have been published and are not reviewed here.

Between 1980 and 1988 the observed coefficient of incidence (new cases per 100,000 population) rose steadily from 1,311 to 3,461, or from a little more than 1% of the population being sick with malaria each year, to almost 3.5%. Since this increase was nearly linear, it was assumed that the same constant rate of increase would prevail in 1989–1996 as in 1980–1988, reaching a level of 5,611 or more than 5.5% of the population suffering an attack of malaria in one year. This is still well below what expert malariologists consider to be saturation levels of incidence, and there is no evidence in the Brazilian data of a cyclic or other non-linear pattern. When incidence is projected separately for each state in the Amazon Basin, the sum of projections rises very rapidly in 1988–1991 before leveling off at a coefficient of more than 7,000 per 100,000 population, more than double the assumption used here for the region as a whole (Akhavan, 1997).

In contrast to the projection, the observed coefficient declined in most years and never exceeded 3.5% of the population. Applying the difference between observed and projected incidence to the population of the Amazon Basin gives the number of cases estimated to have been prevented each year. This is the major source of uncertainty in the analysis; where treatment is concerned, the only uncertainty is how many cases may have occurred and gone untreated, but that does not affect the cost-effectiveness of the program. For 1996, only half the cases treated or estimated to have been prevented are counted, because the project ended in June of that year and the calculation of costs runs through only half the year.

The observed severity, or share of malaria cases due to *falciparum*, reached a peak of 55% in 1986 and stayed in the range 0.53–0.55 from 1984 to 1987. It is assumed that in the absence of the program, severity would have remained at that peak; again, this number appears to be below the saturation equilibrium level. *Falciparum* parasites become available to infect vectors in only about 5.5 days and the incubation period before symptoms begin is 12–14 days; for *vivax* parasites these intervals are, respectively, 8 and 11–12 days.

In consequence of the shorter time before transmission is possible and the longer time when a person is infected but asymptomatic, the basic reproductive rate of *falciparum* is at least double that of *vivax*, which means that severity may saturate at around 60–65%.

Finally, 10% of those sick with *falciparum* are assumed to die within a short period if not treated, while the other 90% of sufferers from *falciparum* and all those infected with *P. vivax* are assumed to be sick for 4 months (0.333 years) before recovering fully. This period is so short that discounting the future at 3% makes almost no difference. Age-weighting, however, makes a substantial difference, because most deaths occur in adolescence or early adulthood, when the weights used to calculate DALYs are near the maximum value of 1.525. The result is that the discounted and age-weighted interval of illness is 0.433 years, longer than the calendar interval; being sick at those ages is worse than average, for any level of disability. Some DALYs may also be lost in the future, because *vivax* malaria can cause relapses (Miller and Warrell, 1990). Since little is known about their frequency or severity, except that they tend to become briefer and less severe, this possible contribution to morbidity is ignored here and discussed briefly later.

The probability of dying from *falciparum* malaria in the absence of any treatment is the third key parameter in the estimate of deaths prevented by the control measures, and therefore in the cost-effectiveness of those measures, and requires some discussion. Beneson (1997, p. 350) states that "prompt treatment is essential, even in mild cases, since irreversible complications may appear suddenly; case-fatality rates among untreated children and non-immune adults exceed 10% by a considerable margin". There are few other published estimates of this rate, so several expert malariologists were consulted (Mangabeira da Silva, 1996; Campbell, 1997; Collins, 1997; Hoffman, 1997); all agreed that 10% is a conservative assumption, their own estimates ranging as high as 30–45%. Case-fatality rates in the range of 25 to 45% have been observed in Africa, but greater malnutrition and higher incidence among children, who are particularly susceptible, may make malaria more lethal there than in Brazil. Death in 10% of untreated *falciparum* cases appears unlikely to overstate the disease risks or the cost-effectiveness of control measures in the Amazon Basin.

Applying the disability weights (0.375 for *falciparum* and 0.22 for *vivax*) to the interval of illness leads to a loss of 0.162 DALYs per non-fatal, untreated case of *falciparum* and 0.095 per case of *vivax*. The total health gain from preventing this temporary disability is some 226,000 DALYs. Although only 5.5% of malaria sufferers would die (10% of the 55% infected with *falciparum*), they would account for a much greater health loss. The average age at death from malaria during this period was 14 years, at which age life expectancy under the life table assumptions employed (Murray, 1994) is still 66 years. Age-weighting and discounting reduce this to 36.27 DALYs lost per death. This value is not very sensitive to the assumption that life expectancy is as high as 66 years, because both discounting and age-weighting greatly reduce the importance of years far in the future. (Varying the assumption about life expectancy would, of course, affect other measures of health gain such as potential years of life lost.) The total health gain from preventing deaths through vector control is about 3.65 million DALYs, and the total gain from prevention of cases, including reduced morbidity, is 3.88 million DALYs, as shown in the bottom line of Table 13.3. Both because of mortality and because morbidity is more severe, nearly all this gain comes from controlling P. *falciparum*; control of P. *vivax* accounts for less than 2% of the total.

Estimating the DALY gains from treatment is simpler, because only the observed incidence and severity matter; these determine the number of sufferers from P. *falciparum* who, if not treated, would have a 10% chance of dying of the disease. Lethality *with* treatment is much lower; it reportedly declined from 0.72 to 0.40% between 1980 and 1988 and continued to fall to 0.15% in 1996. However, it is suspected that overall mortality is substantially under-reported (Akhavan, 1996): some people die without getting treatment and some die even after receiving ambulatory care and these deaths may not be registered. The only study of under-reporting of hospital deaths, undertaken in the state of Rondônia in 1985 (Fiusa Lima and da Silva, 1988), found that actual deaths were 38.8% higher than reported. To take account of this, it is conservatively assumed that on average throughout the period, 0.78% of treated *falciparum* cases would have died; this applies the 1985 under-reporting estimate to the average reported lethality in 1980–1988 (1.388 times the average of 0.40 and 0.72 is 0.78), with no allowance for subsequent decline.

Lives saved by treatment are therefore the number of people sick with *falciparum*, discounted to present value, times the difference between untreated and treated lethality, 9.22% (10.0 − 0.78). Savings from reduced morbidity are similar to those gained by prevention, with the difference that it is assumed the typical patient would still suffer for 12.5 days, 10 before seeking treatment and 2.5 days from the start of treatment to the cessation of symptoms. (This is a very conservative assumption; if malaria victims received care within a few days, the health gain from treatment would be substantially larger.) This means that the interval of health gain drops from 0.333 to 0.299 years, or 0.388 years when discounted and age-weighted. This does not apply to those *falciparum* sufferers saved from death, because they would probably have died quickly rather than being sick for four months.

Tables 13.2 and 13.3 show how the estimates of health gains were constructed, following the assumptions described earlier. The total number of malaria cases which occurred despite the control efforts was 4.1 million, or 3.7 million in 1996 present value. The total number of cases prevented is estimated as 1.97 million, equivalent in present value to 1.83 million cases. Expressing the estimates in present value terms takes account of their occurrence over a span of almost eight years, so as to match the discounted cost estimates. The assumptions about severity and lethality imply that 101,000 more people would have died of malaria had it not been for the preventive component of the project and another 1.7 million would have been sick.

The effectiveness of concentrating vector control in areas where *P. falciparum* was most prevalent shows in the substantial reduction of reported *falciparum* cases, while the number of *P. vivax* cases fluctuated with no trend. Under the assumption about lethality described above, treatment resulted in saving almost 130,000 lives and in reducing the morbidity caused by 1.27 million cases of *falciparum* and 2.19 million cases of *vivax*. All together, some 5.5 million people benefited from the control program, either as patients or because they did not get malaria. Table 13.3 summarizes the savings in lives, cases and DALYs, according to the type of malaria and whether the gains came from prevention or treatment.

The total gain measured in DALYs was 8.97 million: 5.08 million from treatment or 31% higher than the gain of 3.88 million DALYs from prevention. Fully 93% of this health gain derived from preventing deaths, with almost no difference in the share between prevention and treatment.

Table 13.2 Estimated Cases, Lives and DALYs Saved by Preventing and Treating Malaria, 1989–1996. Cases Prevented and Cases Reported and Savings in Lives and Morbidity

YEAR	COEFFICIENT OF INCIDENCE/100,000 PROJECTED	OBSERVED	DIFFERENCE	POPULATION (MILLIONS)	CASES PREVENTED	PRESENT VALUE	CASES REPORTED FALCIPARUM	VIVAX	PRESENT VALUE FALCIPARUM	VIVAX
1989	3730	3478	252	16.04	40,409	32,856	264,469	293,318	215,037	238,494
1990	3999	3331	668	16.40	109,526	91,726	243,622	302,473	204,030	253,316
1991	4268	3183	1085	16.78	181,813	156,833	212,592	320,710	183,384	276,647
1992	4536	3308	1228	17.12	210,207	186,766	237,576	328,703	211,083	292,048
1993	4805	2741	2064	17.48	360,760	330,147	171,698	397,435	157,128	363,709
1994	5074	3089	1985	17.84	354,115	333,787	192,505	358,603	181,454	338,018
1995	5343	3082	2260	18.20	411,329	399,349	198,671	362,354	192,884	351,800
1996	5611	2388	3224	18.56	299,208	299,208	63,871	157,729	63,871	157,729
Totals										
Old Strategy 1989–92					541,955	468,181	958,259	1,245,204	813,534	1,060,505
New Strategy: 1993–96					1,425,412	1,362,491	626,745	1,276,121	595,337	1,211,256
Entire Period: 1989–96					1,967,367	1,830,672	1,585,004	2,521,325	1,408,871	2,271,761

Severity of Cases Prevented: 0.55 falciparum and 0.45 vivax

Number of Cases Prevented: 1,006,870 ... 823,803 ... 1,267,983 ... 2,271,761

Outcome if Untreated: 0.10 Dead ... 0.90 Sick ... 1.00 Sick ... 0.10 Dead ... 0.90 Sick ... 1.00 Sick

Lethality if Treated: 0.0078

Difference (Gain from Treatment): 0.0922

Saving in Lives: 100,687 ... 129,897

Saving in Cases (Reduced Morbidity): 906,183 ... 823,803 ... 1,267,983 ... 2,271,761

258

Table 13.3 Estimated Cases, Lives and DALYs Saved by Preventing and Treating Malaria, 1989–1996. Conversion of Savings in Lives and Cases to Disability-Adjusted Life Years

| | SAVINGS FROM PREVENTION | | | SAVINGS FROM TREATMENT | | | TOTAL (OR AVERAGE) |
| | FALCIPARUM | | VIVAX | FALCIPARUM | | VIVAX | |
	DEATHS	NON-FATAL CASES	NON-FATAL CASES	DEATHS	NON-FATAL CASES	NON-FATAL CASES	
Saving in lives	100,687			129,897			230,584
Saving in cases		906,183	823,803		1,267,983	2,271,581	5,269,550
Disability weight	1.00	0.375	0.22	1.00	0.375	0.22	(0.314)
Duration in years							
Unadjusted	66.19	0.333	0.333	66.19	0.299	0.299	[3.07]
Discounted and age-weighted	36.27	0.433	0.433	36.27	0.388	0.388	[1.91]
DALYs per case (disability weight X adjusted duration)	36.27	0.162	0.095	36.27	0.146	0.085	(1.62)
Total DALYs	3,651,917	147,141	78,475	4,711,364	185,126	193,084	8,967,107
	Total from prevention: 3,877,533			Total from treatment: 5,089,574			

259

This concentration reflects the fact that on average, a beneficiary of the control program saved only three years of life, or less than two DALYs, but someone who would otherwise have died gained 66 years of life and 36 DALYs. In contrast to the results for preventing cases, where *falciparum* was nearly twice as important as *vivax*, the gains from reducing morbidity through treatment are almost equally divided between *falciparum* and *vivax*: this reflects the success of the program in reducing severity when it would otherwise have remained constant.

Estimating Program Costs and Cost-Effectiveness

The estimated health gains just described were derived from both prevention and treatment, so the costs attributable to malaria control include both kinds of expenditures. Spending on prevention (vector control) was partly through the World Bank project (PCMAM), all of which occurred in the Amazon Basin, and partly through the NHF malaria control program, which operated in the whole country; it is estimated that 92% of those expenditures occurred in the Amazon. Capital investment and non-salary recurrent expenditures (insecticides, travel costs and per diem for field workers) of the NHF program were directly recorded and charged to the program. Labor costs are not budgeted to the control program; they were estimated from the number and type of personnel needed for vector control operations and salaries for each level of worker.

Expenditure on treatment was partly for hospitalization and partly for ambulatory care and includes the cost of diagnosis. The number of hospitalizations rose from 7,000 or less before 1987, to over 20,000 in 1988 and to a peak of over 53,000 in 1992. As treatment improved, the average length of stay fell abruptly from around 5.5 days before 1992, to about 4.4 days from that year on. The number of ambulatory treatments rose from around 30,000 in 1984–1985 to around 500,000 in 1992–1995. The cost of ambulatory care was estimated by assuming that all reported but non-hospitalized cases were treated, and applying to each patient the costs of four ambulatory visits, two blood tests and the required medications, equal to US $18.70. 'Costs' of both hospital and ambulatory care are what the federal health system (SUS) paid for treatments, and understate true costs to the extent that they do not cover salaries of staff of the Ministry of Health or NHF, or the capital cost of existing hospitals and clinics. (New investments are included in the cost estimates.) SUS tariffs are believed to be significantly above or below true costs for many interventions, but the fact that it was possible to expand treatment rapidly in the program suggests that for malaria, federal payments were adequate to cover at least all recurrent costs. Since the more severe hospitalized cases were almost entirely due to *falciparum*, ambulatory patients were assumed to be infected with *falciparum* in only 44% of cases and with *vivax* in the rest. However, the cost of medication is only 8% of the cost of ambulatory treatment, so differences in which drugs are administered, reflecting differences in the distribution of the two kinds of malaria, have little effect on total costs.

All financial information was initially reported in Brazilian currency and underwent three transformations to make the numbers comparable in present value. These are (i) conversion from Brazilian currency to US dollars in the current year, using the average of the official buying and selling rates for the dollar in that year; (ii) adjusting to 1996 US dollars by the US GDP deflator for the current year; and (iii) discounting to 1996 present value at 3% per year. These adjustments remove, so far as possible, the effect of inflation in the US and the much more rapid inflation (prior to 1995) in Brazil, and express all values in constant US dollars of 1996 purchasing power. The discount factor (3%) is the same used to discount numbers of cases prevented or occurring, and therefore to discount the sums through times of lives and DALYs saved.

For recurrent expenditures (largely or entirely consumed in the same year as purchased), only these adjustments are necessary. Capital expenditures require two further adjustments. The first is to incorporate depreciation over the useful life of the capital. This is assumed to be constant (linear), with different lifetimes for the three categories; 25 years for buildings, 10 years for vehicles and 5 years for equipment. The cost to the program in a given year is then the value of the capital investment divided by the useful life. Capital entirely depreciated during the project has its cost entirely attributed to the program; capital with a useful life extending beyond 1996 is charged to the program only for 1996 and prior years. The second adjustment is to take account of the opportunity cost of capital. In a stable economic environment this would be given by the rate of interest, but the high inflation in Brazil prior to stabilization in 1994 led to very high nominal and even real interest rates. The US Prime Rate was therefore used as a better approximation (although possibly an underestimate) of the true opportunity cost of capital.

All these steps are shown in the initial evaluation (Akhavan, 1996). Table 13.4 summarizes the final result: expenditures in discounted dollars of 1996

Table 13.4 Costs of the Malaria Control Program, 1989–1996 (Thousands of 1996 US$, Discounted at 3% for 1989–1995) and Cases Treated (Thousands of Hospital or Ambulatory Patients)

CATEGORY	1989	1990	1991	1992	TOTAL 1989-1992	1993	1994	1995	1996	TOTAL 1993-1996	TOTAL 1989-1996
Prevention	123,443	86,636	53,221	77,210	340,510	63,559	34,688	63,878	22,986	185,111	525,620
Investment	6,374	11,800	6,548	10,239	34,961	3,423	4,897	4,726	813	13,859	48,820
Buildings	2,863	1,168	634	1,143	5,808	1,123	240	305	99	1,767	7,575
Vehicles	1,499	611	312	464	2,886	267	348	82	17	714	3,599
Equipment	2,012	10,020	5,602	8,632	26,266	2,033	4,309	4,340	697	11,379	37,646
Recurrent	117,069	74,836	46,673	66,971	305,549	60,136	29,791	59,152	22,173	171,252	476,800
Salaries	10,013	9,407	8,191	8,768	36,379	18,315	7,708	10,669	5,496	42,188	78,567
Other	107,057	65,429	38,482	58,203	269,171	41,821	22,083	48,483	16,677	129,064	398,234
Treatment	10,269	11,096	12,474	13,310	47,149	12,258	13,951	12,238	4,940	43,387	90,534
Hospital	2,132	2,987	4,566	4,789	14,474	4,889	5,159	2,818	1,089	13,955	28,430
No. cases	22.8	28.5	43.2	53.5	148.0	48.6	52.4	42.3	15.7	159.0	307.1
Unit Cost	93.47	104.98	105.72	89.44	97.80	100.53	98.42	66.57	69.22	87.77	92.57
Ambulatory	8,136	8,109	7,908	8,521	32,674	7,369	8,792	9,419	3,851	29,431	62,105
No. cases	535.0	517.6	490.1	512.7	2,055.4	430.5	498.7	518.7	269.7	1,717.6	3,773.1
Unit cost	15.21	15.67	16.14	16.62	15.90	17.12	17.63	18.16	14.28	17.13	16.46
Total costs	133,712	97,732	65,694	90,520	387,658	75,817	48,640	76,115	27,926	228,498	616,155

value. Overall, from 1989 through the end of PCMAM in mid-1996, the malaria control program is estimated to have cost US $616.2 million, divided between US $525.6 million for vector control and related activities and US $90.5 million for treatment. About 30% of treatment cost was for hospitalization and 70% for ambulatory care. Preventive expenditures included US $48.8 million of investment in buildings, vehicles and equipment, US $78.6 million in salaries and US $398.2 million for all other operating costs, including the costs of preparing and managing the project, insecticides, fuel, training and staff travel and per diem.

Since the program is estimated to have prevented some 1.83 million cases of malaria (in present value), it also eliminated the need to treat that number of episodes of disease. Assuming the same distribution between hospitalization and ambulatory care as in the cases actually treated, the unit cost per patient would have been the same, averaging US $22.19 over the period. This implies a total saving in treatment expenditures of US $41.5 million. (Savings would of course be smaller, if some of the prevented cases would not in fact have been treated had they occurred.) Subtracting that from estimated actual expenditures leaves a net cost of the malaria control program of US $574.6 million, and implies that for every dollar spent on prevention, seven cents were saved in treatment.

Comparing the costs to the estimated saving in lives gives overall cost-effectiveness estimates of US $2,672 per life saved, or US $2,492, taking account of savings in treatment costs. These ratios ignore the much smaller health gains from reduced morbidity. If costs and gains are compared for prevention alone, the ratio is higher, because prevention accounted for the bulk of the costs but saved slightly less than half the total lives; the corresponding figures are US $5,200 per life saved without taking account of treatment cost savings and US $4,808, counting those savings. In contrast, treatment appears to have cost only about US $700 to save a life. The last three columns of Table 13.5 summarize the results just presented for cases prevented and lives saved, which are based on the most plausible assumptions discussed in the text and incorporated in Tables 13.2, 13.3 and 13.4. When the savings in morbidity are included and compared to lives saved, using DALYs as the composite measure, the result is an overall cost-effectiveness of US $69 per DALY (US $64, if based upon the cost net of savings in treatment). As with lives saved, the cost is higher for prevention, with ratios of US $136 and US $125, respectively, as savings are or are not taken into account. With treatment, it cost less than US $18 to save one disability-adjusted life year.

Discussion

Since the project helped to introduce a major change in malaria control strategy halfway through the period analyzed, Table 13.5 presents the cost-effectiveness results separately for 1989–1992 and for 1993–1996, considering only lives saved by preventing or treating cases of *falciparum*. The same assumptions about incidence are used as for the analysis of the whole period 1989-1996, because the control efforts in 1989–1992 do not appear to have had much effect on incidence. The cost of saving a life by treatment rose 25% between the early and the later years, presumably as a result of more aggressive care (a higher share of patients hospitalized). However, the cost of saving lives by prevention fell dramatically when preventive efforts were more sharply focused against *falciparum*, from about US $13,000 to between US $2,000 and US $2,500. This improvement in efficiency did not come at the cost of the absolute number of lives saved by preventing cases, which nearly tripled between one period and the other, while expenditures on prevention were cut almost in half. The overall result was to reduce the average cost of preventing a death from nearly US $4,000 to under US $2,000, or as low as US $1,500 when savings in treatment cost are considered. (These savings increased in line with the gain in efficiency of preventive efforts.) This analysis validates the new control strategy and illustrates how wasteful the preventive program previously was, which explains why the epidemic had continued to expand.

In the absence of the preventive effort, incidence was projected to rise linearly and rather rapidly, which could lead to an over-estimate of the number of cases prevented and therefore of lives saved by prevention. (This would not, of course, affect the estimate of how many lives were saved by treatment.) By the same token, the assumption of increasing incidence could bias the comparison between the early and later periods; higher projected numbers of cases in the later years might magnify the apparent gains from the revised strategy. In Table 13.6, incidence is subjected to sensitivity analysis, to see how much overall cost-effectiveness, and the contrast between 1989–1992 and 1993–1996, depend on assumptions as to how many cases of malaria would have occurred in the absence of the project. Expenditures on the program are assumed to be the same as those actually recorded or estimated.

Incidence is first assumed to remain constant at the level of 1988, or 3,361 per 100,000 population. So far as the period 1993–1996 is concerned, this is roughly equivalent to assuming that if the control strategy had not changed, the earlier strategy would have maintained incidence constant at about the 1989–92 level, so that any gains in the later period would

Table 13.5 Cost-Effectiveness of Saving Lives from *Falciparum*, 1989–1992, 1993–1996 (Discounted Present Values). Most Plausible Assumptions (from Tables 13.2 and 13.3 and Text)

CONCEPT	OLD STRATEGY, 1989–1992			NEW STRATEGY, 1993–1996			ENTIRE PERIOD, 1989–1996		
	PREVENTION	TREATMENT	TOTAL	PREVENTION	TREATMENT	TOTAL	PREVENTION	TREATMENT	TOTAL
Cost (thousand US$)	340,510	47,149	387,658	185,111	43,387	228,498	525,620	90,534	616,155
Expenditures prevented (thousand US$)	10,014	—	10,014	31,501	—	31,501	41,515	—	41,515
Net cost (thousand US$)	330,496	47,149	377,644	153,610	43,387	196,997	484,105	90,534	574,639
Falciparum cases prevented	257,500	—	257,500	749,370	—	749,370	1,006,870	—	1,006,870
Falciparum cases treated	—	813,534	813,534	—	595,337	595,337	—	1,408,871	1,408,871
Lives saved	25,750	75,007	100,757	74,937	54,890	129,827	100,687	129,897	230,584
Cost per life saved (US$)									
Based on total cost	13,224	629	3,847	2,470	790	1,760	5,220	697	2,672
Based on net cost	12,835	629	3,748	2,050	790	1,517	4,808	697	2,492

Table 13.6 Cost-Effectiveness of Saving Lives from *Falciparum*, 1989–1992, 1993–1996 and 1989–1996 (Discounted Present Values). Sensitivity Analysis: Cost-Effectiveness of Prevention Related to Projected Incidence (No Change in Severity or Lethality)

CONCEPT	INCIDENCE CONSTANT AT 1988 LEVEL, 3,461			INCIDENCE RISING STEEPLY, TO 7,500		
	1989–1992	1993–1996	1989–1996	1989–1992	1993–1996	1989–1996
Cost (thousand US$)	340,510	185,111	525,620	340,510	185,111	525,620
Expenditures prevented (thousand US$)	983	10,262	11,245	15,955	52,989	68,944
Net cost (thousand US$)	339,527	174,849	514,375	324,555	132,122	456,676
Falciparum cases prevented	45,971	443,848	489,819	745,912	2,291,918	3,037,830
Lives saved	4,597	44,385	48,982	74,591	229,192	303,783
Cost per life saved (US$)						
Based on total cost	74,072	4,170	10,731	4,565	808	1,730
Based on net cost	73,858	3,939	10,501	4,351	576	1,503

represent the improvement over the previous strategy rather than gains with respect to no program at all. The results of the comparison are that if there had been no danger of an expanding epidemic, only 49,000 lives would have been saved by prevention and the cost of saving a life would have been correspondingly much higher, US $10,731. Since fewer cases prevented would also mean smaller savings in treatment, only US $11.2 million, there is little difference according as total or net cost is used. The most striking result, however, is that since observed incidence hardly changed in 1989–1992, very few lives would have been saved under the old strategy, and the cost per life saved would have been as high as US $74,000. Nearly all the gain would have come under the revised strategy, with a cost per death prevented only slightly higher, around US $5,400, than with rising incidence. The apparent improvement in cost-effectiveness therefore is not an artifact of assuming that the epidemic would have continued to grow.

All the indications are that, on the contrary, Brazil faced an explosive epidemic of malaria and that the reorientation and concentration of prevention was crucial in bringing it under control. Applying the projected incidence in each state separately (Akhavan, 1997) would only strengthen this conclusion. If in the absence of the project the coefficient of incidence had risen steadily to 7,500 (which is slightly slower than the sum of state-level projections), the preventive component of the project would have saved 304,000 lives and the overall cost-effectiveness would have been between US $1,503 and US $1,730 per life saved. Savings in treatment cost might also have been much larger, US $568.9 million, although it is less plausible that all this saving could have been realized, since it would imply that Brazil had the capacity to treat an additional three million cases of *falciparum* malaria alone. Assuming very rapid growth in cases is also more favorable to the old strategy, which would have prevented 75,000 deaths during 1989–1992 even without reducing observed incidence, bringing the cost per life saved down to about US $4,500. Even so, the revised strategy continues to appear more cost-effective, saving lives through preventing cases for only US $600 to US $800.

Of the three crucial parameters in those calculations, only the severity or share of *falciparum* cases was both readily observable and nearly constant during the interval of the project. There is therefore no apparent reason to evaluate the project using different estimates of severity. The other important parameter is the case fatality rate, or lethality, for untreated *falciparum*, since that determines the health gains from both treatment and prevention. As indicated above, that rate was assumed to be 10%, but expert opinion suggests that it could be substantially higher. Table 13.7 shows the outcome

Table 13.7 Cost-Effectiveness of Saving Lives from *Falciparum*, 1989–1996 (Discounted Present Values). Sensitivity Analysis: Untreated *Falciparum* Case Fatality Rate 25 or 5%

CONCEPT	PREVENTION	LETHALITY 25% TREATMENT	LETHALITY 5% TOTAL	PREVENTION	TREATMENT	TOTAL
Cases prevented	1,006,870	—	1,006,870	1,006,870	—	1,006,870
Cases treated		1,408,871	1,408,871		1,408,871	1,408,871
Lives saved	251,718	324,744	576,463	50,344	64,949	115,293
Cost per life saved (1996 US$)						
Based on total cost	2,088	279	1,069	10,441	1,394	5,344
Based on net cost	1,923	279	997	9,616	1,394	4,984

of assuming that 25% of untreated *falciparum* sufferers would have died: the number of lives saved increases to 593,000, with the result that the cost of saving a life falls to about US $1,000. Under this assumption, which may be implausibly high for Brazil although not elsewhere, there would be large increases in the gains from both prevention and treatment, and no significant change in their relative cost-effectiveness. The exercise is repeated with a lethality rate of 5% which, holding constant the assumptions about expenditure and cases prevented and treated, simply means one-fifth as many lives saved and five times as high a cost per death prevented. Even so, most of the gain from controlling malaria comes from preventing deaths; if the case fatality rate were near zero, malaria would not be the dreaded disease that it is.

How much did changes in each of the three crucial parameters contribute to the total health gain from the project? Since mortality occurs almost exclusively when a person is infected with *P. falciparum* and dies of it, the probability of death can be expressed as $D = I \times S \times L$, where I is incidence, S is severity and L is lethality. The program apparently succeeded in reducing all three of these factors; how the total effect on mortality is partitioned among them depends on the assumptions about what would have happened to each factor. Comparing deaths actually registered (indicated by R) with the number of deaths to be expected (E) in the absence of the program as estimated in Tables 13.2 and 13.3, using the most plausible assumptions, $D_R / D_E = (I_R/I_E)(S_R/S_E)(L_R/L_E)$.

Expressing this in logarithms,

$$\log D_R - \log D_E = (\log I_R - \log I_E) + (\log S_R - \log S_E) \\ + (\log L_R - \log L_E).$$

The share of mortality reduction attributable to reduction in incidence is then

$$(\log I_R - \log I_E)/(\log D_R - \log D_E)$$

and similarly for reductions in severity and lethality. Table 13.8 shows this calculation.

The coefficient of incidence in 1996 was only 2,388 per 100,000 population, against the projected level of 5,611. Case treatment has not been shown to have any major effect on transmission (Miller and Warrell, 1990), so the reduced incidence is probably due entirely to vector control. However, early, widespread and aggressive treatment of *falciparum* in the Amazon may have reduced the likelihood of mosquitoes acquiring new

Table 13.8 Effects of Reduced Incidence, Severity and Lethality on Mortality Reduction

	COEFFICIENT OF INCIDENCE/ 100,000	SEVERITY (SHARE OF P. FALCIPARUM)	LETHALITY	COEFFICIENT OF MORTALITY
I. Comparison to projections				
Observed (R) 1988	3461	0.51	0.0040	7.0604
Observed (R) 1996	2388	0.29	0.0015	1.0388
Projected (E) 1996	5611	0.55	0.0033	10.1840
Observed/projected 1996	0.4256	0.5273	0.4545	0.1020
Log difference 1996	−0.8543	−0.6400	−0.7885	−2.2827
Contribution to mortality reduction	0.3742	0.2804	0.3454	1.0000
II. Comparison to initial situation				
Observed 1996/observed 1998	0.6900	0.5686	0.3750	0.1471
Log difference 1988–1996	−0.3711	−0.5645	−0.9808	−1.9164
Contribution to mortality reduction	0.1936	0.2946	0.5118	1.0000

infections and thereby contributed to reducing severity, which at 0.29 *falciparum*, was barely half the expected level of 0.55. It is not known what level of treatment coverage might be required for a significant effect.

Observed lethality among those treated had been declining slowly for some years before the project began and was expected to reach 0.33% by 1996; instead, it fell to 0.15%. (Data on actual mortality are incomplete, but since it is only the ratio of lethalities that matters for this decomposition, a constant proportional underestimate makes no difference to the result. If however the project led to reduced under-reporting, then the apparent increase in cases and deaths is overstated and the project was correspondingly more effective in containing the epidemic than it appears.)

Combining these factors suggests that mortality in 1996 was only 10% as high as would have been expected: 191 deaths instead of 1,872 (coefficient of mortality of 1.04 per 100,000 population instead of 10.18). This means that 37.42% of the saving in mortality was attributable to reduced incidence, 28.04% to the decline in severity and 34.54% to improvements in survival. This decomposition gives great weight to incidence, because it was expected to keep on rising in the absence of the project. Lethality is given less weight because it was expected to continue declining slowly. Nonetheless, reducing the likelihood of death once people were infected with *falciparum* seems to have accounted for more than one-third of the total saving in lives.

The same calculation can be performed comparing actual levels in 1996 not with those projected for that year, but with the starting point of 1988. This amounts to assuming that the three factors would have maintained their 1988 levels, in the absence of the project. Over the eight years, incidence fell from 3,461 to 2,388 per 100,000; severity from 0.51 to 0.29; and lethality from 0.40 to 0.15 (constant proportional under-reporting of deaths would not affect the ratio of these rates and therefore would not change the logarithmic differences). These figures imply that deaths per 100,000 population should have fallen to 14.7% of the 1988 level. The number of deaths is registered only through 1995, so it is not known whether the death rate in 1996 matched this decline exactly. Table 13.8 shows the coefficient of mortality consistent with these levels of incidence, severity and lethality; it fell from 7.06 to 1.04.

On this comparison, reduced incidence accounted for only 19.4% of the reduction in deaths, decreases in severity for 29.5% and improved survival for the largest share, 51.2%. As indicated above in the methodological discussion, these assumptions are much less plausible than those used in Tables 13.2 and 13.3; there is no reason to believe that incidence, which had been increasing dramatically before the project started, would not have continued rising. Even with assumptions that give less weight to prevention, however, reducing overall malaria incidence and particularly cutting down the share of *falciparum* cases, accounts for almost half the saving in lives. The fact that treatment appears to have been more cost-effective, on average, than prevention, does not reduce the importance of vector control as a public health measure. And both assumptions about what would have happened to incidence coincide in showing the value of concentrating preventive efforts against *falciparum*, since reduced severity accounted for close to 30% of the overall mortality reduction.

Morbidity results when a person is infected by *P. vivax*, or is infected by *P. falciparum* but does not die. The probability of non-fatal morbidity is then

$$M = I \times (1 - S) + I \times S (1 - L), \text{ which is equal to } M = I \times (1 - (S \times L)).$$

Reducing incidence obviously makes the same contribution to lessened morbidity as it does to reduced mortality, whatever is assumed about incidence in the absence of the project, but the effects of reduced severity and lethality interact and cannot be decomposed as for deaths. In fact, reducing lethality *increases* morbidity, if survivors are sick for a longer interval than those who die. In any case, since morbidity from *falciparum* is more severe than that from *vivax*, simply adding the probabilities of being sick from one or the other does not capture the expected health damage. Table 13.8 therefore does not partition the reduction in morbidity among the three factors.

In summary, the most plausible estimate of the total gain from both vector control and treatment is 1.83 million cases prevented, 230,000 lives saved and a total saving of 8.97 million DALYs. This health benefit is divided about equally between prevention and treatment (43 to 57%), but very unequally between mortality and disability (93 to 7%) and, because *falciparum* causes nearly all malaria deaths, between *falciparum* and *vivax* (97 to 3%). This last distinction is an underestimate of the gains from controlling *vivax*, to the extent that this form of malaria causes relapses in the years immediately following the initial attack. Such relapses usually become less severe with time. Taking account of their contribution to morbidity, therefore, would probably not raise the gains from *vivax* control above 5% of total health benefit. (This estimate corresponds to supposing relapses in three successive years, of the same duration as the initial attack but with the disability weight declining linearly from 0.22 to 0.02 as each relapse is less severe than the one before.)

With respect to mortality versus morbidity, malaria resembles some other diseases such as measles, which present a risk of death but seldom cause long-term disability among survivors. It is clear *a priori* that most of the health gain from a control program will come from preventing deaths, but whether that will be more easily or cheaply accomplished by preventing cases or by treating them, depends on the particular setting and on how well prevention is focused. The experience of the Amazon Basin program also shows that the choice is not only between preventing cases in general, and treating, since there are much greater gains to preventing a case of one strain of malaria than of the other. This is evident in the substantial contribution to reduced mortality of reductions in the share of *falciparum* infections. Previous estimates of the cost-effectiveness of malaria control programs have been made mostly in Africa and Asia and have shown a wide range of costs per DALY which depend strongly in each country on the case-fatality rate (Najera *et al.*, 1993, Table 13.3). The cost estimated here, US $64–69 per DALY, is low compared to the majority of these calculations. It falls at about the median cost-effectiveness of 52 interventions, both public health and clinical, for which some estimate could be made at the time of the project (Jamison, 1993, Table 1A.6). Only a few earlier estimates concern malaria programs that include both vector control and chemotherapy, and from the available information it appeared that case treatment was generally much more costly per year of healthy life saved than vector control measures (Jamison, 1993, Tables 1A.3 and 1A.5). The results for the Amazon Basin suggest, in contrast, that a large share of the total health gain can be achieved by treating patients, and that this need not lead to a very high cost per DALY. In fact, treatment can be a significantly cheaper way to save lives and healthy years. This will be true in particular where P. *falciparum* is prevalent and where frontier conditions, both ecological and social, limit the effectiveness of vector control by insecticide spraying and fogging unless it is sharply targeted. It is easy to waste resources on prevention, with consequent low cost-effectiveness, and reducing that waste by concentrating efforts yields a very high gain. In the case of the Amazon Basin, this is evident in the better cost effectiveness in 1993–1996, after the change in control strategy, than during 1989–1992, when preventive efforts were more diffuse and cost much more per life saved. The most cost-effective control efforts will probably always include both components, in proportions that depend on the distribution and severity of malaria.

References

Akhavan, D., 1996, Análise de Custo-Efetividade do Programa de Controle da Malária na Bacia Amazônica (PCMAM), relatório final, 18 de novembro. National Health Foundation and United Nations Development Program, Brazil.

Akhavan, D., 1997, Cost-Effectiveness Analysis of Malaria Control and Treatment in the Brazilian Amazon: lessons in Strategy. Operations Evaluation Department, the World Bank, Washington, DC.

Beneson, A.S., 1997. Manual para el Control de las Enfermedades Transmisibles, 16th Edition. Pan American Health Organization, Washington, DC (Scientific Publication No. 564).

Brazilian Institute of Municipal Administration (Instituto Brasileiro de Administração Municipal, IBAM), 1996a. Análise do Modelo Gerencial do PCDEN. IBAM, Brazil.

Brazilian Insitute of Municipal Administration (Instituto Brasileiro de Administração Municipal, IBAM), 1996b. Gestão de Políticas Públicas: O Projeto de Controle da Malária na Bacia Amazônica (PCMAM). IBAM, Brazil.

Campbell, C., 1997. Personal communication. Department of Public Health, Faculty of Medicine, University of Arizona, Tucson, AZ.

Collins, W., 1997. Personal communication. Malaria Unit, Centers for Disease Control, Atlanta, GA.

Cruz Marques, A., 1988. Main Malaria Situations in the Brazilian Amazon, SUCAM, Brazil.

Fiusa Lima, J., da Silva, M.A., 1988. Estudo sobre sub-registro de mortalidade por malária em Rondônia, Brasil. In: XXIV Congresso da Sociedade Brasileira de Medicina Tropical, Manaus, 28 February-3 March.

Hoffman, S., 1997. Personal communication. Director, Malaria Program, US Navy, Washington, DC.

Jamison, D.T., 1993. An Overview. In: Jamison, D.T., Mosley, W.H., Measham, A.R., Bobadilla, J.L. (Eds.), Disease Control Priorities in Developing Countries. Oxford University Press, Oxford. pp. 3-34.

Mangabeira da Silva, C.J., 1996. Personal communication. Malaria Control Program of the National Health Foundation, Brazil.

Miller, J.H., Warrell, D.A., 1990. Malaria. In: Warren, K.S., Mahmoud, A.A.F. (Eds.). Tropical and Geographic Medicine. McGraw-Hill, New York, pp. 245-264.

Murray, C.J.L., 1994. Quantifying the burden of disease: the technical basis for disability-adjusted life years. In: Murray, C.J.L. Lopez, A.D. (Eds.). Global Comparative Assessments in the Health Sector: Disease Burden, Expenditures and Intervention Packages. World Health Organization, Geneva. pp. 3-19.

Murray, C.J.L., 1996. Rethinking DALYs. In: Murray, C.J.L., Lopez, A.D. (Eds.). The Global Burden of Disease, World Health Organization, Geneva, pp. 1-89.

Murray, C.J.L., Lopez, A.D., Jamison, D.T., 1994, The global burden of disease in 1990; summary results, sensitivity analysis and future directions. In: Murray, C.J.L., Lopez, A.D. (Eds). Global Comparative Assessments in the Health Sector: Disease Burden, Expenditures and Intervention Packages. World Health Organization, Geneva, pp. 97-138.

Najera, J.A., Liese, B.H., Hammer, J., 1993. Malaria. In: Jamison, D.T., Mosley, W.H., Measham, A.R., Bobadilla, J.L. (Eds.), Disease Control Priorities in Developing Countries. Oxford University Press, Oxford, pp. 281-302.

National Health Foundation (Fundação Nacional de Saúde, FNS), 1996. Relatório de Avaliação: Divulgação de Resultados, Projecto de Controle de Doenças Endémicas no Nordeste, PCDEN [e] Projecto de Controle da Malária na Bacia Amazônica, PCMAM. Ministry of Health, Brazil.

Pan American Health Organization, 1991. Epidemiological stratification of malaria in the region of the Americas. Epidemiological Bulletin of the Pan American Health Organization 12 (4), pp. 1-7.

Sawyer, D., Sawyer, D., 1987. Malaria on the Amazon Frontier: Economic and Social Aspects of Transmission and Control. CEDEPLAR, Federal University of Minas Gerais, Belo Horizonte.

The World Bank, 1993. World Development Report 1993; Investing in Health. Oxford University Press for the World Bank, New York.

The World Bank, Social and Human Development Group, Latin America and the Caribbean Regional Office, 1996. Implementation Completion Report: Brazil,

Amazon Basin Malaria Control Project, Loan Number 3072-BR. The World Bank, Washington, DC.

World Health Organization, 1978. Malaria Control Strategy. Report by the Director General, A31/19. World Health Organization, Geneva.

World Health Organization, 1993. A Global Strategy for Malaria Control. World Health Organization, Geneva.

World Health Organization, 1993. Implementation of the Global Malaria Control Strategy, Technical Report Series No. 839. World Health Organization, Geneva.

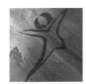

CHAPTER 14

Do the Poor in Brazil
Pay More for Food?

Acknowledgments

Cláudio Castro provided the original inspiration for this project. For help-
ful comments on a previous paper derived from this study, thanks are due to
Clóvis Cavalcanti, Dirceu Pessoa, Hélio Moura, Sónia Lessa, and Yony
Sampaio.

Malnutrition, Poverty, and Food Prices

Research on food consumption and nutritional status in Brazil, based primarily on the large, nationwide Estudo Nacional da Despesa Familiar
(ENDEF) survey of 1974–75, appears to have established that protein-
calorie malnutrition is widespread in the country, and that it is due
principally to poverty rather than cultural or educational factors.[1] Dietary
knowledge and habits do help account for malnutrition, especially among
very young children, but many families' incomes are simply too low to purchase an adequate diet, even if nutrients were obtained at minimal cost and
were adequately distributed among family members. Both malnutrition and
poverty are concentrated in northeastern Brazil and are found among urban
squatter populations as well as in rural areas.

Under these conditions, the prices of basic foodstuffs are of fundamental importance: incomes are low only in relation to prices. If the poor pay

Co-authored with Osmil Galindo. Reprinted, with permission, from "Do the Poor
Pay More? Retail Food Prices in Northeast Brazil," *Economic Development and Cul-
tural Change* 37(1), October 1988, pp. 91–109. ©1988 by The University of
Chicago. All rights reserved.

more for their food than they need to, or more than other consumers, then some part of poverty and malnutrition could be eliminated by enabling or persuading them to buy at lower prices. What may be called the "ideology of malnutrition" in Brazil includes a number of hypotheses about food prices and their role in malnutrition and poverty, [2] some of which are examined in the research reported here. These hypotheses include the following:

1. Food prices are systematically high because of a combination of inadequate storage facilities, high transport costs, and monopsony or monopoly in food marketing, which exploits both farmers and retailers and involves a large number of intermediaries.

2. Poor consumers typically patronize the most expensive retailers, the very small establishments (*varejistas*) whose costs are high because of small volume, shortage of working capital, and ease of exploitation by middlemen who may be the only source of credit as well as of foodstuffs. These establishments are presumed not to compete in price with larger and more modern retailers, such as supermarkets and the "mini-markets" that resemble supermarkets but offer a more limited range of foods, usually excluding those needing refrigeration.

3. If the poor patronize these high-cost retailers, it is presumably because there are compensating advantages. Location is one: the small retailers are widely distributed in poor neighborhoods, saving their customers lengthy trips to the better-off neighborhoods where supermarkets tend to locate. Two other potential advantages are the possibility of buying on credit and of buying in fractional amounts: a handful of rice instead of a full kilogram, or as much manioc flour as the customer has cash to buy.

4. If the poor customers could buy their food for less, without giving up the advantages that compensate them for high prices, they would buy appreciably more food, particularly calorie-rich basic foodstuffs such as rice, beans, sugar, and manioc flour. Thus lower food prices would reduce malnutrition and would not simply constitute an income transfer to be spent on other goods.

These hypotheses range from the most general (that all food prices are higher than they should be) to the most specific (that in some transactions, the poor pay more because they receive a service without which they could not buy at all). The first two hypotheses are partly contradictory, differing as to whether all or only part of the food marketing system is inefficient. And the third hypothesis is necessary to explain why, if the second one is true, the high-cost small retailers have not all been driven out of business. Some such hypothesis is necessary to sustain the view that poor consumers are rational in their food buying and that their problem is poverty rather than ignorance or foolishness. The fourth hypothesis is also "pro-consumer" in this sense.

Together, these ideas about food prices suggest the importance of several variables: location (within individual towns or cities and between one town and another), wholesaling practices (number and type of intermediaries and conditions of purchase by retailers), type of retailer and conditions of sale to final consumers (including the provision of credit and the prevalence of fractional purchases). There has been rather little research on these issues, and much public policy seems simply to have taken one or another hypothesis for granted. The government has invested heavily in roads and in food storage and marketing facilities in order to reduce food costs, with apparent success,[3] although there has been no differential favorable effect on the poor. All customers appear to have benefited equally from increases in market efficiency. The second, third, and fourth hypotheses together are used to justify a subsidy of 11 basic foodstuffs, the Projecto de Abastecimento de Alimentos Básicos em Áreas de Baixa Renda, or PROAB, which operates only in poor neighborhoods, only in large cities of the Northeast, and only through the traditional small retailers. The government's defense of this program, however, does not rest on estimates of high price elasticities, but on the greater ease and lower cost of administration of public assistance when individual clients need not be identified and on the "respect" for consumers' preferences implicit in allowing them to spend their food money as they please rather than giving them fixed amounts of specified foodstuffs, as occurs in two other major nutrition programs.[4] The subsidy program has operated since 1978; starting in 1985, the government launched a much larger program that similarly operates only through small retailers but that aims to lower prices purely by rationalizing the market, without using subsidies.[5]

There are estimates, based on the 1974–75 ENDEF nationwide household survey data,[6] that price elasticities for basic foodstuffs among the poor are in fact very high, so that even small price reductions would have substantial consequences for consumption.[7] More recent research with the same data suggests that these estimates are biased because they are aggregated over income levels and over regions of Brazil where food habits differ. Disaggregated estimates for the Northeast alone yield appreciably lower price elasticities and higher income elasticities.[8] It remains true, however, that the highest price elasticities characterize carbohydrates, so that rice and sugar are the foods for which a subsidy is most justified.

These previous investigations consider the effects of public policy on the general level of food prices, or the supposed effects on consumption and nutrition of reducing those prices, but they do not directly confront the hypothesis that the poor pay more for their food than they need to, or that high food prices are associated with particular retailers or particular selling practices. A partial exception is a study of food marketing in Curitiba, in southern Brazil, which found that poor consumers are not tied to the traditional *varejistas* but also patronize supermarkets and other vendors in search of the lowest prices.[9] In part, the scarcity of relevant research is due to the attention to temporal changes in food prices, which were very rapid until the monetary reform and price stabilization plan that were introduced in March 1986. During 1985, for example, the national consumer price index maintained by the Instituto Brasileiro de Geografia e Estatística, referring to households with incomes of between one and five minimum wages, rose by 228%. The consumer price index for Recife increased by essentially the same amount (230%). Food prices increased slightly faster than other prices during the year. Price data are collected only in major cities, which limits spatial comparisons to those between states or regions of Brazil, and while data are obtained from different types of retail establishments, these are not published separately. All price index data refer to cash purchases of standard quantities of foodstuffs, so they do not allow any test of the third hypothesis stated above.

The June 1985 Northeast Food Price Survey

To study the other dimensions of basic food prices, a survey was conducted in June 1985 by the Fundação Joaquim Nabuco (FUNDAJ), which publishes the monthly consumer price index and other economic indicators for the metropolitan area of Recife, with financial support from the Instituto Nacional de Alimentação e Nutrição (INAN) of the Ministry of Health and with technical assistance from the Pan American Health Organization. To reduce the effects of inflation on price differences between towns surveyed at different times, all prices were collected in a 2-week interval. June turned out to be the lowest inflation month of 1985 in the Recife price index, with an increase of only 5.41%, versus a monthly average that year of 10.46%. Thus, during the fieldwork, food prices probably rose, on average, no more than 3%. Price differences of 10% or more (our limit for economic importance) therefore are most unlikely to reflect only inflation. The survey was conducted in three state capitals (Recife, Fortaleza, and Teresina), six medium-sized cities in those and three other states, and 10 small towns, one or two in each of the six states. A total of 498 retail establishments were surveyed, of which the majority (295) are small outlets in poor neighborhoods. In the three state capitals (where some of these are in neighborhoods served by the PROAB subsidy) and in the large and medium-sized cities, neighborhoods classified as non-poor were also surveyed (in the small towns, no such distinction is possible). Table 14.1 shows the distribution of establishments by city size, neighborhood, and type, including small numbers of supermarkets, mini-markets, and stalls or booths in traditional public markets or "fairs." The sample of outlets is not proportional to the numbers of different types of establishments so as to include as many supermarkets and mini-markets as possible (typically all those existing in the smaller towns). Neither is the sample proportional to volume of purchases; in the absence of a household survey, there is no information on where different classes of consumers shop. Consequently, price averages across different types of establishments are not reported here, as they would need to be weighted.

Table 14.1 Sample Size (Number of Retailers) by City Size, Type of Neighborhood, and Type of Establishment

TYPE OF NEIGHBORHOOD AND ESTABLISHMENT	METROPOLITAN AREAS (3)	MEDIUM-SIZE CITIES (6)	SMALL TOWNS (10)	TOTAL (19)
Poor, served by subsidy:	67	. . . . .	. . . . .	67
Affiliated retailers	49	. . . . .	. . . . .	49
Nonaffiliated	18	. . . . .	. . . . .	18
Poor, not served by subsidy:	68	114	104	286
Small retailer	41	103	84	228
Supermarket	6	1	1	8
Mini-market	11	5	8	24
Market stall	8	2	7	17
Fair stall	2	3	4	9
Nonpoor, no subsidy:	66	79	. . . . .	145
Small retailer	38	28	. . . . .	66
Supermarket	7	10	. . . . .	17
Mini-market	7	17	. . . . .	24
Market stall	12	11	. . . . .	23
Fair stall	2	13	. . . . .	15
All neighborhoods:	201	193	104	498
Small retailer (varejista)	146	131	84	361
Supermarket	13	11	1	25
Mini-market	18	22	8	48
Market stall	20	13	7	40
Fair stall	4	16	4	24

The questionnaire, which in most cases was answered by the owner or manager of the outlet, provides data on the prices of standard quantities of bread (in five sizes), canned meat and fish (seven types), and 13 other non-perishable foodstuffs. For three foods—rice, beans, and manioc flour—prices were also obtained for the amount that would fill a cup supplied by the interviewer. This provided a standard measure for less-than-standard-package amounts. For these and some other foods—sugar, spaghetti, dried beef, soybean oil, margarine, and coffee—the vendor was also asked the weight and price of the smallest quantity he would be willing to sell. Both of these approaches attempt to measure the unit cost of fractional purchases. Data were also obtained on the vendor's suppliers, the criteria used to set prices, the clientele served, the number of employees and of unpaid workers, and the existence of other costs of doing business (rent, utilities, etc.). Prices were collected for credit purchases, along with the criteria for setting them, but since credit transactions often depend on personal acquaintance and are settled in the future, the interviewers could not check the accuracy of the reported prices.

The FUNDAJ has published a full description of the questionnaire, sample, and field procedures, together with a large selection of mean prices classified by various dimensions.[10] We have analyzed a subset of these price comparisons, looking particularly for differences that are both economically important (10% or more) and statistically significant.[11] The principal conclusion to emerge from that analysis is the remarkable homogeneity of prices. Few price differences are large, and fewer still are statistically significant. The latter restriction, of course, reflects the very small number of observations in some categories. If there are only two or three supermarkets, a supermarket/*varejista* comparison may yield large errors of estimate, but it might still make a significant economic difference to the consumer where he or she shopped. The small number of observations also make it impossible to analyze some of the foods considered, particularly the canned items, and here we consider only 14 foods. The next two sections display some further findings, including some derived from regression analysis, and the final section considers the implications of our findings in the light of the hypotheses described above.

Town Size, Neighborhood, and Establishment Type

Since traditional small retailers not affiliated with the subsidy program are by far the commonest outlets in the survey, comparisons across towns are limited to these outlets. These results appear in Tables 14.2 and 14.3.

Table 14.2 Mean Prices, in June 1985 Cruzeiros, of Selected Basic Foods by Municipality for Small Retailers Not Affiliated with Subsidy Program

MUNICIPALITY	RICE (KG)	SUGAR (KG)	MANIOC FLOUR (KG)	CORNMEAL (500 G)	SPAGHETTI (500 G)	BREAD (50 G)	BEANS (KG)	POWDERED MILK (200 G)	DRIED BEEF (KG)	CANNED SARDINES (125 G)	EGGS (DOZ)	SOYBEAN OIL (900 ML)	MARGARINE (250 G)	COFFEE (250 G)
Metropolitan areas:														
Recife	2,880	1,473	1,520	1,269	1,292	158	3,114	2,199	7,447	1,571	2,402	4,612	1,873	4,284
Fortaleza	2,559	1,685	1,289	1,315	1,468	200	1,964	2,215	10,500	1,355	2,704	5,494	1,932	4,744
Teresina	2,016	1,719	1,468	980	1,704	156	2,125	2,424	...	1,365	2,864	5,767	2,169	4,652
Medium-size cities:														
Arapiraca	2,567	1,598	1,242	1,343	1,619	191	2,847	2,517	9,700	1,704	2,495	5,389	2,245	4,463
Palmares	2,896	1,444	949	1,264	1,329	158	3,068	2,390	6,667	1,600	2,588	5,046	2,043	4,060
Campina Grande	2,503	1,578	1,142	1,070	1,305	170	2,200	2,114	8,708	1,443	2,634	5,063	1,921	4,408
Caicó	2,375	1,601	975	1,034	1,426	150	1,426	...	9,500	1,478	2,746	5,307	1,865	4,573
Itapipoca	2,004	1,604	774	1,193	1,404	200	1,696	2,310	...	1,173	2,963	4,975	1,816	4,294
Picos	1,958	1,958	944	1,087	1,575	...	1,700	2,200	...	1,387	2,446	5,276	1,940	4,711

(continued)

Table 14.2 continued

MUNICIPALITY	RICE (KG)	SUGAR (KG)	MANIOC FLOUR (KG)	CORNMEAL (500 G)	SPAGHETTI (500 G)	BREAD (50 G)	BEANS (KG)	POWDERED MILK (200 G)	DRIED BEEF (KG)	CANNED SARDINES (125 G)	EGGS (DOZ)	SOYBEAN OIL (900 ML)	MARGARINE (250 G)	COFFEE (250 G)
Small towns:														
Lagoa da Canoa	2,371	1,763	1,000	1,200	1,675	200	2,500	2,317	10,000	1,825	2,429	5,760	2,313	4,400
Joaquim Nabuco	2,557	1,431	860	1,234	1,325	175	2,950	2,467	6,171	1,475	2,650	5,375	2,134	4,164
Arará	2,467	1,622	750	1,222	1,422	...	2,000	2,067	7,833	1,529	3,275	5,162	1,875	4,300
Soledade	2,133	1,475	1,050	988	1,400	200	1,233	2,100	...	1,400	3,080	5,500	2,000	4,367
Jardim do Seridó	2,313	1,563	850	1,125	1,406	...	1,157	2,000	8,000	1,500	2,680	5,350	1,875	4,550
Ouro Branco	2,325	1,538	988	1,138	...	200	986	...	...	1,370	2,400	5,057	2,063	4,150
São Luis do Curú	2,190	1,620	855	1,138	...	200	1,800	2,217	...	1,225	2,745	5,000	1,830	4,644
Traírí	2,218	1,564	818	1,133	...	200	1,550	2,200	...	1,160	2,891	5,375	1,882	4,730
Inhuma	1,678	1,789	1,000	544	...	275	1,200	2,350	...	1,380	2,280	5,300	2,006	4,556
São José do Piauí	1,850	1,667	900	513	...	...	1,200	2,720	...	1,350	2,400	4,922	2,050	4,628

Table 14.3 Mean Prices, in June 1985 Cruzeiros, of Selected Basic Foods by City Size for Small Retailers Not Affiliated with Subsidy

PRODUCT	UNIT	METROPOLITAN AREAS (3)	MEDIUM SIZE CITIES (6)	SMALL TOWNS (10)
Rice	kg	2,474 (52) **	2,362 (37) *	2,205 (42)
Sugar		1,626 (22)	1,604 (15)	1,611 (23)
Manioc flour	kg	1,425 (29) *	1,006 (20) *	893 (20)
Cornmeal	500 g	1,157 (32)	1,137 (25) *	997 (45)
Spaghetti	500 g	1,479 (21)	1,457 (18)	1,483 (21)
Bread[a]	50 g	159 (7)	167 (3) *	200 (7)
Beans	kg	2,390 (74)	2,236 (89) *	1,593 (118)
Powdered milk	200 g	2,287 (40)	2,320 (32)	2,314 (41)
Dried beef	kg	8,029 (420)	8,314 (233)*	7,131 (343)
Canned sardines	125 g	1,389 (30)	1,427 (25)	1,388 (33)
Eggs	dozen	2,658 (35)	2,657 (25)	2,737 (50)
Soybean oil	900 ml	5,341 (121)	5,200 (41)	5,262 (54)
Margarine	250 g	1,995 (24)	1,968 (22)	1,991 (30)
Coffee	250 g	4,545 (40)	4,437 (45)	4,470 (44)

Note: Numbers in parentheses are standard errors of estimate.
[a]Prices sometimes differ in the opposite direction for different sized loaves (e.g., 100 or 200 g).
*Price difference significant, with 95% confidence.
**Price difference significant, with 90% confidence.

Comparisons among types of retailers are limited to large and midsize cities, respectively, in Tables 14.4 and 14.5, and all three variables are treated together in Table 14.6. All these results refer to the standard packages or quantities, commonly a kilogram or a regular fraction (one-half, one-fourth, one-fifth, or one-eighth) thereof.

When mean prices are shown separately for all 19 towns (Table 14.2), there is a great deal of geographic variation. The highest price exceeds the lowest by more than 70% for rice and for bread, by 100% for manioc flour, 160% for cornmeal, and over 200% for beans. The only pattern visible in these large differences is that traditional foodstuffs produced in the interior of the Northeast (all of the above except for bread) seem to vary much more in price than more modern—and often more highly industrialized-products, particularly spaghetti, powdered milk, and soybean oil, which tend to be imported from other parts of the country. The lowest price for each of the traditional foodstuffs always occurs in one of the small towns and the highest price in a larger city. Thus, for these products, local supply seems to be very important.

This pattern persists when prices are averaged across towns in each size class, as Table 14.3 shows. Mean prices are significantly lower in small

Table 14.4 Mean Prices, in June 1985 Cruzeiros, of Selected Basic Foods by Type of Establishment: Three Metropolitan Areas

PRODUCT	UNIT	AFFILIATED SMALL RETAILER (49)	NONAFFILIATED (97)	MINI-MARKET (18)
Rice	kg	2,009 (31)*	2,474 (52)	2,463 (119)
Sugar	kg	1,398 (31)*	1,626 (22)**	1,742 (65)
Manioc flour	kg	1,101 (30)*	1,425 (29)	1,344 (82)
Cornmeal	500 g	901 (46)*	1,157 (32)*	1,332 (32)
Spaghetti	500 g	1,195 (23)*	1,479 (21)	1,583 (71)
Bread	50 g	155 (8)	159 (7)	. . .
Beans	kg	2,115 (109)	2,390 (74)	2,304 (138)
Powdered milk	200 g	1,768 (10)*	2,287 (40)	2,282 (108)
Dried beef	kg	6,424 (422)*	8,029 (420)	. . .
Canned sardines	125 g	1,374 (29)	1,389 (30)	1,431 (66)
Eggs	dozen	2,256 (33)*	2,658 (35)	2,716 (102)
Soybean oil	900 ml	4,510 (62)*	5,341 (121)	5,587 (222)
Margarine	250 g	2,011 (38)	1,995 (24)	2,093 (71)
Coffee	250 g	4,499 (66)	4,545 (40)	4,670 (97)

Note: Numbers in parentheses are standard errors of estimate. Ellipses indicate too few observations for comparison.
*Price difference significant, with 95% confidence.
**Price difference significant, with 90% confidence.

Table 14.5 Mean Prices, in June 1985 Cruzeiros, of Selected Basic Foods by Type of Establishment: Six Medium-Size Cities

PRODUCT	UNIT	SUPER-MARKETS (11)	SMALL RETAILERS (131)	MINI-MARKETS (22)
Rice	kg	2,468 (158)	2,362 (37)	2,456 (124)
Sugar	kg	1,503 (61)	1,604 (15)	1,548 (57)
Manioc flour	kg	1,203 (161)	1,006 (20)	1,067 (68)
Cornmeal	500 g	1,032 (81)	1,137 (25)*	1,017 (51)
Spaghetti	500 g	1,343 (61)	1,457 (18)*	1,340 (52)
Bread	50 g	. . .	167 (3)	. . .
Beans	kg	1,763 (167)*	2,236 (89)	2,500 (181)
Powdered milk	200 g	. . .	2,320 (32)	2,305 (72)
Dried beef	kg	8,216 (518)	8,314 (233)	7,619 (349)
Canned sardines	125 g	. . .	1,427 (25)	1,348 (51)
Eggs	dozen	2,668 (72)	2,657 (25)	2,526 (54)
Soybean oil	900 ml	4,925 (130)	5,200 (41)	5,115 (4)
Margarine	250 g	1,886 (73)	1,968 (22)	1,930 (38)
Coffee	250 g	4,282 (96)	4,437 (45)*	4,284 (69)

Note: Numbers in parentheses are standard errors of estimate. Ellipses indicate too few observations for comparison.
*Price difference significant, with 95% confidence.

Table 14.6 Prices as Functions of City, Neighborhood, and Type of Establishment: Regression Coefficients

PRODUCT/R^2	CITY SIZE		SUBSIDY NEIGHBORHOOD		SMALL RETAILER		MODERN RETAILER
	Large	Medium	Yes	No	Subsidy	No	
Rice (kg)/.113	321*	203*	−83.5	−131	−430	31.3	59.4
	(65)	(62)	(117)	(52)	(137)	(63.2)	(75.1)
(in cup) .033	66.9	37.7	−18.3	4.09	−25.4	49.0	−4.07
	(44.7)	(42.5)	64.0	(37.5)	(72.3)	(40.3)	(78.8)
Sugar/.123	113*	27.3	−145*	−44.3	−182*	−17.2	−71.9
	(32)	(30.3)	(56)	(24.9)	(66)	(31.1)	(37.2)
Manioc flour (kg)/.417	602*	200*	−210*	−120*	−244*	−51.0	−67.5
	(43)	(42)	(68)	(32)	(82)	(40.8)	47.8
(in cup) .283	269*	135*	−60.0	−60.1*	−24.3	34.6	−83.0
	(35)	(35)	(43.1)	(27.3)	(51.1)	(30.8)	(53.7)
Cornmeal/.096	178*	79.5	−14.9	60.1	−254*	−9.09	−20.5
	(49)	(46.5)	(91.0)	(38.8)	(106)	(48.5)	(56.7)
Spaghetti/.154	49.1	−14.4	−125*	−30.9	−189*	21.6	−41.9
	(31.1)	(29.7)	(57)	(24.3)	(67)	(30.5)	(36.0)
Beans (kg)/.116;	807*	562*	−224	−4.5	32.8	141	199
	(136)	(136)	(225)	(97.6)	(263)	(122)	(138)
(in cup) .150	284*	203*	2.1	76.9	−5.3	13.7	−67.9
	(74)	(74)	(89.2)	(54.3)	(104)	(59.7)	(106)
Powdered milk/ .349	23.4	48.1	−64.7	−58.0	−476*	26.3	9.87
	(59.0)	(55.4)	(100)	(46.8)	(115)	(61.4)	(66.5)
Dried beef/.141	1,054*	870*	−1,262	−528	−102	848	603
	(483)	(434)	(870)	(324)	(1011)	(529)	(522)
Eggs/.198	24.2	−23.2	−216*	−34.6	−236*	22.1	−37.2
	(51.8)	(51.4)	(85)	(38.6)	(113)	(73.4)	(79.4)
Soybean oil/ .069	36.8	−60.6	−240	−123	−396	135	165
	(142)	(134)	(288)	(110)	(322)	(136)	(154)
Margarine/.014	32.9	−28.0	−50.3	13.0	71.9	24.3	45.3
	(37.3)	(36.3)	(66.6)	(29.4)	(79.4)	(38.2)	(44.6)
Coffee/.032	105	−17.4	129	−8.53	−151	34.5	−64.2
	(62)	(59.8)	(113)	(49.3)	(132)	(60.5)	(71.3)

Note: Numbers in parentheses are standard errors.
*Distinct from zero, with 95% confidence.

towns than in midsize cities for five traditional foodstuffs, including dried beef. For rice and manioc flour, there is a further price increase in the three large cities, but otherwise prices differ little between large and medium-size urban areas. Only bread seems to be systematically more expensive in small towns.

The urban poor appear to pay more than their rural counterparts for certain basic foods (although they pay less for bread), but this says nothing about whether there are cheaper alternatives to the small urban retailers, or whether all outlets' prices are higher in larger towns. Table 14.4 examines this question within the three metropolitan areas, and Table 14.5 within the six medium-size cities. Table 14.4 shows clearly that retailers who participate in the PROAB subsidy have systematically lower prices than those who do not, indicating that nonaffiliated retailers cannot or at least do not match the subsidized prices. For some products—rice, sugar, cornmeal, dried beef, eggs, and soybean oil—the unsubsidized metropolitan area price was higher than that in the small settlements. This can be seen by comparing the last column of Table 14.3 with the first two columns of Table 14.4. This result does not mean, however that the full amount of the subsidy is passed on to the consumer, since the final price difference may be smaller than the subsidy. Because of difficulties in financing and managing the subsidy program, final subsidized prices have often been based on needlessly high wholesale prices, so that the participating retailers have been selling at or above the prices of supermarkets and mini-markets. This was particularly true in 1984, as studies in Recife and throughout the PROAB system have shown, and the problem persisted in 1985. Typically, less than half the subsidy is actually transferred for at least one-fourth of the time.[12] According to Table 14.4, unsubsidized retailers have generally been able to compete with more modern outlets such as mini-markets. In fact, where there are significant price differences (for sugar and cornmeal) it is the *varejistas* whose prices are lower. A similar pattern obtains in the midsize cities, where there is no subsidy (Table 14.5). The small retailers are more expensive for a few products (cornmeal, spaghetti, and coffee), and the lowest price for beans was in supermarkets, but generally the *varejistas* compete with more modern establishments and sometimes they have the lowest prices (manioc flour).

Table 14.6 tests simultaneously for price differences according to city size, type of neighborhood, and type of retailer, comparison being made to small towns, non-poor neighborhoods, and traditional markets or fairs. The results confirm the tendency for prices of traditional foodstuffs to be higher in the larger towns (higher still in the largest cities, for sugar and cornmeal), to be lower in subsidized shops, and otherwise not to differ among outlets. They also show some tendency for prices to be lower in poor neighborhoods, even when these are not reached by the subsidy. Overall, there is no evidence that the poor pay more than their non-poor neighbors simply because of where they live or where they shop, at least so long as they pay in cash and purchase the standard amount of a foodstuff.

Credit and Fractional Purchases

As was indicated earlier, it is difficult to be sure of the price in a credit transaction; it would be necessary to record what a real customer pays when settling accounts with a retailer and to know for how long credit had been extended. Such data cannot be collected on a single visit by an interviewer who is not a regular client. The most that was possible in this survey was to classify sales as cash or credit and compare the prices declared by the vendor.[13] This comparison shows significant differences only for rice, beans, and manioc flour, and for these products the declared cash price is higher, not lower, implying a negative nominal interest rate and a still more negative real rate. The comparison is not, however, limited to the same establishments and is not controlled for city size, so there is no evidence that individual vendors subsidize credit sales.

We are on firmer ground in considering the other service traditional small retailers provide their customers, namely, selling fractional amounts of a product. First, prices were recorded for a cupful of rice, of beans, and of manioc flour, which weighed much less than a kilogram. The results in Table 14.6 show that these prices also went up in larger cities and down in subsidized stores, but because the quantity was smaller the price differences were also smaller, and in roughly the same proportion. In the case of beans, a cupful sold for more on average in an unsubsidized store in a poor neighborhood than in a non-poor neighborhood, but the difference is not significant. The regression coefficients do not suggest that unit prices are systematically higher when a cupful rather than a kilogram is bought.

The second approach to fractional-purchase prices was to estimate the regression:

$$P = b_0 + b_1 Q + b_2 Q^2,$$

where Q is the smallest amount a retailer would agree to sell, and P is what he charged for it. If the amount has no effect on the unit price, then b_0 and b_2 should be zero, and b_1 should equal the price per gram of the standard quantity (or the price per milliliter for cooking oil). If instead customers pay more to buy in fractional amounts, then both b_0 and b_2 should be positive, while b_1 can be of either sign. The results are shown in

Table 14.7 Quadratic Regression of Price versus Quantity for Fractional Purchases of Eight Basic Foods, in all Establishments and Small Retail Outlets only

PRODUCT AND ESTABLISHMENT	CONSTANT	QUANTITY (GRAMS)	(QUANTITY)^2 X 10^{-5}
Rice:			
All establishments	43.1 (44.4)	2.05 (.35)*	28.0 (53.8)
Small retailers only	34.4 (46.4)	2.10 (.36)*	23.2 (56.0)
Sugar:			
All establishments	.94 (22.3)	1.63 (.18)*	−2.07 (29.0)
Small retailers only	.17 (24.8)	1.61 (.21)*	4.66 (32.1)
Manioc flour:			
All establishments	7.50 (34.6)	1.18 (.25)*	−8.18 (38.3)
Small retailers only	26.1 (32.3)	1.03 (.24)*	7.81 (35.7)
Spaghetti:			
All establishments	413 (845)	2.81 (9.39)	−671 (2,416)
Small retailers only[a]	. . .	. . .	. . .
Beans:			
All establishments	115 (90.7)	1.43 (.71)*	83.1 (112)
Small retailers only	119 (91.3)	1.37 (.73)**	95.5 (115)
Dried beef:			
All establishments	−141 (111)	9.55 (1.16)*	−296 (200)
Small retailers only	−322 (126)	11.7 (1.38)*	−681 (234)*
Soybean oil:			
All establishments	370 (84.8)*	−.08 (1.38)	1,397 (298)*
Small retailers only	378 (89.5)*	−.19 (1.44)	1,410 (319)*
Coffee:			
All establishments	47.2 (61.9)	18.4 (2.05)*	−1,223 (1,421)
Small retailers only	53.0 (68.2)	18.5 (2.31)*	−1,435 (1,608)

[a]Minimal quantity same for all retailers.
*Distinct from zero, with 95% confidence.
**Distinct from zero, with 90% confidence.

Table 14.7 for all vendors who agreed to fractional sales and also for *varejistas* only, who were always the great majority of such vendors. For every product except soybean oil, the hypothesis is confirmed that fractional sales are charged the same price per gram as the standard package. The coefficient of quantity is indistinguishable from the mean price in Table 14.3, and the other two coefficients are not distinct from zero, except for the quadratic for dried beef. Only when buying oil in small amounts does the customer face a higher unit price, perhaps because the remaining oil in an open bottle or can goes rancid quickly (the Northeast climate is very hot), whereas this does not happen so easily to rice or other dry products when the package is opened.

Conclusions and Implications

The results presented here do not directly confront the first hypothesis, described in Section 1, that food prices are systematically higher than they need to be, but they nonetheless cast doubt on it. The hypothesis of inefficiency, if true, should apply particularly to the traditional small retailers who have no control over the wholesale purchase, transport, or storage of foodstuffs. Supermarkets, because they bypass many intermediaries and take on many wholesaler's functions, should then achieve lower prices than retailers bound to an exploitative or wasteful supply system. The fact that supermarket and *varejista* prices do not differ greatly or systematically makes it appear, then, that the food marketing system functions fairly well. An important corollary of this conclusion is that there is probably little or no room to lower food prices by public intervention in that system: the government's belief that it can bring down prices to consumers simply by acting as a wholesaler, which is the assumption of the Programa de Abastecimento Popular (PAP), is almost surely wrong. Subsidies will be required, explicitly, and the experience with the existing subsidy program indicates considerable inefficiency in achieving increased food consumption.

The principal conclusions we reach concern hypotheses 2 and 3: there is little or no evidence that in patronizing traditional small retailers, consumers are paying too much for their food, and this is true even when allowing for their practice of buying on credit or in smaller than standard amounts. The *varejista* typically does not appear to be exploiting his customers nor to be charging them significantly for services they cannot get elsewhere. Thus, persuading poor customers to buy elsewhere, or to pay cash, or to buy in standard amounts would have little or no effect on their food bills or their consumption. Only by some more substantial step, such as taking over the retailing function through cooperatives, could they benefit. This finding reinforces the largely ideological argument that poor consumers are economically rational and that they are not to blame for their poverty and malnutrition. They may be of course still be nutritionally irrational, buying cheaply but not buying well.[14] It also means that in operating a subsidy program through *varejistas*, the government is not necessarily supporting high-cost retailers and thus reducing the benefits of the subsidy.

So far as urban-rural differences are concerned, we find that for certain traditional staples, the rural poor generally face lower prices, which does not occur for more modern and more processed foods. This may help explain the finding that at a given income level, the rural poor suffer less protein-calorie malnutrition than their urban counterparts—their real incomes are in fact slightly higher.[15] This advantage is partly offset by the smaller variety of foods available in rural areas and small towns of the interior, as shown in Table 14.2. And this narrower diet probably contributes to the higher prevalence of some specific dietary deficiencies, such as vitamin A shortage, in rural areas.[16] The rural advantage in prices is also offset by the subsidy program for those urban poor who live in the areas it serves. The subsidy program is, in this sense, working in the right direction, acting to lower prices to consumers where they are naturally highest, although this is a geographic difference rather than one that is due to the high costs of particular outlets.

If the evidence in favor of these hypotheses is so weak—that is, if price differences seem to contribute so little to poverty and malnutrition—how did such hypotheses ever come to be part of the ideology about this issue in Brazil? The question is of practical importance, because very large sums have been spent and continue to be spent on food and nutrition programs inspired by this belief.[17] If the suppositions are misguided, then some of that expenditure is wasteful or ineffective.

We can find three possible explanations for the hold these ideas have on the thinking about malnutrition in Brazil. The first is casual empiricism, or scattered and anecdotal evidence that the hypotheses are correct. At a sufficiently detailed level, such as comparing one small town with another, there is in fact much price variation. The same is doubtless true of some detailed comparisons of cash versus credit prices, of some fractional-purchase costs (as we find for soybean oil), and of some comparisons among establishments. It takes only a hasty generalization to go from such observations to a belief that the poor systematically pay more for their food. Such careless generalization may be especially easy in a time of rapid inflation, because when all prices are changing, comparisons are difficult, and when the relative price of food is in fact rising, inflation is systematically more burdensome to the poor.

The trouble with this explanation is that casual empiricism might just as easily have made the opposite observation, seeing only small price differences in general, which often serve to benefit rather than work against the poor. And casual observation, even if correct, does not explain why these hypotheses were so thoroughly accepted and incorporated into public policy despite the flimsiness of the evidence. This suggests a second explanation, which depends more on theory than on facts. It is theoretically plausible to suppose that a market characterized by thousands of small producers and of small retailers could be dominated by middlemen, who would supply scare credit as well as transportation and storage services; that partly for this reason and partly because of small scale, such small retailers would necessarily have to charge more than supermarkets; and that consumers might nonetheless patronize them, obtaining such facilities (which in themselves would appear to raise costs) as purchases on credit or in small amounts. Unless confronted by firm evidence to the contrary, all these propositions could seem self-evident. And this consistency could even discourage the search for evidence by making it seem unnecessary. Investigation would then be directed to the consequences of public food and nutrition programs rather than to their suppositions, and this seems to be what occurred.

Neither the explanation via casual empiricism nor that based on theoretical plausibility takes any account of the temporal dimension of the issue. Our price data refer to mid-1985, but the hypotheses under attack were formulated and accepted in the mid-1970s. The INAN launched its first nutrition program in 1974 and its subsidy program in 1978; the chief source of data on malnutrition refers to 1974–75, and the most influential analyses of those data were completed in 1977–79. During this period, no one collected or analyzed price data of the sort presented here. It may be that a third explanation is correct: the hypothesis that the poor paid too much for their food could have been valid, or more nearly valid, a decade or more ago than it is today. If that is the case, we are not showing that the ideology of malnutrition was wrong from the start on this question, but only that is mistaken now.

It is not hard to imagine how the reality could have changed while beliefs did not. On the one hand, public investments in infrastructure have reduced transport and storage costs, thereby reducing price dispersion. Public programs of price support may have had the same effect. On the other hand, there has been a great expansion of supermarkets and mini-markets in the last 10 years. These are no longer confined to rich neighborhoods in larger cities but have penetrated poorer neighborhoods and even some small towns in the interior. The buying habits of poor consumer shave shifted accordingly, and the traditional retailers have had to compete or go out of business. There is in fact anecdotal evidence that many of them have disappeared, and that there has been an even greater reduction in the other traditional vendors to the poor, the fairs and markets composed of many small retailers, each specializing in a few products. For those *varejistas* who remain in business, offering credit and allowing fractional purchases may be a way not to exploit customers, but simply to retain them, without charging more for those services. Anecdotal evidence suggests that both credit and fractional sales are less prevalent than they used to be. (This trend is partly offset by some supermarkets allowing credit or fractional sales to regular customers.) In almost every respect, the market for food has become more modern and more homogeneous. Part of this change is the shift to more industrialized foods, typically produced outside the Northeast, which vary less in price than the traditional rice, beans, and manioc flour. All these changes started in south-central Brazil and may have begun to affect the Northeast only within the last decade.

Consequently, there seems to be little scope for benefiting poor consumers without cost to the government by persuading them to buy at different outlets or in large amounts, or by improving the competitiveness of the food market and reducing price dispersion. Both of these beneficial transformations are already well advanced. This emphatically does not mean that price differences do not matter to food consumption and thus to nutritional status. It means only that the reduction of food prices for the poor requires subsidies, at considerable public cost. We also find that subsidies have less of a role to play than has been believed in "correcting" regional price differences. The question is whether a given cost in the form of a subsidy yields more or less nutritional benefit than the same expense in a program of direct distribution of foodstuffs, and here the evidence for Brazil is incomplete and inconclusive.[18] Comparisons of subsidy and donation programs do not show a clear superiority of either; still less clear is how far both types of programs could be replaced by measures to generate more income for the poor or to reduce the cost of growing food, relative to the incomes they now have. What is clear is that price differences now play only a minor part in explaining the country's burden of malnutrition.

Notes

1. World Bank, *Brazil: Human Resources Special Report* (Washington, D.C.: World Bank, 1979). This is a principal summary of information derived from the ENDEF 1974–75 household budget survey.
2. Philip Musgove, "Ideología, pesquisa y realidad de la situación almentaria y nutricional del Brasil," *Cadernos de Estudos Sociais 2*, no. 1 (1986); 329–48.
3. Dirceu Pessoa, *Alimentação no Nordeste: Da carência crónica às centrais de abastecimento*, Trabalhos para Discussão no. 24 (Recife: Fundação Joaquim Nabuco, June 1986).
4. Instituto Nacional de Alimentação e Nutrição (National Food and Nutrition Institute), "Subsídio para o encontro de avaliação da execução do *Projecto de Abastecimento de Alimentos Básicos em Áreas de Baixa Renda PROAB*," vols. 1 and 2 (Brasília: INAN, August 1984).

5. Philip Musgrove, "Que los pobres coman major: Evaluación de programas destinados a mejorar el consumo alimenticio de familias pobres en el Brasil" (So the poor can eat better: Evaluation of programs intended to improve food consumption of poor families in Brazil) (Washington, D.C.: Pan American Health Organization, January 1987), chaps. 4 and 7. There is no evidence yet that this aim can be achieved and sustained.

6. Fundação Instituto Brasileiro de Geografia e Estatística (IBGE), *Estudo nacional da despesa familiar: Consumo alimentar, antropometria; dados preliminares*, 4 vols. (Rio de Janeiro: IBGE, 1977, 1978). This publication provides the tables of aggregated data from which many subsequent researchers have worked.

7. Cheryl Williamson Gray, *Food Consumption Parameters for Brazil and Their Application to Food Policy*, Research Report no. 32 (Washington, D.C.: International Food Policy Research Institute, September 1982).

8. Philip Musgrove, "A despesa familiar e os preços dos alimentos como determinates do consumo alimentício no Nordeste Brasileiro," (Washington, D.C.: Pan American Health Organization, August 1986). The estimates reported here appear to be the first consumption functions estimated directly from the household-level data. The effect of family size on food consumption is treated in a companion paper: Philip Musgrove, "Demografia e bem-estar: Tamanho familiar e consumo alimentício no Nordeste Brasileiro" (presented to the 5th national meeting of the Associação Brasileira de Estudos Populacionais, Águas de São Pedro, São Paulo, Brazil, October 12–16, 1986).

9. Instituto Paranaense de Desenvolvimento Econômico e Social (IPARDES), *Abastecimento alimentar básico: Formas e fontes de suprimento; resultados finais* (Curitiba: IPARDES, July 1985).

10. Osmil Galindo, *Quanto pagam os pobres? Estudo de comparação espacial de preços de alimentos no Nordeste Brasileiro* (Recife: Fundação Joaquim Nabuco, 1985).

11. Osmil Galindo and Philip Musgrove, "Quanto pagam os pobres? Determinantes geográficos e comerciais dos preços dos alimentos no Nordeste," *Revista Econômica do Nordeste* 17, no. 2 (April–June 1986): 305–30.

12. The failures of the system in Recife are described in Cleide Galiza de Oliveira and Rejane Pinto de Medeiros, *O Projeto de Abastecimento de Alimentos Básicos em Áreas de Baixa Renda: Uma avaliação*, (Recife: Fundação Joaquim Nabuco, 1985). For a summary of experience in several cities served by the program, see note 4, above.

13. Galindo and Musgrove, table 7.

14. Elca Rosenberg, "Consumer Behavior in Relation to Nutrition: A Brazilian Case Study" (Ph.D. thesis, Vanderbilt University, Department of Economics, Nashville, May 1976.).

15. World Bank (see n. 1 above), annex 3, p. 49.

16. Malaquias Batista Filho and Nize de Paula Barbosa, *Alimentação e nutrição no Brasil, 1974-1984*, (Brasília: Instituto Nacional de Alimentação e Nutrição, 1985).

17. Musgrove, "Que los pobres coman mejor," table 9.

18. Ibid., Chaps. 6 and 8.

CHAPTER 15

Do Brazilian
Nutrition Programs
Make a Difference?

Acknowledgments

So many people helped in the research on which this article is based that it is impractical to thank them all by name. I am grateful to numerous colleagues in the Pan American Health Organization, the World Bank, the International Food Policy Research Institute, the Instituto Nacional de Alimentação e Nutrição, the Legião Brasileira de Assistência, the Fundação Joaquim Nabuco, the University of São Paulo, and the Federal Universities of Pernambuco and Minas Gerais. For encouragement to condense a monograph into this short article, I am especially grateful to Vicente Navarro and Alberto Valdés.

Introduction

Among Latin American countries, Brazil has undoubtedly had the most varied and extensive experience with food and nutrition programs meant to improve food consumption and nutritional status of the children of poor families (1). In contrast to many countries where such programs have depended on foreign aid, usually in the form of donated foodstuffs, Brazil's programs have been financed almost entirely from internal sources; and in

Reprinted, with permission, from "Do Nutrition Programs Make a Difference? The Case of Brazil," International Journal of Health Services 20(4), 1990. This is a translation of an article originally prepared at the invitation of the journal *Cuadernos de Economía*, published by the Institute of Economics of the Catholic University of Chile, Santiago, Chile.

contrast to the experience of some countries such as Chile, a variety of approaches have been tried, in circumstances of competition among public agencies and among different diagnoses or explanations of malnutrition, which give rise to different ways to attack it.

The Pan American Health Organization has been studying this experience since 1983, with the objectives of giving technical assistance to Brazil and of deriving lessons applicable to other countries. The study began with a comparison of two approaches–a subsidy to basic foodstuffs versus direct distribution to beneficiaries–and then expanded to cover five programs that operated during some part of the period 1974–86. The analysis was published at the end of 1989 (2): the present article summarizes some of the most interesting findings, concentrating on the four programs for which the most empirical information is available. These and some other programs have been described and evaluated in other comparative studies (3–5), which do not analyze the programs' results relative to their objectives. Individual programs have also been subject to particularly valuable evaluations (6–16). This study draws heavily on these analyses, as well as on operational information made available by the Brazilian public agencies responsible for the programs.

Table 15.1 summarizes some features of these institutions, the population coverage and operational mechanisms of each program, and the underlying diagnosis or "ideology" (17), which determines the kind of foods provided and the means of transferring them to beneficiaries. The principal difference among the programs is that two of them distributed food directly to identified beneficiaries, while the other two subsidized foodstuffs. There is a secondary difference between the donation programs, in that one provided specially formulated foods, directed at specific family members (the PCA or Complementary Food Program), whereas the other used traditional commercial foods (the PNS or Nutrition through the Health System Program, later renamed the PSA or Food Supplement Program). There was also a difference between the subsidy programs: the PINS or Integrated Nutrition and Health Program was an experiment that registered beneficiary families, where the PROAB or Program of Basic Food Supply in Low Income Areas was open to any consumer patronizing the shops that participated in the program. In this last case, it is impossible to measure directly any impact on the beneficiaries. Three programs were administered by INAN, the National Food and Nutrition Institute, which is part of the Ministry of Health, and the fourth by the LBA or Brazilian Assistance Legion, which is part of the Ministry of Social Welfare.

It is estimated that up to the end of 1986, the three permanent or non-experimental programs had cost the government a total of $767 million

Table 15.1 Principal Characteristics of Four Nutrition Programs, Brazil, 1974–86[a]

	COMPLEMENTARY FOOD PROGRAM (PCA)	NUTRITION THROUGH THE HEALTH SYSTEM PROGRAM/ FOOD SUPPLEMENT PROGRAM (PNS/PSA)	INTEGRATED NUTRITION AND HEALTH PROGRAM (PINS)	PROGRAM OF BASIC FOOD SUPPLY IN LOW-INCOME AREAS (PROAB)
Institutional[b]				
Executing agency	IBA	INAN	INAN/World Bank	INAN
Ministry responsible	MPAS	Health	Health	Health
Physical distribution of food	MPAS	COBAL	COBAL	COBAL
Coverage	North and Northeast (15 states), Federal District, Espirito Santo, Minas Gerais and Rio de Janeiro, urban areas	Nationwide, urban areas and municipalities	Recife	Northeast (8 states), large urban areas
Point of delivery	Health posts, churches, community centers, etc.	Health posts[c]	COBAL establishments	Participating retailers
Mechanism	Monthly donation	Monthly donation	Quantitatively restricted subsidy	Unrestricted subsidy
Problem and beneficiaries				
Determinants of malnutrition				
Low income	Family	Family	Family, within neighborhood or zone	Neighborhood or zone
High prices	No	No	Yes	Yes
Poor intrafamily distribution	Yes: Specific foods for family members	(Partial: includes milk)	Partial: includes anthropometry for children	No

(continued)

Table 15.1 continued

	COMPLEMENTARY FOOD PROGRAM (PCA)	NUTRITION THROUGH THE HEALTH SYSTEM PROGRAM/ FOOD SUPPLEMENT PROGRAM (PNS/PSA)	INTEGRATED NUTRITION AND HEALTH PROGRAM (PINS)	PROGRAM OF BASIC FOOD SUPPLY IN LOW-INCOME AREAS (PROAB)
Nutritional deficiencies				
Calories	Yes	Principal	Principal	Principal
Protein	Yes	Secondary (milk)	Secondary (milk)	Secondary (milk, meat, eggs, fish)
Micronutrients	Yes: blends	No	No	No
Target population			Entire family	Entire family without individual rations
Pregnant women	Yes: equal ration	Yes: equal ration		
Nursing mothers	Yes	Yes		
Children 6–12 mo	Yes	Yes		
Children 1–3 yr	Yes	Yes: equal ration		
Children 4–6 yr	No	Yes[d]		
Health care	Yes	Yes	Yes, some families	No

[a]Source: reference 2, Table 1.
[b]Abbreviations: LBA, Brazilian Assistance Legion; MPAS, Ministry of Social Assistance and Insurance; INAN, National Food and Nutrition Institute; COBAL, Brazilian Food Company (a state enterprise).
[c]In Sao Paulo, consultations at health posts and physical distribution elsewhere.
[d]Eliminated in the PSA; age limit of three years.

300

Table 15.2 Aggregate Estimates for Physical Distribution of Foods, Total Cost, and Total Public Expenditure at Constant June 1984 Prices, for the PNS, PROAB, and PCA, from the Beginning of Each Program through the End of 1986[a]

| | PHYSICAL DISTRIBUTION, TONS | | | UNIT VALUE, CR$/KG, JUNE 1984 | TOTAL COST, CR$ MILLION, JUNE 1984 | | | | | COST, US$ MILLION, 1986 | |
| | PNS, 1976-86 | PROAB, 1980-86 | TOTAL | | PNS, TOTAL COST | PROAB | | TOTAL 2 OR 3 PROGRAMS | | TOTAL COST | PUBLIC EXPENDITURE |
						TOTAL COST	SUBSIDY	COST	PUBLIC EXPENDITURE		
Natural Products											
Rice	405,550	120,657	526,207	586	237,652	70,705	16,705	308,357	254,608	188	156
Sugar	243,452	131,723	385,175	569	144,214	74,950	16,837	219,165	161,051	134	98
Dried meat	—	9,813	9,813	3,196	—	31,362	7,414	31,362	7,414	19	5
Beans	203,093	29,671	232,764	1,118	227,058	35,172	8,654	260,230	235,712	159	144
Maize meal	140,256	23,218	163,474	614	86,117	14,256	3,228	100,373	89,345	61	55
Cassava meal	94,848	30,103	124,951	709	67,247	21,343	5,551	88,590	72,798	54	44
Powdered milk	50,750	5,565	56,315	3,942	200,057	21,937	4,657	221,994	204,714	136	125
Pasta	885	16,283	17,168	655	580	10,665	2,141	11,245	2,721	7	2
Soya oil	6,288	16,829	23,117	2,440	15,343	41,063	10,795	56,406	26,138	34	16
Eggs	—	20,347	20,347	1,845	—	37,540	8,245	37,540	8,245	23	5
Salt fish	—	1,448	1,448	2,978	—	4,312	1,291	4,312	1,291	3	1
Total 11 products	1,155,122	405,657	1,550,779	—	978,268	363,268	85,769	1,339,574	1,064,037	818	651
Unit cost, Cr$/kg or US$/kg					(821)	(939)	(245)	(854)	(701)	(0.52)	(0.43)
PCA blends, 1977-86			111,105	1,702 (US$1.05)				189,101	189,101	116	116
All products			1,671,884					1,528,675	1,253,138	934	767

[a]Source: reference 2, Table 19.

(1986 U.S. dollars) (Table 15.2). The largest share of this was due to the PNS, both because of its large coverage and because it began much earlier than the PROAB. These factors offset the higher unit cost of the foods distributed through the PCA, about $1.00 per kilogram versus approximately 50 cents per kilogram for the nonformulated foods. The total value during these years of donated and subsidized food reached $934 million, including the beneficiaries' contribution to buying the subsidized products. These estimates are based on the quantities distributed, amounting to some 1,662,000 tons, of which three-fourths correspond to the PNS. Nonetheless, the dollar estimate is very close to calculations based on annual budgets in *cruzados* (Cr$), adjusted for inflation and exchange rates (5). During 1984–86, expenditure on the programs ran about 0.1 percent of Brazil's gross domestic product, and a much larger share of total public spending.

Data on the programs' operations and outcomes can be interpreted in various ways. Here, they will be used to test a series of hypotheses or expectations related to the objectives of food and nutrition interventions and the determinants of their success or failure. Specifically, evidence will be presented concerning beneficiaries' participation, program costs and their relation to benefits actually transferred to clients, and nutritional impact, as determined by anthropometry. This last subject can be further divided, depending on whether the data refer to all participating children, to those initially malnourished, to those less than one year old, or to those born to beneficiary mothers.

Beneficiaries' Participation

The "ideology" of all the programs presumes that malnutrition is caused chiefly by poverty, being due to low incomes or high food prices or both. In the case of the PROAB, which merely subsidized foodstuffs, this was effectively the only cause considered, whereas the donation programs (PNS and PCA) admitted a role for medical care and for nutrition status and health. The emphasis on economic factors carries with it the implicit assumption that the beneficiaries—provided they are correctly chosen—will be too poor not to take advantage of the subsidy or donation, so they can be expected to participate regularly in the program benefits. The available evidence suggests, however, that participation can be interrupted or abandoned for various reasons, due to the program itself or to clients' behavior.

Table 15.3 shows what happened to the number of participants (families with the right to buy subsidized food) and the number of users (families

Table 15.3 PINS: Number of Families Entitled to Purchase Subsidized Food ("Participating") and Number of Families that Actually Bought, by Subsidy Model, 1978–80[a]

	1978[b]				1979				1980			
	I	II	III	IV	I	II	III	IV	I	II	III	IV
Model A (initially 2,500 families)												
Participating	2,251[c]	2,500	2,500	2,406	2,203	2,295	2,234	2,173	2,104	2,115	2,132	2,138
Buying	1,880	2,068	2,093	1,998	1,862	1,858	1,920	1,928	1,917	1,947	2,014	1,860
Model B (initially 2,500 families)												
Participating	2,488[c]	2,500	2,500	1,378	1,292	1,400	1,114	1,113	1,154	1,128	1,083	1,081
Buying	1,497	1,351	1,234	1,135	974	919	942	936	949	951	981	928
Model C (initially 2,563 families)												
Participating	2,266	2,563	2,563	2,085	1,894	1,909	1,786	1,638	1,710	1,562	1,619	1,619
Buying	1,317	1,525	1,575	1,512	1,357	1,323	1,365	1,372	1,410	1,427	1,475	1,381
Model D (initially 2,508 families)												
Participating		1,543[c]	2,508	2,508	2,305	1,091	850	878	880	772	781	782
Buying		630	1,271	1,512	976	745	740	875	786	661	694	625
Total (initially 10,071 families)												
Participating	7,005	9,106	10,071	8,377	7,694	6,695	5,984	5,802	5,848	5,577	5,615	5,620
Buying	4,694	5,574	6,173	6,155	5,169	4,845	4,967	5,111	5,062	4,986	5,164	4,794

[a]Source: reference 2, Table 6; from 6, pp. 169–172.
[b]Each year is divided into four 3-month periods, denoted I through IV.
[c]During the first period (January–March 1978 for Groups A, B, and C, and April–June 1978 for Group D), not all the families had yet been registered; the total of 10,071 families registered was reached in July–September 1978.

actually purchasing) during the three years of operation of the PINS. The total of more than 10,000 families registered in 1978 fell rapidly during 1979, to stabilize at about 5,600 in 1980. The number of users fell less markedly, but still substantially. The loss was smallest for Group A, which could buy at a 60 percent subsidy, and greatest for Group D, which received only a 30 percent subsidy. This shows that the subsidy had to be quite high to offset the obstacles the program posed for its clients—limited quantities, restricted times when they could buy (which did not always coincide with times when the families had money to buy), and poor quality products. The discrepancy between results for Groups B and C is explained by the fact that beneficiaries in the former had to take their children once a month to be weighed and measured: both groups received a subsidy of 45 percent, but the bother of the anthropometry session reduced participation in Group B. The differences in participation between one group and another, due to different subsidy rates and requirements for consultation, were not reflected in differences in the purchase of foods per person and per month among those remaining in the program. This amount was stable at 4 to 5 kilograms in all groups throughout the experiment (2, Table 7).

Some related evidence concerning the PNS is presented in Table 15.4. During a period of two years, the beneficiaries were entitled to receive food 24 times; however, as the "total" column shows, fewer than 20 percent of them took advantage of this right as many as 18 times, and more than 10 percent of them received food on six or fewer occasions. Among the reasons given by participants for not participating regularly in the program were the poor quality and small amounts of foodstuffs, and the variation in their own economic circumstances (11). They accepted the donation when the alternative was to go hungry, but did without it when their own resources permitted. This may be entirely sensible behavior for beneficiaries, but it illustrates again how being "poor" is not enough to guarantee stable participation in a nutritional program, if the benefits appear quite small.

Costs and the Transfer of Benefits

One of the chief justifications offered for the experimental subsidy program, the PINS, was that it should be cheaper to administer a subsidy than a donation program, allowing for a larger share of costs to consist of food and to reach the beneficiary. It is very difficult to obtain comparable data on the structure of costs of the different programs, but the slight evidence

Table 15.4 Changes Observed in Weight for Age in Children Participating in the PNS in Two Municipalities in São Paulo, March 1980–April 1982, According to Frequency of Visits to Receive Food; Expressed as Number of Children[a]

NO. OF VISITS/ INITIAL NUTRITIONAL STATUS	FINAL NUTRITIONAL STATUS[b]				CHANGE OF STATUS		
	NORMAL	I	II & III	TOTAL	NONE	IMPROVED	WORSENED
Fewer than 6 visits							
Normal	271	114	9	394	271	—	123
Malnourished I	84	199	57	340	199	84	57
II and III	20	56	83	159	76	79	4
Total	375	369	149	893	546	163	184
6–11 Visits							
Normal	1,188	342	30	1,560	1,188	—	372
Malnourished I	184	641	143	968	641	184	143
II and III	22	119	132	273	117	149	7
Total	1,394	1,102	305	2,801	1,946	333	522
12–17 Visits							
Normal	713	261	31	1,005	713	—	292
Malnourished I	170	473	105	748	473	170	105
II and III	29	99	100	228	87	137	4
Total	912	833	236	1,981	1,273	307	401
18–More Visits							
Normal	506	166	21	693	506	—	187
Malnourished I	131	327	62	520	327	131	62
II and III	20	60	69	149	61	84	4
Total	657	553	152	1,362	894	215	253

[a] Source: reference 2, Table 32; from 12, Tables 1–4.
[b] I, II, and III are grades of malnutrition: I, mild; II, moderate; and III, severe.

available offers little support to the expectation that a subsidy is more efficient in concentrating expenditure on foodstuffs. There was no systematic
difference in this regard between the PINS and the food donation programs
(Table 15.5). Including some health care service greatly reduces the share of
cost in food, both in the PINS and in one model of the PNS that incorporated such services; but when these are not included, expenditures on food
generally account for 80 to 90 percent of total spending.

The PINS identified its clients, and limited the places where they could
buy at subsidized prices; in addition, the experimental design required some
administrative expenses for data collection and analysis. All these features
were discarded in the PROAB, which sold at a subsidy to retailers, who in
turn promised to sell to the public at the prices fixed by the program. This
simplification, as well as the use of already established retailers who must
compete with other sellers (at least for nonsubsidized products), created the
expectation that a larger share of total expenditure should reach the consumer in the form of reduced prices. The need to control not only prices
but also the quantity sold to each participating retailer (to avoid resale at
wholesale prices) still implies substantial administrative costs. Even so, it
was to be expected that the program would reduce food prices by the same
amount as the subsidy, if the government were no less efficient than the private sector in marketing foods.

Tables 15.6 and 15.7 show to what degree this expectation was not ful-
filled. First (Table 15.6), the nominal subsidy (which varied from 15 to 30
percent, according to the product and the moment) is compared with the
effective subsidy or the reduction in the final price to the consumer relative
to prices in supermarkets. There were intervals when the effective subsidy
exceeded the nominal one, but there were also many times when a nominal
subsidy of 20 percent succeeded in lowering the retail price by only 5 or 10
percent. On many occasions, indicated by the plus signs in Table 15.6, the
final price would have exceeded that of the supermarkets, were it not for the
subsidy. This shows that the program was unsuccessful in competing with
the wholesale private sector.

In Table 15.7, a shorter period (23 weeks instead of seven years) is examined to estimate the degree of effective transfer of the subsidy. Although
during many weeks it was possible to transfer all or nearly all of the nominal subsidy, there were also many weeks in which only half or less of the
program's expenditure on the subsidy reached the consumer. If the comparison is made with the minimum price observed during the week, the
results are of course still worse. This does not by itself demonstrate the

Table 15.5 PNS, PCA, and PINS: Cost Structure in Percentage Terms (Data for One or More Years between 1978 and 1980)ᵃ

EXPENDITURE ITEM	PNS, 1978–79 MODELS E, Fᵇ			PCA, JANUARY–JUNE 1980ᶜ				PINS, JANUARY 1978–DECEMBER 1980ᵈ				
	1979 TOTAL	WITH HEALTH	WITHOUT HEALTH	RIO DE JANEIRO	BELO HORIZONTE	FEDERAL DISTRICT	TOTAL, 3 REGIONS	A	B	C	D	TOTAL
Food: total subsidy value	86.86	25.16	73.72	84.26	90.11	80.95	86.12	90.69 (151.15)	66.24 (147.20)	83.40 (165.33)	66.50 (221.67)	80.40 (161.84)
Food transportation and storage	10.74			1.79	1.22	1.79	1.55					
Personnel		1.39	4.07	10.81	7.01	12.04	9.44	1.58	4.74	2.93	6.27	3.19
Transportation of personnel				1.89	1.03	4.10	1.91					
Consumption material		0.17	0.50	0.03	0.06	0.37	0.10	0.07	0.10	0.12	0.27	0.12
Third-party services and other costs	2.40	7.40	21.68	1.21	0.57	0.76	0.87	7.67	13.77	13.56	27.03	12.75
Health activities		65.87							15.07			3.53

ᵃSource: reference 2, Table 11; from 6, p.164, and 10, section 4.23, with arithmetic corrections.

ᵇTwo PNS evaluation experiments were included, up to January 1980, in the PINS project (models E and F). The calculations refer to the sum of the models; the "without health" figures show the percentages of total expenditure excluding the 65.87 percent spent on health activities.

ᶜThe costs of personnel in the central administration are distributed among the three regions in proportion to the cost of food, which should be proportional to the number of beneficiaries. The costs of transportation of central administrative personnel are distributed between Rio de Janeiro and Belo Horizonte only in proportion to food costs in these regions, on the assumption that this item mainly represents travel between one of these regions and the Federal District.

ᵈA, B, C, D, indicate subsidy models.

ᵉFor the PINS, the value of the food exceeded the total subsidy cost to the government, as indicated by the figures in parentheses.

ᶠTransfers by INAN to pay the costs of the state secretariats of health; these may be regarded as administrative costs, principally for personnel.

Table 15.6 Recife, Pernambuco: Subsidy Level (Percentage) and PROAB Prices (Percentage Difference from Supermarket Price, with and without Subsidy) for Six Products, June 1980–July 1986[a]

Top panel

	Rice			Beans			Manioc Flour		
	Percentage Subsidy	Consumer Price Without Subsidy	With Subsidy	Percentage Subsidy	Consumer Price Without Subsidy	With Subsidy	Percentage Subsidy	Consumer Price Without Subsidy	With Subsidy
1980 Jun	20	−28.2	−42.4	20	−1.8	−21.5	20	+10.6	−11.5
Nov	20	+4.8	−16.3	23	+6.6	−18.0	15	+1.0	−14.2
1981 Jun	20	−9.6	−27.7	23	+13.0	−12.1	20	−0.7	−20.8
Nov	20	−10.1	−27.7	23	−0.1	−22.1	20	+3.1	−18.1
1982 Jun	15	−6.4	−20.6	20	+5.5	−15.6	20	−1.5	−22.1
Nov	15	−1.1	−16.3	13	−3.1	−15.7	20	+8.4	−12.7
1983 Jun	30	+7.5	−25.0	10	−8.4	−26.5	25	−12.9	−34.9
Nov	25	+11.2	−16.7	30	−1.4	−31.1	30	+10.7	−22.6
1984 Jun	25	+11.2	−16.5	30	+10.2	−22.8	30	+8.0	−24.4
Nov	20	−2.1	−21.7	—	—	—	—	—	—
1985 Jan	20	+7.1	−14.3	20	+7.1	−14.3	20	+3.3	−17.4
Jun	20	−2.4	−21.9	20	+10.3	−11.8	20	+8.1	−13.5
1986 Jan	20	−9.1	−27.3	20	−40.0	−52.0	20	−10.8	−28.6
Jul	—	—	—	—	—	—	—	—	—

Bottom panel

	Sugar			Powdered Milk			Soya Oil		
	Percentage Subsidy	Consumer Price Without Subsidy	With Subsidy	Percentage Subsidy	Consumer Price Without Subsidy	With Subsidy	Percentage Subsidy	Consumer Price Without Subsidy	With Subsidy
1980 Jun	10	−5.1	−14.4	15	−16.8	−28.5	17	−1.3	−11.0
Nov	10	−1.7	−8.5	17	+4.7	−13.2	20	+10.2	−5.2
1981 Jun	10	−7.0	−3.4	20	+8.3	−13.9	20	+6.7	−14.4
Nov	10	−7.0	−3.4	20	+10.6	−11.8	25	+7.1	−19.5
1982 Jun	10	+0.9	−9.2	15	+0.9	−14.6	20	−7.4	−26.2
Nov	15	+3.5	−11.9	15	+5.0	−10.7	20	+3.7	−16.9
1983 Jun	20	+5.0	−15.7	30	+9.7	−23.4	30	+10.3	−23.0
Nov	25	+1.6	−23.9	25	+13.5	−15.8	30	+9.4	−23.5
1984 Jun	25	+5.4	−20.9	25	+6.7	−19.9	30	+8.9	−23.8
Nov	20	+9.0	−12.9	—	—	—	—	—	—
1985 Jan	—	—	—	—	—	—	20	+8.6	−13.1
Jun	20	+7.1	−14.3	20	−0.1	−20.1	20	−3.4	−22.7
1986 Jan	20	+2.6	−17.9	20	+5.1	−15.9	20	−1.9	−21.5
Jul	20[b]	—	—	—	—	—	—	—	—

[a] Source: reference 2, Table 15; data from INAN. Dash indicates product not sold by the PROAB.
[b] Product unavailable in the supermarkets; there is no information on prices.

Table 15.7 Actual Transfer of the PROAB Subsidy to the Consumer, in Relation to Minimarket Prices, Recife, March-August 1984[a,b]

PERCENTAGE OF SUBSIDY TRANSFERRED	NO. OF WEEKS PER TRANSFER INTERVAL					
	RICE	BEANS	MANIOC FLOUR	SUGAR	POWDERED MILK	SOYA OIL
IN RELATION TO THE MINIMUM PRICE DURING THE WEEK						
100 and more	0	3	0	0	2	0
75–99.9	3	1	1	2	6	1
50–74.9	5	3	10	6	5	5
25–49.9	3	3	12	13	1	9
0–24.9	9	3	0	1	4	6
Negative	3	10	0	1	5	0
IN RELATION TO THE AVERAGE PRICE DURING THE WEEK						
100 or more	4	12	0	6	9	0
75–99.9	6	5	6	2	6	4
50–74.9	7	1	9	12	4	5
25–49.9	1	3	8	2	3	11
0–24.9	4	0	0	0	1	1
Negative	1	2	0	1	0	0

[a]Source: reference 2, Table 16; from 15, Tables 7 and 10, pp. 86 and 90. Prices were obtained over 23 weeks for all the products except soya oil (21 weeks).

[b]A "minimarket" is a small supermarket with a limited range of foods; those requiring refrigeration are not sold. Prices in such an establishment are normally no higher than those in a full supermarket.

309

inferiority of a subsidy compared with a donation, but it does show how difficult it is to assure that a dollar of public expenditure on food becomes a dollar of benefit to the participant.

Another reason given to justify the PROAB was that the poor paid artificially or unnecessarily high prices for their food. It has been shown that the government's intervention as a wholesaler did not produce retail prices comparing favorably with those of the private sector. Beyond that result, a direct examination of prices in June 1985 found no support for that hypothesis (18–20). It may have been true a decade earlier, when the assumptions that guided the programs were formed, but it was no longer true. Poverty is a problem of low incomes, not of high prices.

Additional Consumption and Physical Growth

The ultimate goal of all the programs was a normal nutritional status for the beneficiary; the justification for pursuing this end through a free or subsidized transfer of food was the assumption that without the program, food consumption would be insufficient, and that the transfer would serve to raise consumption. However, none of the programs had any way to determine, directly, whether this increase occurred. If the beneficiary relies on the program for only a small fraction of total intake (typically 20 to 25 percent of estimated needs, and an unknown share of actual consumption), then the change in consumption need not correspond to the amount of the transfer. In consequence, the only way to estimate the increase in consumption is to calculate food consumption functions based on survey data, taking account, in principle, of the most important determinants of intake such as income, family size and composition, and food prices. Estimates of this kind have been extensively used to evaluate the programs analyzed here (21, 22), but it must be emphasized that the data were not generated within a nutritional intervention. For this reason, and in addition to the difficulties of estimating such functions, these estimates may be a poor guide to the impact of any program other than a pure donation or subsidy, with no educational or health care components. They would thus be more helpful for evaluating the PROAB than for any other program.

The most complete and most valuable information on the impact of the programs was generated in several evaluative exercises, which measured the height and weight of beneficiary children before and after their participation in a program, and related the changes in nutritional status to age, initial nutritional situation, and length of participation. (In the case of birth weights, the comparison was not before-and-after, but between a group of beneficiary mothers and similar group who did not participate in the program.) Four examples of this kind of analysis are discussed in what follows, corresponding to four hypotheses or expectations about what a food and nutrition program should be able to accomplish.

Change of nutritional status

The most general expectation is that participating in a program should improve the status of a malnourished child, and keep normal those who enter the program normal. At the group level, this means more normal children and fewer malnourished children after some interval of participation than before. The first expectation corresponds to a curative, and the second to a preventive, criterion; program ideology does not emphasize one of these criteria over the other.

Table 15.8 summarizes the results of the three most complete anthropometric evaluations, referring respectively to the PCA, PNS, and PINS, and to weight for age. In these cases (although not in all the available information about the programs) the initial and final nutritional status are known for each individual child, so that the instances of improvement and worsening can be counted, rather than just knowing whether the number of children in each category grew or shrank. Four findings, more or less common to all three programs, are worth mentioning. First, the majority of participants showed no change in status: whether well nourished or malnourished, they tended to stay in the same category during intervals as long as 48 months. A large share of this stability is due to children who started out normal, but many malnourished children—especially those with first-degree (grade I) malnutrition—also did not change.

Second, there was a marked recovery for those children who began with moderate or severe malnutrition. In this curative sense, the programs show an impact. It is not clear whether this was due simply to the transfer of food, or whether the transfer of information about the danger to the child and the way of saving him or her was more important; the lack of evidence from the PROAB program does not allow a comparison with a pure physical transfer. Consistent with this finding, a child with moderate malnutrition rarely deteriorated further. Data in Table 15.9 are limited to children initially underweight for age, in the PNS and the PINS. The information distinguishes according to age at entry into the program and length of participation, as well as separating cases of improvement according to

Table 15.8 Changes Observed in Children Participating in the PCA, PNS, or PINS, According to Anthropometric Criterion, Duration of Participation, and Initial Nutritional Status, 1976–80, Expressed as Number of Children[a]

| | NORMAL | FINAL NUTRITIONAL STATUS[b] | | TOTAL | NONE | CHANGE OF STATUS | |
		I	II & III			IMPROVED	WORSENED
Weight for Age							
PCA (6 months)							
Normal	598	56	6	651	589	—	62
Malnourished I	170	196	12	378	196	170	12
II & III	12	33	12	57	12	45	—
Total	771	285	30	1,086	797	215	74
PNS (6–24 months)							
Normal	693	203	7	903	693	—	210
Malnourished I	198	509	66	773	509	198	66
II & III	21	148	167	336	135	197	4
Total	912	860	240	2,012	1,337	395	280
PNS (24–28 months)							
Normal	480	121	8	609	480	—	129
Malnourished I	296	558	71	925	558	296	71
II & III	68	272	155	495	113	376	6
Total	844	951	234	2,029	1,151	672	206
PINS (12 months)							
Normal	2,261	849	48	3,158	2,261	—	897
Malnourished I	477	2,141	248	2,866	2,141	477	248
II & III	36	350	510	896	451	426	19
Total	2,774	3,340	806	6,920	4,853	903	1,164

PINS (24 months)						
Normal	1,636	843	65	2,544	1,636	—	908
Malnourished I	467	1,456	224	2,087	1,456	407	224
II & III	55	333	310	698	261	426	11
Total	2,098	2,632	599	5,329	3,353	833	1143
Weight for Height						
PNS (6–24 months)						
Normal	985	63	6	1,054	985	—	69
Malnourished I	145	34	9	188	34	145	9
II & III	31	20	13	64	7	56	1
Total	1,161	117	28	1,306	1,026	201	79
PNS (24–28 months)						
Normal	450	32	6	488	450	—	38
Malnourished I	128	26	2	156	26	128	2
II & III	35	4	—	39	—	39	—
Total	613	62	8	683	476	167	40
Height for Age						
PNS (6–24 months)						
Normal	303	210	72	585	303	—	282
Malnourished I	58	209	146	413	209	58	146
II & III	18	65	225	308	152	114	42
Total	379	484	643	1,306	664	172	470
PNS (24–28 Months)						
Normal	125	89	17	231	125	—	106
Malnourished I	70	110	44	224	110	70	44
II & III	30	64	134	228	91	118	19
Total	225	263	195	683	326	188	169

[a]Source: reference 2, Table 30; from 10, section 7.25; 14, pp.23–25; and 16, Tables 47, 48, and 51–54.
[b]See footnote b, Table 4.

Table 15.9 Changes in Weight for Age in Initially Underweight Children Participating in the PNS or PINS, by Program, Initial Age, and Duration of Participation, Expressed as Number of Children[a]

	IMPROVED		TOTAL IMPROVED	NO CHANGE	DETERIORATED	TOTAL
	TO NORMAL	PARTIALLY				
PNS, participation 6–24 months						
Age 6–12 months	82	62	145	263	41	449
Age 12–36 months	137	113	250	381	29	660
PNS, participation 24–48 months						
Age 6–12 months	81	82	163	179	31	373
Age 12–36 months	283	226	509	492	46	1,047
PINS, participation 12 months						
Age 0–12 months	54	58	112	214	88	414
Age 12–72 months	459	332	791	2,378	179	3,348
PINS, participation 24 months						
Age 0–12 months	64	64	128	193	77	398
Age 12–72 months	398	307	705	1,524	158	2,387

[a]Source: reference 2, Table 35; from 16, Table 66; and 14, pp. 23–26.

whether the child reached normal nutritional status (full recovery) or remained malnourished (partial recovery). Cases of improvement were more frequent than stability only for children initially older than one year who participated in the PNS for at least two years. The results in Table 15.9 indicate that recovery—especially complete recovery—when it occurred, did not tend to happen quickly. They also suggest that the programs were more successful with children aged over one year than with younger infants: cases of deterioration are concentrated among infants. At older ages, a lack of change in nutrition status was more common. The question of children younger than one year is treated in more detail below.

Third, at least in the donation programs, improvement was more frequent than deterioration. That is, the net impact was for improvement. This did not happen, however, with the PINS subsidy. It is not clear whether this was the fault of the program which brought only a fraction of the beneficiaries to a health post and therefore could not obtain the potential medical and educational benefits of such intervention, or whether it was due to differences between Recife, where the PINS operated, and the cities of Brasília and Salvador. The different evaluations were conducted in essentially the same period, so it is unlikely that the general economic conditions of the country can account for this phenomenon.

Finally, the programs were only partly successful in maintaining normal status for those children who entered with no nutritional problems. In all cases a substantial fraction of the beneficiaries worsened, usually to a state of mild malnutrition. Apparently these interventions are more effective at cure than at prevention. However, the lack of observations on changes of nutritional status in a control group makes it impossible to attribute success or failure to a program.

Table 15.8 includes information on two other indicators, height for age and weight for height, just for the PNS and for only a subset of the children whose weight was recorded. Table 15.10 also provides data on all three indicators in the case of the PINS, but without registering the individual transitions. In both cases, one sees a tendency to retardation in growth, giving rise to an increase in the number of children who were slightly short for age and a decrease in the number of normal height. On the other hand, curative results were obtained in weight, but it is difficult to recover losses in height. In consequence, the data on weight for height show few cases of deterioration; slowed growth in stature is not accompanied by a proportional slowing in weight gain, so that weight is usually adequate in relation to height although low relative to age.

Table 15.10 Number of Children Initially Aged Under Six Participating in the PINS, According to Initial and Final Nutritional Status, by Anthropometric Criterion and Duration of Participation, 1978–80[a]

| | NUTRITIONAL STATUS[b] | | | | |
	NORMAL	I	II	III	TOTAL
Weight for Age					
Start	3,658	3,545	1,027	122	8,452
12 months	3,547	3,473	813	81	7,914
24 months	3,212	3,340	755	57	7,364
Weight for Height					
Start	6,788	1,380	202	77	8,447
12 months	6,600	1,228	149	37	8,014
24 months	4,967	1,930	389	78	7,354
Height for Age					
Start	5,312	1,286	1,411	341	8,350
12 months	5,412	1,131	1,187	275	8,005
24 months	4,516	2,166	447	226	7,355

[a]*Source:* reference 2, Table 31; from 14, pp. 16, 18, and 20.
[b]See footnote *b*, Table 4.

Length and regularity of participation

The data in Tables 15.8, 15.9, and 15.10, like those of Table 15.4, throw some light on the relation between changes in nutritional status and the interval of participation in a program, or the frequency with which food was received. The expectation in every program is that the benefit will be greater, and the outcome better, when the client participates regularly and for a long enough time to take full advantage of the benefits. Returning to Table 15.4, one can see that there is no relation between the number of times food was received during two years of participation and the relative frequencies of improvement and worsening. The reason is simple: The children who participated most frequently came from the families with the worst food situation at home, which offset the benefit or more regular participation. (In contrast to comparisons by age or initial nutritional status, frequency is not compared among random subsamples of the population of beneficiaries: frequency is endogenous to the experiment.)

In the case of the PNS there are data on children participating between six and 24 months and on another group participating between 24 and 48 months, without registering the number of times they actually received food during those intervals (Table 15.8). The evidence conforms to expectations for all three anthropometric indicators—the longer the interval, the better the results. The data in Table 15.9, referring only to children initially malnourished, confirm the findings of Table 15.8. Note that this result cannot be due to differential abandonment of the program, because the children who withdrew after a few months would tend to have better nutritional status, which would show up as greater success over shorter intervals. On the other hand, withdrawal from the program after less than two years could be due to greater age at entry: the data do not control simultaneously for age. The data on the PINS in Tables 15.8, 15.9, and 15.10 show less of a pattern: the frequency of worsening tends to rise, as the interval of participation is longer. However, these typically are transitions from normal to mildly malnourished. Reduction in the frequency of moderate and severe malnutrition continues in evidence.

Infants younger than one year

Infants present more of a problem for the success of food and nutrition programs than children at least one year old on entry: that is, the program seem less effective for the younger children, particularly in preventive terms (Table 15.9). This question is examined in Tables 15.11 and 15.12, which are limited to infants initially less than 12 months old and six months or older in the PNS but with no minimum age in the PINS. (The PINS registered families rather than individual children, so there was no minimum age for participants—as there is in the donation programs, so as not to interfere with breastfeeding.) In both tables, the individual transitions of nutritional status are recorded.

Table 15.11 shows two alarming results. First, there were many more cases of deterioration than of improvement among the infants supposedly benefited by the PINS; second, the absolute number of cases of moderate and severe malnutrition increased. This means that the worsening was not limited to children initially normal, although these were the most frequent instances. This result may not be surprising, because the PINS included health check-ups for only one group of infants, and it was in this group that the most families abandoned the program. It seems evident that a pure food subsidy, without any medical or educational intervention, is ineffective against deterioration of nutritional status in the first year of life. This worsening is almost surely due to the tendency not to breastfeed, or to stop nursing after only a few months, which leaves the child exposed to illness

Table 15.11 Changes in Weight for Age Observed in Children Initially Aged Under 12 Months, Participating in the PINS, According to Duration of Participation, 1978-80, Expressed as Number of Children[a]

DURATION OF PARTICIPATION/ INITIAL NUTRITIONAL STATUS	FINAL NUTRITIONAL STATUS[b]				CHANGE OF STATUS		
	NORMAL	I	II & III	TOTAL	NONE	IMPROVED	WORSENED
One year of participation							
Normal	501	383	36	920	501	—	419
Malnourished I	46	173	84	303	173	46	84
II and III	8	47	56	111	56	55	—
Total	555	603	176	1,334	730	101	503
Two years of participation							
Normal	357	411	47	815	357	—	458
Malnourished I	50	169	75	294	169	50	75
II and III	14	56	34	104	24	78	2
Total	421	636	156	1,213	550	128	535

[a]Source: reference 2, Table 34; from 14, pp. 23–26.
[b]See footnote b, Table 4.

and therefore to weight loss or, at best, inadequate growth. The PNS, in contrast, included health and education components, in the form of a monthly check-up for clients, and this probably explains its greater success in protecting infants. As Table 15.12 shows, cases of worsening were relatively less frequent; and for children who participated for two years or more, worsening was absolutely less frequent than improvement. This contrast does not invalidate the assumption that malnutrition is caused principally by poverty, but it clearly indicates that a small economic transfer, with no intervention in health or family behavior, is insufficient to protect or cure infants.

Weight at birth

The donation programs (PCA and PNS) gave free food not only to the children registered as beneficiaries, but also to pregnant women and nursing mothers, as a means to improve birth-weight and prevent malnutrition at early ages. Table 15.13 presents data comparing the experience of

Table 15.12 Changes Observed in Children Participating in the PNS, Initially Aged between 6 and 12 Months Old, According to Anthropometric Criterion and Duration of Participation, 1976–80, Expressed as Number of Children[a]

	WEIGHT FOR AGE	WEIGHT FOR HEIGHT	HEIGHT FOR AGE
Initial Distribution			
Normal	822	734	521
Malnourished I	567	142	266
Malnourished II	205	43	108
Malnourished III	50	16	40
Total	1,644	935	935
Changes with 6–24 months of participation:			
Total	992	644	644
None	651	504	285
Improved	145	101	37
Worsened	196	39	322
Changes with 24–48 months of participation:			
Total	652	240	240
None	388	170	107
Improved	163	50	47
Worsened	101	20	86

[a]Source: reference 2, Table 33; from 16, Tables 2, 9, 12, 60, 62, and 63.

Table 15.13 Weights of Live Births to Mothers who were Beneficiaries of the PNS and PCA, Compared with Non-Beneficiaries[a]

WEIGHT AT BIRTH	PNS, Salvador, 1974-78		PCA, Rio de Janeiro and Ceará, 1984				Total, Both States	
			Rio de Janeiro		Ceará			
	NO. OF BIRTHS	%	NO.	%	NO.	%	NO.	%
2,500 g or less								
Non-beneficiaries	136	15	1,467	10.3	850	11.1	2,317	10.6
Beneficiaries: total	129	15	624	8.3	647	9.8	1,271	9.0
For 3 months or longer	72	11						
2,501–3,000 g								
Non-beneficiaries	316	35	3,878	27.1	1,701	22.2	5,579	25.4
Beneficiaries: total	223	26	1,997	26.5	1,513	22.8	3,510	24.8
For 3 months or longer	112	17						
3,001–3,500 g								
Non-beneficiaries	316	35						
Beneficiaries: total	309	36						
For 3 months or longer	257	39						
Over 3,500 g								
Non-beneficiaries	136	15	8,941	62.6	5,119	66.7	14,060	64.0
Beneficiaries: total	198	23	4,904	65.2	4,464	67.4	9,368	66.2
For 3 months or longer	217	33						
Total births								
Non-beneficiaries	904	100	14,286	100.0	7,670	100.0	21,956	100.0
Beneficiaries: total	859	100	7,525	100.0	6,624	100.0	14,149	100.0
For 3 months or longer	658	100						

[a]Source: reference 2, Tables 27 and 28.

mothers who were beneficiaries of each program with women in nonpartici-
pating control groups. The implicit hypothesis, corresponding to a purely
preventive criterion, is that there should be fewer cases of low birth-weight
in the beneficiary group. The results appear to confirm this expectation,
although the differences are never substantial. In the PCA, for example, the
frequency of births with weight below 2.5 kilograms differed by no more
than two percentage points in the control group. (This difference can be as
large as 19 percent, but that happens because all the percentages are small,
not because the program achieved a large change.) The data on the PNS
provide additional information, by distinguishing women who participated
for three months or more before giving birth from those who were clients
for shorter periods. The frequency of low birth-weight does not differ from
that in the control group when all beneficiaries are considered together, but
it falls by four points, from 15 to 11 percent, when counting only those who
participated for at least a trimester. One may suspect the results for the PCA
would improve if the same distinction were made.

Concluding Remarks

It is difficult to reach any conclusion about the apparently simple comparison that initially motivated this study—that is, whether it is preferable to
attack childhood malnutrition through direct food donations or through a
subsidy to basic foodstuffs consumed by poor families. The results do not
disconfirm the underlying hypothesis that malnutrition is, above all, a consequence of poverty, and that therefore it cannot be prevented or corrected
without an economic transfer. Nonetheless, the analysis of two donation
and two subsidy programs leads to rejection, or at least weakening, of a
series of associated secondary hypotheses or expectations. Thus for example, it is not the case that the poor pay too much for their food; nor that
they are so poor as to guarantee their regular, long-term participation in a
program; nor that a subsidy is cheaper to administer; nor that a nominal
subsidy is automatically transformed into a real benefit for the client; nor
that the beneficiaries of a subsidy reach a final nutritional status as good as
or better than that of those who participate in a donation program.
In summary, the economic diagnosis of malnutrition justifies a direct
intervention just as well. It also appears that this diagnosis is incomplete,
as it does not adequately value the medical and educational components
that characterize a donation program. Particularly when the results are

compared for infants under one year old, it is evident that these components may be crucial.

Aside from the comparison between these two approaches, the empirical
analysis leads to a series of other conclusions, of greater or lesser solidity. It
is shown that despite the small economic value of the transfers, either type
of program can help to reduce the frequency of malnutrition. It is also
evident—and sad—that this impact is quite small, and that the majority of
beneficiaries experience no change in their nutritional status. The changes
that are produced tend to be more curative than preventive, with the obvious exception of the results for birth weight. Given a system to identify
beneficiaries and know when they suffer moderate or severe malnutrition,
recovery is possible for many if not all of them. It is much more difficult to
prevent the decline of a normal child to a state of mild under-nutrition.
Finally, the programs are successful primarily with respect to weight (in
relation to height or to age), and for children older than one year. They are
less effective in maintaining or increasing children's height in relation to
age; and they are relatively ineffective in protecting infants from the risks to
which the first year of life, and premature weaning, expose them. This finding reinforces the importance of regarding malnutrition as a health problem, and not merely as a deficit of food consumption.

Despite the extensive, rich, and varied experience accumulated in Brazil
during the last decade and a half, it takes some daring to draw recommendations for the design of operation of nutrition programs in that country,
and still more so for other countries. These experiments say nothing about
the value of interventions of the types studied relative to other potential
interventions—changes in wages or employment opportunities, expansion
or reorientation of health services, educational campaigns about breastfeeding or other practices, and so forth. (Several of these interventions have
been tried in Brazil; what is lacking, but would not be easy to provide, is a
comparative evaluation among programs of very different natures.)
Nonetheless, it seems legitimate to draw a few lessons, with emphasis on:

- The value of combining food transfers with health interventions and
  educational efforts;

- The importance of operating programs efficiently, so that the supposed
  benefits actually reach the client, a question of particular importance when
  the program is intended to compete with the private commercial sector;

- Attention to the quality and acceptability of foodstuffs, without relying on the assumption that the beneficiaries are too poor for such things to matter to them;

- Minimizing the costs the program imposes on the client, in time, distance, or other obstacles, assuring that for every cost or difficulty there corresponds a real gain for the beneficiary; and

- Abandonment of ideological or predetermined ideas, in order to take advantage of real experience and learn from it in practical circumstances.

In the absence of data and analyses, there is no alternative to trusting in the most plausible assumptions one can reach; but once empirical information exists—as it does, abundantly, in Brazil—this should be the basis for any decision about food and nutrition interventions.

References

[1] Pan American Health Organization. Estudio Sobre Intervenciones Alimentario-Nutricionales para Poblaciones de Bajos Ingresos en Latinoamérica y el Caribe. Resumen del Proyecto Colaborativo OPS-INTA. Unpublished Document HPN 89.9. Washington, D.C., 1989.
[2] Musgrove, P. Fighting Malnutrition; An Evaluation of Brazilian Food and Nutrition Programs. Discussion Paper No. 60. The World Bank, Washington, D.C., 1989.
[3] Campino, A.C. A Review of Nutrition Programs in Brazil. Fundação Instituto de Pesquisas Econômicas (FIPE), São Paulo, 1987.
[4] Carvalho da Silva, A. A summary of programs related to food and nutrition in Brazil. Annex 2 of Population, Health and Nutrition Department, the World Bank, Brazil: Nutrition Sector Review. The World Bank, Washington, D.C., 1983.
[5] McGreevey, W.P. Brazil—Public Spending on Social Programs; Issues and Options. Report No. 7086-BR, The World Bank, Washington, D.C., 1988.
[6] Cavalcanti, C., et al. Avaliação Socio-Econômica do PINS e do PNS em Pernambuco : II Relatório Parcial. Fundação Joaquim Nabuco (FUNDAJ), Recife, Brazil, 1980.
[7] Cavalcanti, C., et al. Pobreza, Carestia, Subalimentação; Relatório Final da Avaliação Socio-Econômica do Projeto Integrado de Nutrição e Saúde. Fundação Joaquim Nabuco (FUNDAJ), Recife, Brazil, 1981.

[8] Cavalcanti, C., *et al.* Pobreza, Carestía, Subalimentação: Avaliação Socio-Econômica de uma Intervenção Nutricional em Pernambuco. Editora Massangana, Recife, Brazil, 1984.

[9] Chaves, S., *et al.* Avaliação do estado nutricional de pre-escolares beneficiários do Programa de Nutrição em Saúde. Alimentação e Nutrição 5(15), 1984.

[10] Fundação Legião Brasileira de Assistência and UNICEF, Projeto de Avaliação do Programa de Complementação Alimentar: Relatório Final. Brasília, Brazil, 1982.

[11] Kalil, A.C., *et al.* Causas do abandono do Programa de Nutrição em Saúde. Alimentação e Nutrição 5(15), 1984.

[12] Kalil, A.C., *et al.* Estudo da freqüênça de gestantes na ativadade de suplementação alimentar em São Paulo. Alimentação e Nutrição 5(15), 1984.

[13] Lerner, B.R., *et al.* Estudo de evolução do estado nutricional de pré-escolares segundo sua freqüênça em um programa de suplementação alimentar. Alimentação e Nutrição 6(22), 1985.

[14] Nunes da Silva, R.M. Avaliação antropométrica do PINS: resultados preliminares obtidos por tabulação manual. Unpublished manuscript. Centro Integrado de Saúde Amaury de Medeiros (CISAM), Recife, Brazil, 1985.

[15] Oliveira, C.G., and Medeiros, R.P. O Projeto de Abastecimento de Alimentos Básicos em Áreas de Baixa Renda: uma Avaliação. Fundação Joaquim Nabuco (FUNDAJ) and Instituto Nacional de Alimentação e Nutrição (INAN), Recife, Brazil, 1985.

[16] Rios, I.M.E. Nutrition Intervention: An Anthropometric Evaluation of Changes in Nutritional Status, with Reference to the National Nutrition Programme in Bahia, Brazil. Ph.D. Thesis, London School of Hygiene and Tropical Medicine, 1981.

[17] Musgrove, P. Ideología, pesquisa y realidad de la situación alimentaria y nutricional del Brasil. Cadernos de Estudos Sociais 2(1), 1986.

[18] Galindo, O. Quanto Pagam os Pobres? Estudo de Comparação Espacial de Preços de Alimentos no Nordeste Brasileiro. Fundação Joaquim Nabuco (FUNDAJ), Recife, Brazil, 1985.

[19] Galindo, O., and Musgrove, P. Quanto pagam os pobres? Determinantes geográficos e comerciais dos preços dos alimentos no nordeste. Revista Econômica do Nordeste 17(2), 1986.

[20] Musgrove, P., and Galindo, O. Do the poor pay more? Retail food prices in northeast Brazil. Economic Development and Cultural Change 37(1), 1988.

[21] Musgrove, P. Demografía e bem-estar; tamanho familiar e consumo alimentício no Nordeste Brasileiro. In: Anais do V Encontro da Associação Brasileira de Estudos Populacionais. Águas de São Pedro, São Paulo, October 12–16, 1986.

[22] Musgrove, P. A despesa familiar e os preços dos alimentos como determinantes do consumo alimentício no Nordeste Brasileiro. Estudos Econômicos 18(1), 1988.

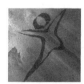

CHAPTER 16

Economic Aspects
of Food Fortification

Acknowledgment

I am grateful to my colleague Judith McGuire for very helpful discussion, but she is not to blame for any of the paper's faults.

Introduction: Is Food Fortification Economically Interesting?

Since this note deals primarily with the economic aspects of fortifying foods with micronutrients, rather than with the nutritional consequences of doing so or the technical issues of how foods are fortified, it is reasonable to begin by asking whether there is anything about the subject which is intrinsically interesting from an economic point of view. That is, would it attract the professional attention of an economist who was not also interested in the results for people's health? Since the most salient fact about fortification is that it costs very little compared to the value of the food being treated—independently of the specific foodstuff and the particular micronutrient(s) employed—the short answer would appear to be no, fortification is not economically interesting. It does not seem to pose any special problems or to require any deep or unusual analysis.

The interest in fortification expressed by the World Bank and other agencies concerned with reducing micronutrient malnutrition in poor countries is consistent with this view. Essentially all the emphasis is on the cost-effectiveness of the technique, compared to other ways of dealing with

Paper presented to the Ninth World Congress of Food Science and Technology, 30 July–4 August 1995, Budapest, Hungary. Reprinted from *International Journal of Food Science and Technology*, with permission from Blackwell Science, Ltd.

micronutrient deficiencies and, in general, other interventions to improve health, educability and productivity. It is this emphasis which led the Bank to sponsor the study of *Disease Control Priorities in Developing Countries* [Jamison, Mosley, Measham and Bobadilla, 1993] and to include in it a chapter on various interventions against micronutrient deficiencies [Levin, Pollitt, Galloway and McGuire, 1993]. The effectiveness of all the interventions studied is measured in units called Disability-Adjusted Life Years, or DALYS, which take into account the age at incidence of a health problem and—if it results in permanent or temporary disability rather than premature death—how severe the disability is [Murray, 1994]. The disabilities caused by severe deficiencies of iodine and vitamin A include cretinism or milder mental retardation, and blindness, and they strike at early ages, so the burden of disease associated with them is substantial, even when the future is discounted so that long-term disability is not simply summed through time. Iron-deficiency anemia tends to strike also at later ages and typically causes less severe health damage, but it affects far more people, so the health burden it causes is still very large, greater in fact than the direct burden due to deficiencies of either iodine or vitamin A [Murray, Lopez and Jamison, 1994]. Since vitamin A deficiency increases the risk of young children dying from other causes [Humphrey, West and Sommer, 1992], there is also a large indirect burden of mortality which can be reduced by preventing or curing the deficiency [World Bank, 1993: Table 4.3]. Iron-deficiency anemia poses a risk of mortality in childbirth, but otherwise iron and iodine deficiencies do not appear to cause appreciable indirect disease burdens.

The combination of the low cost of fortification with these three micronutrients and the large potential health gains in populations where deficiencies are prevalent mean that food fortification can be among the most cost-effective health interventions known, costing as little as $5–$20 per DALY gained, whereas many other interventions yield health improvements only at a cost of $100 or more per DALY [Jamison, 1993: Tables IA-3 and IA-6]. These findings are the basis for the World Bank's recommendation that micronutrient interventions, including fortification, be included in an "essential package" of public health and clinical services which governments should ensure are available to the whole population and should subsidize for the poor [World Bank, 1993: Table 4.7; Bobadilla, Cowley, Musgrove and Saxenian, 1994]. The conclusion that "No other technology offers as large an opportunity to improve lives . . . at such low cost and in such a short time" is the basis for Bank policy on overcoming vitamin and mineral malnutrition in developing countries [World Bank, 1994], with or without the development of a complete essential package of services. What is economically interesting in this approach is the very high value for money that can be obtained when deficiencies are prevalent enough and can be effectively reduced by supplementation, fortification or changes in diet.

This narrow view of the economic aspects of fortification arises from several limiting factors which are of particular relevance in very poor countries:

- Prevalence is quite high (the cost-effectiveness estimates are based on 15% of the population being vitamin A-deficient, 24% iodine deficient, and 50% suffering from iron deficiency anemia, with the share rising to 63% among pregnant women);

- Only three well-studied micronutrients are considered, and no account is taken of interactions among them or between any of them and other trace elements or compounds: there are thus no complicated questions of what is happening to the entire diet;

- The objective is always to *increase* consumption of the nutrient, never to decrease it or simply to inform consumers so that they can choose to control their intake; and

- Fortification is most often applied to relatively unprocessed foods (or, in the case of iodine, to well water) such as sugar, salt, rice or flour, which most of the population already eats, although more industrialized foods are sometimes used [World Bank, 1994: Table 4.1].

One result of these limitations is that deficiencies can be considered a public health problem justifying or even requiring strict government intervention, typically by mandating that all commercial supplies of a food be fortified, with sanctions for noncompliance by producers [World Bank, 1994: 31–32 and 46–47]. The same conditions may justify government financing of the additional costs imposed by fortification, including the costs of protecting the food from nutrient loss, informing the public, and monitoring compliance with the mandate. Poor consumers may reduce their consumption in response to even very small price increases, while poor, artisan producers may find fortification more costly than large industrial producers. As a result, fortification may provide micronutrients preferentially to those consumers who need them least, and may discriminate against small, low-income producers unless the costs are subsidized. Another consequence is that fortification is rather sharply distinguished from dietary change, because while the fortified foods may be perceived by the population as different from traditional, unfortified foods and it may be necessary to gain public acceptance of the fortification, the object is not to introduce any completely new foods or to change markedly the characteristics of what people already eat. In fact, if it were not for the possibility that consumers will perceive—or imagine—such differences and avoid the fortified foods, there would be no reason to explain fortification to them or to incur the costs of labeling and experimentation to gain public acceptance.

All these limiting assumptions change as a population becomes richer and more educated. The economic questions change accordingly. It is still important to know whether fortification or other modification of a foodstuff is cost-effective in improving health, but both the costs and the effects can be quite different when the health consequences may be primarily changes in cardio-vascular disease or cancer rather than blindness, anemia or mental retardation, and the costs are increasingly related to information and monitoring. Such costs can be much larger relative to the costs of modifying the food itself, than in the simpler situation of poor countries and minimal information expense [US Food and Drug Administration, 1991]. As fortification becomes less a uniform procedure applied to a small number of foods and more a way for producers to differentiate their products in a highly competitive market, retailers as well as producers may adopt particular strategies to expand or defend their market shares, to protect themselves against liabilities and to affect government regulation in favorable ways [Caswell, 1991]. Both because prevalence of micronutrient problems is likely to be lower and because consumers and producers are better able to bear the costs of fortification, it becomes less clear that public subsidy is justified, and the question of who should pay to fortify foods becomes more important.

The Relation of Fortification to Poverty, Ignorance and Disease

It is convenient to identify these three factors as the crucial causes of malnutrition, whether that refers to protein-calorie undernutrition or to micronutrient deficiencies [Musgrove, 1993: 27–28]. There are of course factors which may be considered more fundamental, such as iodine-poor soils which lead to iodine shortage in foodstuffs—but for that to lead to iodine deficiency disease, people have to be too poor to buy foods grown or caught elsewhere, or too ignorant to know that they need such foods in addition to those produced locally. Illness is least important as a source of micronutrient deficiency disease where iodine is concerned, and probably most important for iron-deficiency, since infection by malaria or intestinal helminths can cause iron-deficiency anemia even when the diet contains enough iron [Jamison, Mosley, Measham and Bobadilla, 1993: 132–38 and 282; Warren and Mahmoud, 1990: 252]. Diarrheal disease also contributes to deficiency of both iron and vitamin A. Poverty is arguably most significant in the case of iron, since the foods richest in readily available iron, such as meat, are also relatively expensive. And ignorance is perhaps the chief cause of vitamin A deficiency, since foods rich in the vitamin or its precursors are available almost everywhere and often are not expensive. However, there is no one-to-one connection between particular micronutrient problems and particular causes.

The economics of food fortification is partly a matter of how fortification is related to these three causes of malnutrition, since the different causes have different economic implications. Fortification appears to be least relevant where disease is concerned: the low, regular doses of micronutrients in fortified foods are too small for therapeutic purposes—in contrast to supplementation with vitamin A as part of the treatment of measles, for example [Jamison, Mosley, Measham and Bobadilla, 1993: 165–6]—although they might reduce the severity of infection. This means that fortification will never entirely supplant supplementation where there is a short-term need for appreciably larger doses, which may be the case not only for disease treatment but also for iron supplementation during pregnancy. Supplementation of pregnant women appears to be cheaper per life saved than fortification for the entire population [Levin, Pollitt, Galloway and McGuire, 1993: Table 19E-3], since the risk of death associated with iron-deficiency anemia is highest for that group, because of the chance of hemorrhage. However, fortification for the whole population is more cost effective in total DALYs gained per dollar, when anemia is also highly prevalent among men and children. Expressing health gains in DALYs or a similar measure is more consistent with economic theory than simply counting deaths averted, since DALYs are integrated through time, incorporate judgements about the disutility associated with disability at different ages, and take account of non-fatal losses. Economics says that all these factors matter, but does not dictate the values of several subjective parameters; different values for these parameters yield different estimates of disease burdens and therefore different rankings of health interventions [Murray, Lopez and Jamison, 1994; Musgrove, 1994]. The relation among the three major strategies for micronutrient deficiency control is treated further in the next section.

In contrast to the situation with respect to disease, fortification is clearly an important response to the problems of poverty and ignorance. Poverty is most relevant where it keeps people from eating more expensive foods supplying the needed micronutrients, so that fortification of cheaper foods is the equivalent of a price reduction for the micronutrient. Thus iodized salt is, so far as iodine deficiency *alone* is concerned, equivalent to a reduction in prices of seafood and other iodine sources, and iron fortification of flour is equivalent, with respect to iron-deficiency anemia, to a reduction in the price of meat. If the consumer were actually buying iron, iodine, vitamin A and other micronutrients separately from the foods which serve as vehicles, these effects would be potentially very important, because the lower a consumer's income, the greater is the response to price changes. Richer consumers can afford to respond less. The price effects need not be constant: the availability of a food fortified with vitamin A, available at a fixed price, could lower the cost of the vitamin at those times when the prices of leafy green vegetables are high, offsetting seasonal price and consumption fluctuations [Bouis, 1990]. This effect should in principle be unimportant for nutrients like vitamin A which the body can store for long periods; however, if average intake is too low to build up adequate stores, fortification can prevent deficiency during periods of low consumption, even for vitamin A.

Price decreases are relevant, of course, only if the food is available and the consumer is accustomed to buying it. The main reason poverty is relevant to the economics of fortification is that being poor is associated with subsistence food production and low cash incomes. This is probably the chief limitation to the market for fortified foods, since there is no way to fortify what people grow on their own small plots and eat with little or no processing. However, simply being poor does not put people beyond the reach of commercial fortification, because the degree to which poverty is associated with non-market food consumption varies greatly among places and populations. For example, extremely poor peasants in the mountains of Peru obtain about half their income in cash, partly from the sale of agricultural produce, and spend about half that cash on food [Figueroa, 1981]. This exchange serves mostly to increase dietary variety, and incidentally creates opportunities for micronutrient fortification of such foods as salt, sugar, oil and processed cereal products.

In practice, the consumer buys the foods and not their individual characteristics, so the effect on micronutrient consumption is the increase due to fortification, less any decline in consumption of the fortified food caused by the consumer having to pay part of the increased cost of fortifying it, plus any increase in consumption motivated by the knowledge that the food is now worth more because it has been fortified. Estimates of the cost effectiveness of fortification generally ignore both the latter effects, assuming that if the fortification program is properly designed and implemented, consumption will not be affected. People will simply buy and consume as much of the fortified food as they formerly did of the unfortified food: no one will eat more sugar in order to get more vitamin A, the demand for sugar being determined rather by its caloric content, price and other bulk features. The crucial question is not whether consumers will want to eat more sugar or flour because they know it to be better for their health, but whether they will continue to prefer the traditional, unfortified food because the fortified alternative tastes different or must be cooked differently, or because they believe there is some danger in eating it.

This way of looking at the demand for a fortified foodstuff is equivalent to supposing that poverty is the main source of malnutrition, and that ignorance is a problem primarily so far as people believe untruths about fortified foods that would reduce the willingness to eat them. Perfect ignorance, in which people do not know that they need the nutrient but also do not know that the food has been fortified, would have no effect on consumption, and "thus, even those consumers who may be unaware of the diet/health revolution may inadvertently eat a better diet" [US Food and Drug Administration, 1991: 60857]. However, such perfect ignorance is probably rare or nonexistent, and fortification programs almost invariably assume that people should be educated about the benefits of the fortified food, since "the creation of demand [is] the indispensable factor for success" [World Bank, 1994: 19]. Even if there is no net effect on consumption, such education at least will counteract the risk of reduced demand because of incomplete or erroneous beliefs. Thus food fortification is intimately linked to ignorance as a cause of malnutrition and—although this is not intrinsically necessary—is often one of the means to reduce that ignorance.

In the terms of economic theory, a fortified food is a different product, not simply the old product at a possibly higher price, and in order for it to provide utility and therefore be demanded, its benefits have to be known. In the long run, these benefits might be learned empirically by ignorant consumers, just as people have learned the health value of traditional, unfortified foods. Those populations which eat *capsicum* peppers as part of their regular diet do not need to know anything about vitamins in order to avoid vitamin deficiencies. But there is no reason to wait for that slow learning: a great part of the attraction of micronutrient fortification is that it can improve health rapidly.

The Relation of Fortification to Supplementation and to Dietary Change

The question of how fortification is related to the three causes of malnutrition helps to understand how it is related to the other two principal strategies for combating that malnutrition—individual supplementation apart from foods, and changes in diets to include more natural sources of the micronutrients. Much of the discussion of cost-effectiveness concerns the relative costs and likely relative outcomes of these strategies, from which to determine in what proportions they should be used for lowest overall cost per DALY gained in a particular population. The answer depends, among other things, on the particular deficiency, its prevalence and severity in different sub-populations, the current diet, people's knowledge of food and health, and the structure of the industry producing the foods which are candidates for fortification.

This variety of factors makes it impossible to specify a uniform strategy for controlling micronutrient deficiencies: in particular, the approach that appears to be cheapest is not necessarily the best for the whole population because of variation in the effectiveness. For example, the cost of protecting one person from deficiency for one year may be 3–4 times as high with vitamin A capsules as with fortification of sugar [Levin, Pollitt, Galloway and McGuire, 1993: Table 19.6], but if some children are severely vitamin-deficient or live in such poor or remote places that they do not eat purchased sugar, then supplementation with capsules may be the most cost-effective approach *for them*. Despite these complications, there is a general pattern of recommendations [World Bank, 1994: Table 7.1]. Supplementation is most appropriate for dealing with severe deficiencies, especially in defined and easily reached sub-populations. For iron deficiency, it is expected that supplementation may be justified for a long time, at least for pregnant women, because of the difficulty of providing them adequate iron through either fortification or dietary change. Supplementation is regarded as only a short-term remedy for most situations of iodine or vitamin A deficiency, to be supplanted by fortification (particularly for iodine) or changes in diet (particularly for vitamin A). Fortification comes closest to being *the* crucial strategy for iodine, since iodine deficiency in the soil will show up in whatever foods are produced, and dietary change has to involve not simply differences in what people eat but differences in where the food is grown or caught. For iron and vitamin A deficiency, it is often assumed that dietary change can take over some (iron) or nearly all (vitamin A) of the scope for fortification.

Of course, this comparison is limited to those three micronutrients: there is little discussion of the relative scope of the three mechanisms for dealing with deficiencies of other nutrients such as calcium, zinc or vitamins other than A. In part, this reflects less complete knowledge of the economics of other micronutrients and their deficiencies. More to the point, it reflects the fact that concern with poor countries is concentrated on the tropics, and on populations which until recently had such short life expectancies and such a disease pattern that most of the easily-correctable disease burden falls on young children [World Bank, 1993: Tables B6.7; Murray, Lopez and Jamison, 1994]. Thus there is no concern with possible deficiency of vitamin D, in populations exposed to strong sunlight all year long—although fortification of dairy products with vitamin D produced dramatic health gains by eradicating rickets in northern Europe. And concern with deficiencies of such minerals as calcium or zinc has been overshadowed by the dominant problem of what is usually called protein-energy malnutrition—even though the low weight and height by which that condition is measured may actually be due, in large part, to micronutrient shortages which are not expressed as disease but which interfere with growth [Golden, 1991].

Fortification of foods that people already eat, and persuading people to eat (more of) different foods, clearly are different approaches to micronutrient deficiencies in several respects—in the degree to which consumers need to be educated, in the involvement of food producers, and in the extent to which food is bought or produced at home. There also seems to be, in some discussions, a belief that dietary change is more "sustainable" than fortification, because it depends more on a permanent change in people's beliefs about food and health. Fortification is seen as more vulnerable to reversal, whether because in economic downturns people would withdraw from the market for purchased food, or because producers would find compliance onerous and evade it, or because governments can change and abandon their commitment to controlling deficiencies. It is partly in response to this possibility, that fortification programs are accompanied by education of the public about the beneficial health consequences—even though that would not be necessary in the situation of perfect ignorance described earlier.

As fortification depends more on information, and as consumers become richer and more educated, and produce less of what they eat and buy more of it, the sharp distinction begins to blur. In richer countries, fortification is not so much an *alternative* to dietary change as it is one *kind* of dietary change. People need to be persuaded to consume the product in both cases, and they must be able to afford it: after that, it hardly matters whether the micronutrients in the food were put there by nature or in a factory. It is abundantly clear that people value variety in the diet, and expand the diversity of foods eaten as they get richer—suggesting, among other things, that they do not consider calorie shortage to be their main nutritional problem, since they will spend additional income on other food characteristics and increase their caloric intake only very slowly unless they are acutely hungry [Behrman and Deolalikar, 1989]. This increased dietary diversity does not seem intrinsically to favor either natural or processed foods; tastes, knowledge and prices will determine which foods are consumed and therefore what happens to nutrient intakes. In fact, so far as micronutrients are concerned, the principal factor working against the expansion of fortification may be that voluntary, unsubsidized supplementation—in the form of oral vitamin and mineral supplements—also becomes much more available and affordable.

"Dietary change", as a strategy to control micronutrient deficiency, means "change for the better." But of course much dietary change in the world is neutral, or even change for the worse; it is driven by changes in tastes, income and relative prices, not simply by a search for better health [Popkin, 1992]. This is the case not only for increased consumption of sugar and fat, with the attendant risks of diabetes, caries, cardiovascular disease and possibly cancer. It is also the case for reduced consumption of some traditional foods of the poor, such as pulses, which are a relatively rich vegetable source of iron. In the quarter century from 1961 to 1986, worldwide availability of pulses fell by about one-third [World Bank, 1994: Figure 5.1], with most of the decline being replaced by increased consumption of cereals. This may have been largely an unintended consequence of the "green revolution". Such changes can contribute to decreased availability of micronutrients, especially iron but—at least in the Sahel and in West Africa over the last two decades—also of vitamin A [World Bank, 1994: Figure 1.1; UN Subcommittee on Nutrition, 1992: Figures 3.2, 3.4 and 3.5]. (Estimates of these average availabilities are based on food balance sheets and say nothing about the distribution of a micronutrient in the population, so they may or may not be correlated with evidence of increased deficiency. In some countries, they reflect increased poverty as well as income-neutral dietary change.) Fortification of the foods being consumed in greater quantities to replace those foods people are eating less is a protective reaction to dietary change which threatens health by reducing nutrient availability.

There has been so much dietary change, in most of the world, in the last couple of decades, and such dramatic health progress, that any guesses about the future of food fortification must be very speculative. But it seems reasonable to expect, based both on the experience of richer countries and on the needs and opportunities in poor populations, that fortification will be a natural and substantial part of any long-term dietary equilibrium. The disappearance of deficiency disease is not going to remove the need for micronutrient intakes, but only reduce the need for large-dose interventions; increased health knowledge will probably continue to expand the scope for fortifying with other nutrients; and modern retailing will reach more and more of the population. For example, the expansion of supermarkets has already done away, in middle-income countries such as Brazil, with price differences that in the past may have penalized poor consumers and contributed to their malnutrition [Musgrove and Galindo, 1988] The people at risk of being left out of this process will be those who continue to live by subsistence farming in remote rural areas, or whose mistaken beliefs about food and health are, for whatever reason, especially resistant to change. Everyone else should end up largely protected from micronutrient deficiencies, either because of deliberate dietary choices or just because so many of the inexpensive foods available to them contain adequate amounts of those nutrients.

Who Can and Should Subsidize Whom?

In economics, it is seldom enough to show that on some criterion of benefit, a good or service is worth buying: the analysis is not complete unless one also knows who should bear the cost. Thus an important part of the discussion of food fortification in poor countries concerns who should pay for it—the consumer, the producer or the government. This may seem odd, because at first glance it appears that even a very poor consumer should be willing to pay the small extra cost of protection against micronutrient deficiency diseases, given the very large potential health benefits. For example, at an income level of $1 per person per day, such protection could be had, for iron, iodine and vitamin A deficiencies, for about $1 per year, or one day's income in the year. (This is the level at which the World Bank's recommended essential health service package would cost about $12 per person per year [Bobadilla, Cowley, Musgrove and Saxenian, 1994: Table 2], including the cost of vitamin A supplementation; adding supplementation or fortification for iron and iodine would still account for only a small share of the total package cost.) Considered purely as an investment in their children, preventing micronutrient deficiency disorders is one of the best-paying things poor parents could spend their limited money for. In high-prevalence environments, such expenditure can often mean the difference between a healthy child who can contribute to the family's income, and a blind, cretinous or severely anemic child who is a drain on his or her parents' resources. Immunization is probably the only comparable low cost insurance against a major health loss [Jamison, 1993: Table IA.3].

However, as the example of immunization shows, parents do not spontaneously demand and buy this insurance: if close to 80% of the world's children are protected today against the six EPI diseases, it is only because of sustained public expenditure, both to cover the cost of immunization and to educate and mobilize parents to take advantage of the subsidy. It is probably illusory to suppose that people will be any more rational or willing to spend their own money on micronutrient protection than on protection against communicable disease. They may even be less willing, when supplementation or fortification represents a repeated expense, whereas immunizations are few and long-lasting.

In economic terms, there are three quite distinct reasons for governments to intervene in the health sector rather than leaving it to private markets. One is to assure the adequate provision of public goods or services with large externalities. Private markets cannot exist for pure public goods since people can benefit from them without paying for them; and markets will under-produce goods with positive (beneficial) externalities since those paying do not obtain all the benefits. Another reason has to do not with the nature of the intervention but with a characteristic of the beneficiary: governments subsidize health services, just as they subsidize other services, for poor people when this is more efficient than transferring income. Finally, in the domain of expensive, private goods, it makes sense for governments to intervene to correct or offset market failures, particularly in the market for health insurance [Musgrove, 1996: Part 2]. Clearly the last of these reasons is irrelevant where micronutrient deficiencies are concerned, since they cost so little to prevent. Any argument in favor of public intervention must depend on poverty or on some public good or externality. And, as indicated above, poverty should not really be an obstacle to people paying the cost of fortification, provided they are already eating one or more of the foods that can be cheaply and easily fortified. There is perhaps even less of a public goods reason to subsidize fortification: micronutrient deficiencies are not communicable, so protecting one person does not protect anyone else even partially, and if the cost of a fortified food is passed on to the consumer, then no one can benefit without also paying for it. (Fortifying a communal water source, such as a well, with iodine is an exception: the water is a public good unless people are required to pay to use the well.)

Nonetheless, it is common for governments to subsidize micronutrient deficiency control programs, and common to argue that this should be done. This is particularly the case for supplementation, which has to be provided individually, so that unwillingness to pay on the part of the beneficiary may be more of a problem—payment is exclusively for the supplement rather than going predominantly for a desired food. It is also common for governments to pay for consumer education and demand-creation programs, as part of dietary change programs, but here the public-good argument does apply; markets are unlikely spontaneously to generate that information and change of habits. Where fortification is concerned, it is usually argued that even if governments do not pay for the process, they should intervene to require all producers to comply and to educate the public so that demand for the product is not affected [World Bank, 1994].

Where governments actually subsidize the fortification, two arguments are probably most important. One is that the cost is so low that even if it is theoretically inappropriate, there is no harm in spending public money, and much health gain to be had. In the same way, it may be a mistake in theoretical economic terms for the state to subsidize the Expanded Program of Immunization, but that error is surely justified by the results. In both cases, government action makes up for the ignorance or indifference of parents, which leads them to be inadequate agents for the health of their children—who, not yet being sovereign adults, cannot choose for themselves whether to buy fortified foods, pay for immunizations, and so on. In market-failure terms, this is a "principal-agent problem", possibly the most serious one in the health sector.

The other argument for subsidy is that until consumers fully understand the value of fortification and are willing to pay for it—in fact, until they come to reject unfortified foods as not being worth the cost saving—it is better not to let even a small price difference separate the traditional, unfortified food and the new, fortified substitute. Initially, producers are not sure they can pass on the cost to consumers, and so ask for subsidy or try to evade the requirement to fortify; governments cannot easily enforce compliance on the industry, particularly if it includes many small producers; and consumers will be more willing to try the changed food if there is no cost to them. Spending more to subsidize the fortification may actually even save a government money, if less has to be spent on enforcement, and in any case fortification may be cheaper than the associated cost of monitoring the quality of the product at the retail level. (There is even more potential saving, if the government would otherwise have to pay for the medical care of the victims of micronutrient deficiency diseases.) Arguments like these explain, for example, why the government of Brazil has chosen to pay the cost of fortifying salt with iodine, and thereby virtually eliminating a previously serious problem of cretinism and endemic goiter in some parts of the country [Medeiros-Neto, 1988].

These obviously are transitional arguments, justifying public subsidy in order to launch fortification and assure that customers will become accustomed to it and eventually demand it. Once that happens, there is much less reason for subsidizing fortification (although there may continue to be a case for subsidy to supplementation, and there will always be a case for public finance of information that contributes sufficiently to better health.) Subsidies to fortify traditional foods such as salt or sugar, with the most important micronutrients—especially iodine and vitamin A—may continue just because it becomes politically difficult to do away with them, but the rest of the industry can evolve toward the current situation in richer countries. Fortified foods, like foods processed in other health-related ways, such as by reducing the content of fat, salt or cholesterol, will have to pass a market test and be paid for by consumers, while the government role becomes primarily one of setting standards and assuring compliance with them [US Food and Drug Administration, 1991]. It becomes particularly important for the government not to subsidize any and every instance of fortification, as more and more foods are fortified and there are multiple sources of individual micronutrients and also more than one micronutrient added to an individual food product—it would be neither cost-effective nor cheap to subsidize whatever producers offer in the market, and so it is crucial to pass the cost to the private market, to be divided between producers and consumers according to the price elasticity of demand.

Finally, since some people continue to be poor even in richer countries, and should not be condemned to micronutrient deficiency diseases just because they are poor, there may be continued occasion for public subsidy for them. But if poverty is a serious problem, the solution probably is not to subsidize only the cost of improving foods' micronutrient content, but (part of) the total cost of the fortified food. Government policy is then a mixture of subsidizing some foods for the poor, and of setting nutritional standards for which foods can be subsidized. This is the case in the United States, for example, where the Women, Infants and Children (WIC) Program subsidizes only certain foods, determined by their nutrient content, whereas the more general Food Stamp Program of income supplementation pays part of the cost of a wide variety of foods and does not discriminate among them according to health criteria (apart from such limitations as excluding alcoholic beverages). To return to the question of the evolution of fortification, the natural trend is toward less subsidy and control of micronutrients as such, but governments will continue an active role in assuring information and product quality. And the costs of those activities will still have to be justified by their consequences for health, including the effects on food safety.

References

Behrman, Jere R. and Anil Deolalikar. 1989. "Is Variety the Spice of Life? Implications for Calorie Intake." *Review of Economics and Statistics* XX: 666–672.

Bouis, Howarth E. 1990. "The Determinants of Household-Level Demand for Micronutrients: an Analysis for Philippine Farm Households." Washington, DC: International Food Policy Research Institute (processed).

Bobadilla, José-Luis, Peter Cowley, Philip Musgrove and Helen Saxenian. 1994. "Design, Content and Financing of an Essential National Package of Health Services." In Murray and Lopez, *GCAHS*.

Caswell, Julie A. and Gary V. Johnson. 1991. "Firm Strategic Response to Food Safety and Nutrition Regulation." Chapter 13 of Caswell, Julie A., ed., *Economics of Food Safety*. New York: Elsevier.

Figueroa, Adolfo. 1981. *La Economía Campesina de la Sierra del Perú*. Lima: Pontificia Universidad Católica.

Golden, Michael H. N. 1991. "The Nature of Nutritional Deficiency in Relation to Growth Failure and Poverty." *Acta Pediatrica Sandinavica*, Supplement 374: 95–110.

Humphrey, J. H., K. P. West, Jr. and Alfred Sommer. 1992. "Vitamin A Deficiency and Attributable Mortality among Under-5-Year-Olds." *Bulletin of the World Health Organization* 70(2): 225–32.

Jamison, Dean T. 1993. "Disease Control Priorities in Developing Countries: An Overview." Chapter I of Jamison et. al., *DCPDC*.

Jamison, Dean T., W. Henry Mosley, Anthony R. Measham and José Luis Bobadilla, eds. *Disease Control Priorities in Developing Countries*. New York: Oxford University Press for the World Bank.

Levin, Henry M., Ernesto Pollitt, Rae Galloway and Judith McGuire. 1993. "Micronutrient Deficiency Disorders." Chapter 19 of *DCPDC*.

Medeiros-Neto, Geraldo A. 1988. "Towards the Eradication of Iodine-Deficiency Disorders in Brazil through a Salt Iodination Programme." *Bulletin of the World Health Organization* 66(5): 637–42.

Murray, Christopher J. L. 1994. "Quantifying the Burden of Disease: the Technical Basis for Disability-Adjusted Life Years." In Murray and Lopez, *GCAHS*.

Murray, Christopher J. L., Alan D. Lopez and Dean T. Jamison. 1994. "The Global Burden of Disease in 1990: Summary Results, Sensitivity Analysis and Future Directions." In Murray and Lopez, *GCAHS*.

Murray, Christopher J. L. and Alan D. Lopez, eds. 1994. *Global Comparative Assessments in the Health Sector: Disease Burden, Expenditure and Intervention Packages [GCAHS]*. Collected reprints from the *Bulletin of the World Health Organization*. *Geneva*.

Musgrove, Philip, and Osmil Galindo. 1988. "Do the Poor Pay More? Retail Food Prices in Northeast Brazil." *Economic Development and Cultural Change* 37(l): 91–109.

Musgrove, Philip. 1993. "Feeding Latin America's Children." *The World Bank Research Observer* 8 (January): 23–45.

Musgrove, Philip. 1994. "Cost-Effectiveness and Health Sector Reform." HRO Working Paper No. 49. Washington, DC: World Bank.

Musgrove, Philip. 1996. "Public and Private Roles in Health." Human Development Department, the World Bank. Washington, DC. Discussion Paper No. 339.

Popkin, Barry M. 1992. "Development and the Nutrition Transition." Chapel Hill, NC: Carolina Population Center, University of North Carolina (processed).

United Nations Administrative Committee on Coordination, Subcommittee on Nutrition. 1992. *Second Report on the World Nutrition Situation. Volume I: Global and Regional Results*. Geneva.

United States Food and Drug Administration. 1991. "Regulatory Impact Analysis of the Proposed Rules to Amend the Food Labeling Regulations." *Federal Register 56(229)*: 60856–77.

Warren, Kenneth S. and Adel A. F. Mahmoud. 1990. *Tropical and Geographic Medicine* 2nd Edition. New York: McGraw-Hill.

World Bank. 1993. *World Development Report 1993: Investing in Health*. Washington, DC.

World Bank. 1994. *Enriching Lives: Overcoming Vitamin and Mineral Malnutrition in Developing Countries*. Washington, DC.

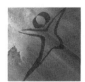

CHAPTER 17

Malnutrition and Dietary Protein

Acknowledgments

We are indebted to George Graham, who convinced us of the importance of the question addressed in this paper and inspired us to proceed with the work. Alan Berg and Richard Steckel made valuable comments on preliminary drafts. The authors would also like to acknowledge the valuable comments from Robert Black and anonymous referees. The research reported here was supported in part by a grant from the Royal Norwegian Ministry of Foreign Affairs to the World Health Organization (WHO). The conclusions of the paper are those of the authors and do not necessarily reflect those of the Norwegian Ministry, WHO, or the institutions with which the authors are affiliated.

Introduction

The mean heights and weights of individuals of a given age and sex vary substantially across countries; it is common to find the difference in means between two national populations to be several times the standard deviation of the distribution within a reference population [1]. In high-income populations, the parent–child correlation in height is high, and it is well established that genetic differences between individuals account for most of the individual variation in anthropometric status in such populations [2]. That said, available evidence suggests that differences across ethnic groups in the

Co-authored with Dean T. Jamison and Joanne Leslie. Reprinted with permission from *Food and Nutrition Bulletin*, vol. 24, no. 2 © 2003. The United Nations University.

distribution of genetic potential account for a relatively small part of the observed differences among populations in anthropometric indicators. The more important share of variation across populations results from differences in the proportion of individuals in each population who fail to reach their genetic potential and in the magnitude of that growth failure [1-3]. Factors influencing the magnitude of growth failure within a population include dietary adequacy, disease patterns, and variations in nutrient requirements induced, for example, by variation in required activity levels or ambient temperatures.[1]

Understanding the determinants of malnutrition—and how they vary from one environment to another—is of central importance to health policy: in a recent quantitative assessment, fully 50% of the total number of deaths in children under five years of age were associated with malnutrition [4]. Better understanding of the magnitude and nature of dietary and other risk factors for malnutrition would provide a valuable avenue for improving disease-prevention strategies relevant to the needs of the poor. Recent research points to a substantial contribution of disease to malnutrition [5]. Easterlin presents historical evidence suggesting that reduction in disease accounted for the rapid rise in the rate of increase in male stature that occurred in Europe from around 1800 to around 1900 [6] (from an average 1.1 cm per century increase to an average 7.7 cm per century increase). While acknowledging the importance of infectious diseases, this paper focuses on the role of diet as a determinant of malnutrition, and in particular, it utilizes several aggregate-level data sets to assess the quantitative significance of dietary quality, particularly the protein content of the diet, as a risk factor for malnutrition.

Although dietary protein can be utilized by the body for energy, with 1 g of protein providing 4 kcal of energy [7], high-protein foods tend to be several times more expensive per kilocalorie of energy provided than foods that are low in protein or relatively inadequate in one or more essential amino acids.[2] It is generally accepted that when diets are low in energy, available protein will in fact be used for energy, although the empirical evidence for this seems to be strongest for severe reductions in energy intake. The important empirical question is how variation around current levels of energy and protein availability influences levels of malnutrition. Just as diets that are low in cost per kilocalorie of energy are low in protein, diets that are low in cost per gram of protein are relatively low in energy. This tradeoff underscores the reason for quantifying the relative importance of increasing the energy content of diets versus improving their quality in reducing malnutrition.

Nutrient Intake and Growth: Data and Methods

We specified a simple function relating an anthropometric indicator to a number of potentially determining variables. Multivariate regression is then used to estimate the parameters of this function. The first data set contains information on average adult heights and weights (both male and female), income, and energy and protein availability from urban areas of 13 provinces of China. The second set also comes from China and refers to 64 largely rural counties. Nutrient availability (energy, protein, lipids, and fiber) is measured from a population sample of actual dietary composition and intake at the county level, rather than from aggregate food balances. Estimates of income were also available. The third data set contains information on national averages from 41 populations in 40 countries of adult male height (but not weight) and from 33 populations in 32 countries of adult female height, energy and protein availability (from aggregate balances), per capita gross national product (GNP), and predominant ethnic group. The sources, methods of analysis, and main results for each data set are first discussed. The final section compares the three sets of results and draws some conclusions concerning the relative importance of energy and protein as determinants of achieved growth. The contribution of this paper lies in the inclusion of dietary energy and protein levels among the determining variables. A previous study also utilized a regression approach to assessing determinants of adult height and included a broader range of variables in its analysis [8].

A number of caveats accompany our analyses. First, available data do not include a number of variables that are potentially important determinants of growth, and the variables they do include are averages rather than individual values.[3] The data also refer to one moment in time rather than to the interval over which people grow, resulting in their final adult height (and, with much more variation, their adult weight). In all three data sets, the estimates of nutrient availability refer to the approximate time when adult heights and weights were measured; we assume that these contemporary measures provide indicators of relative availabilities during the preceding two or three decades. This assumption is most defensible for the second analysis, because "dietary patterns in these rural areas of China, being simple in food variety, have probably remained simple and similar for many years, since foods consumed in each area are produced locally under reasonably stable local crop conditions" [9]. We also assume that few people in the sample populations have migrated to or from the province, county, or country in which they grew up, so that the nutrient availability in the place where they lived when surveyed is probably similar to the nutrient availability when they were growing up.

Growth Failure and Health

Our principal dependent variable, stature, is increasingly used in many fields as an indicator of general well-being [8]. Evidence from a wide range of studies suggests that malnutrition impairs mental development, in the most severe cases by a direct effect on brain cells and in more moderate cases by lowering the child's motivation and energy level and thereby reducing the amount of effective learning time [10, 11]. There is also evidence that malnutrition reduces the activity levels of poor children in developing countries [12], and that malnourished children are less likely to attend school and less likely to succeed if they do attend [13, 14].

The mortality consequences of malnutrition are probably mediated through a cyclic interaction among dietary inadequacy, malnutrition, immune status, and infectious diseases. Malnourished children are more susceptible to disease, and they are more likely to die if infected. Children who are ill eat less and are less able to absorb what they do manage to eat [15–20] at a time when their nutrient requirements are actually increased.

Quantitative estimates have been developed of the extent to which infection accounts for observed levels of malnutrition in a broad range of environments [5], and such estimates vary greatly (10% to 80%) across environments, suggesting that the entry points for intervention to break the adverse cycle will also vary.

Data Set 1. Height and Weight of Young Urban Adults in 13 Chinese Provinces

A concern with the identification and development of sports talent among the youth of China gave rise to a detailed study in 1979 of 183,414 school-age children and young adults from 13 provinces and the three provincial-level metropolitan areas of Beijing, Shanghai, and Tianjin [21]. This study reported heights and weights of urban males and females in the age range 18 to 25 years in each province. The variables used to explain these anthropometric data came from several other sources. An early World Bank policy paper on the health sector in China used the 1979 data, data from other published sources, and data collected specifically for the report to document levels and trends in nutritional status [22, 23]. These reports describe an environment of rapidly improving nutritional status, particularly in urban areas, and of possibly worrisome inequality in the distribution of protein consumption.

We used the official Chinese estimate of total industrial and agricultural output per capita in 1981 [24] to measure provincial income. Provincial-level data on energy and protein production were obtained from another World Bank study of trends in food and nutrient availability in China [25]. These data on income and on nutrient availability cover another 13 provinces besides those for which anthropometric indicators are available. All data were for the year 1979, except the total value of industrial and agricultural output, which was for the year 1981. Table 17.1 gives the definitions, means, and standard deviations of all the variables, over all provinces for which they were available.

Although there were 16 observed locations for adult heights and weights (including the metropolitan areas), the relations between energy and protein, and between height and weight, are based on only 13 observations. The figures for the urban areas of Beijing, Shanghai, and Tianjin could not be included, since the data on nutrient availability excluded all interprovincial and international trade in food crops and hence resulted in gross underestimates of nutrient availability. For the 26 nonmetropolitan provinces,

Table 17.1 Variables for Urban China in 1979

VARIABLE	NO. OF OBSERVATIONS (PROVINCES)	MEAN	SD
Male height, age 18–25 yr (cm)	16	170.3	1.43
Female height, age 18–25 yr (cm)	16	159.0	1.22
Male weight, age 18–25 yr (kg)	16	58.9	2.70
Female weight, age 18–25 yr (kg)	16	51.5	1.24
Income: industrial and agricultural output per capita (1981) (yuan)[a]	26	646	264
Energy: net dietary energy available from provincial production (kcal/capita/day)	26	2,300	386
Protein share: fraction of available dietary energy from protein (%)	26	10.7	2.1

Sources: heights and weights from Keusch [18]; income from Jamison et al. [23]; energy and protein share from State Statistical Bureau [24].
[a]1.7045 yuan = US$1 (1981).

exclusion of trade in grain probably leads to only small errors in estimates of provincial nutrient availability [25]. All analyses are based on multiple linear regressions using height or weight as the dependent variable.

To provide context, relations between income and nutrient availability (for total energy and for energy from protein) were calculated from the logarithms of the provincial averages. Although the demand for and supply of nutrients cannot be distinguished in these data, we assumed that demand determines availability and interpreted the coefficients as demand elasticities. Not surprisingly, the income elasticity of demand for protein (0.68) was much greater than that for energy (0.40), but both were substantial and statistically significant, suggesting that the poor derive a smaller percentage of their total dietary energy from protein sources.

Results

A previous analysis used univariate regressions to relate each of these variables separately to male and female heights and weights for both urban and rural areas of each province [25]. It found that male anthropometric status was systematically more closely related to all the explanatory variables than was female status, and that urban heights and weights were better explained than those in rural areas—much better, when energy and protein availability were used as explanatory variables.

Univariate regressions say nothing about whether protein availability affects adult height or weight, given a particular level of energy availability, nor do they distinguish the nutrient effects from those of income and other variables. Table 17.2 therefore shows multiple regression relations between height

Table 17.2 Determinants of the Height and Weight of Young Adults (Age 18–25 Years) in Urban China in 1979

INDEPENDENT VARIABLE	HEIGHT[a]		WEIGHT[a]	
	MALE	FEMALE	MALE	FEMALE
Income (1981)	0.0025 (2.88)**	0.0005 (0.39)	0.0009 (0.19)	0.0004 (0.33)
Energy	0.0006 (0.93)	0.0008 (0.87)	0.0021 (1.74)*	0.00096 (1.00)
Protein share	0.46 (4.50)**	0.44 (3.00)**	0.618 (3.25)**	0.470 (3.08)**
Constant	162.0	151.8	46.13	43.80
R^2 adjusted[b]	0.78	0.43	0.53	0.44
No. of observations	13	13	13	13

[a]The t-statistics are given in parentheses after the coefficients.
[b]R^2 is the (adjusted) percentage of variance accounted for.
*$p < .10$, **$p < .05$.

and weight and all the hypothesized determining variables. Because rural anthropometric status appears much harder to explain with these variables, our analysis is limited to urban areas. By itself, higher income was found to affect male height positively and significantly and to have a positive but not statistically significant effect on female height (these simple regressions are not reported in table 17.2). When available energy and the proportion of energy from protein were entered together with income, protein, but not energy, was found to have a positive and highly significant effect on height for both sexes.

The effects on weight were, not surprisingly, quite similar to the effects on height. The effect of income on weight was less strong than its effect on height, whereas the effect of protein on weight was almost as strong as its effect on height. In contrast to the effect on height, total energy availability was also found to have a marginally significant positive effect on the weight of males but not of females.[4]

Data Set 2. Adult Height and Weight in 64 Rural Chinese Counties

In 1976 a major study was conducted of the causes of death in China, covering some 20 million deaths during the period 1973 to 1975. Primarily in order to relate cause-specific mortality, and particularly mortality from several different cancers, to a variety of lifestyle factors, including diet, a supplementary survey was undertaken in 1983 in 65 mostly rural counties. Attained height and weight for both male and female adults were also measured. Some 1,950 families participated, and three-day dietary intake measurements were made for 13,000 individuals [9].

As in the provincial-level study, the estimate of income refers to the total value of industrial and agricultural output per capita in 1982 at the county level. Average food intake in these data refer to average consumption in the specific communities studied. Relations were again estimated between the anthropometric variables and income, total dietary energy, and the share of energy obtained from protein.

Table 17.3 shows the means and standard deviations of the variables analyzed. These differ slightly between men and women—apart from the sex-specific differences in height and weight—because we used data for 64 counties for females and only 63 counties for males. Both men and women are shorter and weigh less in rural than in urban areas. Rural energy intakes appear to be very slightly higher and rural protein intakes somewhat smaller, but the comparison is complicated by the difference in the way

Table 17.3 Variables for Rural Chinese Counties in 1983

	MALES		FEMALES	
VARIABLE	MEAN	SD	MEAN	SD
Male height (cm)	163.4	2.64	—	—
Female height (cm)	—	—	153.3	2.40
Male weight (kg)	54.16	2.97	—	—
Female weight (kg)	—	—	48.13	3.06
Income: industrial and agricultural output per capita (1982) (yuan)[a]	646	671	642	666
Energy: net dietary energy available from provincial production (kcal/capita/day)	2,624	392	2,461	411
Protein share: fraction of available dietary energy from protein (%)	9.88	1.27	10.02	1.66
No. of observations (counties)	63	—	64	—

Source: ref. 20.
[a] 1.7045 yuan = US$1 (1981).

intakes were estimated—by province-level availability (table 17.1) and by direct household-level observation (table 17.3).

Results

Table 17.4 shows the regression results for male and female heights and weights. For both sexes and for both anthropometric measures, total dietary energy is never significant, whereas the share obtained from

Table 17.4 Determinants of Adult Height and Weight in Rural Chinese Counties in 1983

INDEPENDENT VARIABLE	HEIGHT[a]		WEIGHT[a]	
	MALE	FEMALE	MALE	FEMALE
Income (1982)	$-9.82(-4)$ (0.21)	$6.78(-5)$ (0.16)	$-1.50(-4)$ (0.27)	$8.36(-5)$ (0.15)
Energy	0.001 (1.62)	$8.45(-4)$ (1.24)	0.001 (1.29)	0.001 (1.45)
Protein share	1.013 (3.75)**	0.595 (3.51)**	0.968 (3.07)**	0.665 (3.02)**
Constant	149.8	145.1	41.3	38.0
R^2 adjusted[b]	0.16	0.15	0.10	0.11
No. of observations	63	64	63	64

[a] Coefficients < 0.001 are shown in scientific notation, with the exponent (power of 10) in parentheses after the coefficient. The t-statistics are given in parentheses after the coefficients.
[b] R^2 is the (adjusted) percentage of variance accounted for.
*$p < .10.$, **$p < .05.$

protein is always highly significant. Income is not significant in any of the regressions.

The only notable difference between the results for men and those for women is that the coefficient on the share of protein in total energy is only about 60 percent as large for female height as for male height and about two-thirds as large for female weight as for male weight. In the provincial-level urban analysis, these coefficients do not differ between the sexes for height, but the female coefficient is appreciably smaller for weight. Male-female differences in predictors of attained weight may result from differences in the typical percentage of body mass in fat.

Data Set 3. Intercountry Differences in Adult Height

The source for adult anthropometric data in the third analysis was Eveleth and Tanner [1]. The authors of this compendium draw on an enormous range of scientific studies, some based on national samples but most based on regional samples or samples drawn from particular ethnic groups; they describe the variation in growth, adult size, and body proportions found across countries and between different genetically similar groups. The four main groups into which samples were divided were Indo-Mediterranean, European, African, and Asian. Among adults, the European and African populations were the tallest: Indo-Mediterraneans were on average shorter than Europeans by approximately 5 cm, and Asians were shorter by approximately 7 cm.

Data

For adult males, data on average heights from 41 populations were used as the dependent variable. (These correspond to 40 countries, since Surinamese of African and Asian origin were treated as separate populations.) Data on female heights were available for 33 populations (32 countries). There was considerable variation among the years in which the data were obtained, but the majority of the studies were from the 1960s (with a few from the late 1950s and a few from the early 1970s). Also included was an indicator of major ethnic group—taking a value of 1 for either Indo-Mediterranean or Asian, the two shorter populations—in order to control at least partly for possible genetic variation in potential height across countries. Since the data include only four European countries and none from North America or northern Europe, this variable serves mostly to

Table 17.5 International Comparisons

VARIABLE	MALES MEAN	MALES SD	FEMALES MEAN	FEMALES SD
Male height (cm)	166.9	5.00	—	—
Female height (cm)	—	—	154.5	4.45
1960 income: GNP/capita (1977 US$)	507	468	510	431
Energy: net dietary energy available (kcal/capita/day)	2,207	349	2,207	364
Protein share: fraction of available dietary energy from protein (%)	10.61	1.67	10.64	1.71
Ethnic group: Asian or Indo-Mediterranean = 1; European or African = 0	0.54	0.50	0.48	0.51
No. of observations (populations)	41	—	33	—

Sources: height, weight, and ethnic group from Eveleth and Tanner [1]; income and energy from Piazza [25]; protein share calculated from energy and World Bank [26].

distinguish these two groups from African populations. The other hypothesized determining variables—per capita GNP and energy and protein availability per capita—were obtained from two World Bank documents: the World Development Report 1979 [26] and the Social Indicators Data Sheet [27].

Table 17.5 shows the means and standard deviations of the variables in the regressions seeking determinants of cross-country variation in average height of adult males. A comparison of the values in table 5 with those in tables 17.1 and 17.3 shows that the average height of males in the 41 populations (166.9 cm) falls between the values for urban (170.3 cm) and rural (163.4 cm) males in China. The average per capita availability of energy was slightly lower (2,207 kcal) than in the Chinese samples (2,300 kcal in urban areas and more than 2,500 in rural areas); the average percentage of energy available from protein was nearly identical in the 40 countries (10.6%) to that in urban China (10.7%).

Results

Table 17.6 shows the results of regressions of the average height of adults in the 41 (or, for women, 33) populations on two different combinations of explanatory variables, using the same formulations for nutrient availability as in the analysis of the Chinese data. For males, the total available energy is not a significant determinant of height, but the percentage of energy

Table 17.6 Determinants of Adult Male Height (41 Populations in 40 Countries) and Adult Female Height (33 Populations in 32 Countries), ca. 1960

INDEPENDENT VARIABLE	URBAN		RURAL	
	MALES	FEMALES	MALES	FEMALES
1960 income	−0.001 (0.82)	−0.002 (1.08)	−0.001 (0.66)	−0.002 (0.86)
Energy	0.001 (0.41)	0.004 (1.35)	0.001 (0.06)	0.002 (0.84)
Protein share	1.155 (2.37)**	0.619 (1.27)	1.073 (2.39)**	0.654 (1.50)
Ethnic group; Asian or Indo-Mediterranean			−3.858 (2.80)**	−3.941 (2.92)**
Constant	153.0	141.1	157.8	145.8
R^2 adjusted	0.12	0.09	0.25	0.28
No. of observations (populations)	41	33	41	33

[a]The *t*-statistics are given in parentheses after the coefficients.
[b]R^2 is the (adjusted) percentage of variance accounted for.
*$p < .10$, **$p < .05$.

available from protein is highly significant; this result is the same whether or not the (significant) ethnic distinction is included. For female heights, the coefficient on the share of energy from protein is only about 60 percent as large as that for male heights, while the standard error of the estimate is unchanged, so the variable is not significant. (The ratio of the coefficients for men and women is about the same as for the analysis of rural Chinese heights: protein seems systematically to make less difference in female height, except in purely urban populations.) Total energy intake continues to be nonsignificant, and ethnicity highly significant, for women.

We also tried a specification different from that used for China, which included per capita GNP, energy available from protein sources in the diet, and energy available from nonprotein sources. Energy available from protein sources was a significant predictor of adult height of males, whereas energy available from nonprotein sources was unrelated to height. These results are not reported here. Adding a control variable for ethnic group indicates that belonging to the Indo-Mediterranean or Asian group has a significantly negative effect on height (about 4 cm) relative to that of Africans or Europeans, but controlling for this component of variation in height does not reduce the significance of energy available from protein (nor does it alter the nonsignificance of per capita GNP). When dietary composition is controlled, the estimated differences between ethnic groups in adult height are much reduced, to slightly less than 4 cm for both males and females.

Conclusions

Substantial differences exist across population groups in the average values of adult malnutrition as measured by anthropometric status. Only a small part of this can be accounted for by genetic differences among populations. It is well established that disease accounts for varying (but often large) proportions of malnutrition in different environments. The analyses presented in the three preceding sections attempt to explain the extent to which levels of nutrient availability can further account for growth retardation. Controlling for average incomes and—when populations are ethnically different—for differences in genetic potential, the analyses address the question of the extent to which energy availability in the average diet (in kilocalories per capita per day) and protein availability (in percent of total energy from protein) are associated with differences in the anthropometric status of population groups.

Limitations of the Analyses

Several caveats are important. First, the numbers of observations are small, particularly for the first (urban) analysis of China; undue importance might therefore be given to a few observations. Second, our international data were collected at different times, in different ways, and with differing sampling frames. Although these shortcomings are in principle more likely to obscure than to illuminate the relations we examine, the heterogeneity of the data is cause for concern. However, neither of these limitations matters for the analysis of rural China, for which the data are most numerous and also most uniform, and where we find the same results.

A third caveat is that individual diets—and disease patterns—determine individual growth, and our data concern only average diets and average growth. Individual, longitudinal data on nutrient intake, disease episodes, and growth allow for more definitive assessments of the relative contributions to growth failure of energy and protein deficiency in diets that are typical of those found in today's developing countries. An example of such an analysis is a longitudinal study of 123 children 2 to 19 years of age from low-income families living in Lima, Peru. It found the percentage of protein from animal sources, but not total energy intake, to be strongly associated with achieved male height and weight [28]. (Our analyses do not distinguish animal and plant sources of protein.) Another study followed 70 much younger children for over a year in Bangladesh; it concluded that dietary inadequacy accounted for perhaps 50% more of the observed retardation of weight gain in the sample than did infections, but it was unable to apportion the dietary effect among nutrients [29]. Other studies (Chernichovsky [30] and Deolalikar et al. [50]) have modeled individual growth trajectories for different samples of children in India, and Bhargava [31] has done the same for a sample of Filipino children, again finding that protein but not energy intake is important. These individual-level longitudinal analyses complement the much more aggregated ones we present and, reassuringly, reach broadly similar conclusions.

Synthesis of Findings

Despite the aggregated and cross-sectional nature of our data, the results consistently suggest that protein rather than energy deficiency is the principal dietary cause of growth failure in the populations studied, as indicated by attained adult height and weight. These findings not only complement similar ones from the limited number of studies using data on individuals, but are consistent with the observations of economic historians that high levels of animal protein availability—and therefore probably total protein intake—may have accounted for the earlier increase in average height in the United States than in Europe [32] and that periods when protein-dense food was relatively costly may have been associated with lower attained heights [33, 34]. A recent assessment [35] concluded that the Native Americans of the Great Plains in the United States were probably the world's tallest population in the mid-19th century, with males being 1 to 2 cm taller than American soldiers of European descent. The authors attribute this in part to diets with high diversity and high animal protein content.

Increases in protein availability thus appear to be more important than increases in energy availability for ameliorating growth failure. One possible reason for this is that the distribution of energy and of protein to individuals within a population almost certainly differs substantially, with protein (especially animal protein) much more unequally distributed than energy. Thus, a larger proportion of the population is likely to be in protein deficit than in energy deficit if the average availability of the two nutrients is at the same percentage of estimated requirements. Energy requirements are expressed as average population needs, on the assumption that individuals will consume more or less than the average, depending on need. The population requirements for protein are given as the average requirement plus 2 SD to cover nearly all of the population.

In contrast to Steckel [8], we found that per capita income levels were generally unassociated with anthropometric outcomes (except for male height in urban China). Our finding of low association appears after controlling for nutrient intake, and, to the extent that the effects of income are mediated through increased protein consumption (and the income elasticity of demand for dietary protein is very high), the positive results concerning income in Steckel and ours concerning protein are consistent. To the extent that protein content correlates with other potential determinants of nutritional status and growth (e.g., disease and micronutrients), this paper's conclusions on the importance of protein would need to be qualified.

Our findings suggest that an increase of one percentage point in the proportion of total energy accounted for by protein would raise adult heights by about half a centimeter in urban China, by 0.60 to 1.01 cm in rural China, and by 0.65 cm (females) to 1.16 cm (males) across a large sample of countries.[5] Except in urban China, the effect would be much larger for men than for women. For Chinese men, these increases amount to 0.32 to 0.38 SD in height, indicating that they are fairly large relative to the natural variation in the population. The increase is smaller relative to the variation across countries (0.23 SD), because in that comparison ethnic differences make the total variation much larger.

As we have stressed, there are many other possible correlates of protein availability that are potential determinants of growth. Examples of other influences include water supplies, education levels, health services, general sanitation levels, and so forth. (In a sufficiently broadly specified model, these would be endogenous.) We have partly controlled for these other potential influences by including income in our regressions; however, the possibility remains that some of the effect attributed to protein availability in our regressions is due not to protein itself but to correlates of protein availability that are less well correlated with energy availability. This might be the case particularly for micronutrient deficiencies that can cause growth failure without causing specific signs of disease [36], even when protein and energy availability are adequate. If that is the case, then dietary variety may be crucial to growth because it increases access to all essential nutrients. That said, the results from each of our three data sets suggest that energy availability is usually not the problem and that protein availability may be.[6]

Notes

1. Several lines of evidence suggest the importance of nongenetic determinants of variation in anthropometric status. Historical records indicate dramatic increases over time in anthropometric indicators for European populations, increases that have reached a limit as adequate levels of nourishment and health have extended to virtually all members of the populations studied [3]. Alternative sets of interacting variables have been proposed to account for the observed improvements [37, 38]. Evidence is available on increased height and also better health, as a result of more and better food consumption, in Europe and the United States in the 18th and 19th centuries [39], and there are studies of individuals from one country growing up in another (e.g., Japanese in California) who showed substantial anthropometric improvements [1].

2. Proteins are composed of different combinations of 20 amino acids, of which 9 are essential for humans in the sense that they cannot be synthesized but must be ingested [40]. In order for protein to be used for growth, rather than for energy, all the essential amino acids must be present in adequate amounts. Generally speaking, foods of animal origin supply needed amino acids in approximately the required proportions, and foods of plant origin are relatively deficient in one or more essential amino acids. Therefore, the amount of available protein that can be utilized from animal sources is in the range of 80% to 90%, whereas the amount of protein that can be utilized from an individual plant source is in the range of 45% to 55%. In consequence, individuals consuming only foods of plant origin must usually consume more protein or a carefully balanced mix of foods in order to meet their protein requirements.

3. The disadvantages of utilizing data aggregates to estimate production processes that occur at an individual level (person, firm, farm, or household) are well known; see Jamison and Lau [41] for an extended discussion of the advantages and disadvantages of using aggregated data in empirical work and Stoker [42] for a discussion of empirical approaches to the aggregation problem. King [43] presents a novel approach for utilizing aggregate data to illuminate relations at the individual level, along with computational algorithms. Because relative income elasticities indicate protein consumption to be much more unequally distributed within populations than is energy consumption, aggregate per capita availabilities of energy and protein that are equally satisfactory for an individual diet will result in a larger proportion of the population being short of protein than short of energy. Scrimshaw [44] presents evidence suggesting that utilizable protein is even more unequally distributed. Whether this means that aggregated data would result in higher or lower estimated elasticities of growth with respect to protein consumption than would be estimated from individual data depends on where the aggregate observations are concentrated along the true, individual relation, since that curve is likely to rise steeply at low levels of protein consumption but level off as protein intake becomes

adequate for reaching one's genetic potential growth. Unfortunately, dietary information obtained at the individual or household level is costly and often highly unreliable, although some individual-level studies (e.g., Graham et al. [28]) allow estimation of the impact of specific nutrients on growth. Other studies [45] often are restricted to utilization of much less precise determinants, such as food-consumption frequencies, or to inferences concerning relative inadequacies of particular nutrients from body composition data [46].

4. Data have also been published on anthropometric indicators of nutritional status for children between 7 and 17 years of age from the 1979 Chinese survey. Preliminary analysis of the data for seven-year-olds found neither energy nor protein availability to be a significant determinant of nutritional status. One plausible explanation is that diarrheal disease (and other health factors) are more important as determinants of children's growth than of attained adult stature.

5. This increase is comparable to the increase in the average height of native-born white males in the United States in the two centuries following the mid-1700s, which was approximately 1.2 cm [47]. Heights increased much more rapidly in the United States than in European countries, so that by the mid-1700s, male heights in the United States already exceeded those in Europe by 2.5 to 5 cm [34].

6. A recent econometric assessment [48] found further effects, in that both energy and protein in the diet remained important for worker wages (in Brazil), even after individual height and body mass index were controlled for, but with energy important only for the very malnourished, whereas increased protein content was important for a much broader range of individuals. A recent broad overview of the relation between nutrition and poverty may be found in Svedberg [49].

References

[1] Eveleth PB, Tanner JM. Worldwide variation in human growth. Cambridge, UK: Cambridge University Press, 1976.
[2] Mueller WH. Parent-child correlations for stature and weight among school-aged children: a review of 24 studies. Hum Biol 1976; 48: 379–97.
[3] Tanner JM. Foetus into man: physical growth from conception to maturity. Cambridge, Mass, USA: Harvard University Press, 1978.
[4] Rice AL, Sacco L, Hyder A, Black RE. Malnutrition as an underlying cause of childhood deaths associated with infectious diseases in developing countries. Bull WHO 2000; 78: 1207–21.
[5] Black RE. Would control of childhood infectious diseases reduce malnutrition? Acta Paed Scand Suppl 1991; 374: 133–40.
[6] Easterlin RA. Growth triumphant: the twenty-first century in historical perspective. Ann Arbor, Mich, USA: University of Michigan Press, 1996.

[7] Wood-Dahlström C, Calloway DH. Nutritional needs and evaluation. In: Warren KS, Mahmoud AFH, eds. Tropical and geographical medicine. New York: McGraw-Hill, 1990.

[8] Steckel RH. Stature and the standard of living. J Econ Lit 1995; 33:1903–40.

[9] Chen J, Campbell TC, Li J, Peto R. Diet, life-style and mortality in China: a study of the characteristics of 65 Chinese counties. Oxford, UK: Oxford University Press, 1990 (published in the United States by Cornell University Press and in China by People's Medical Publishing House).

[10] Lloyd Still JC. Malnutrition and mental development. Littleton, Mass, USA: Publishing Sciences Group, 1976.

[11] Read MS. Malnutrition and behavior. Appl Res Ment Retard 1982; 3:279–91.

[12] Beaton GH, Ghassemi H. Supplementary feeding programs for young children in developing countries. Am J Clin Nutr 1982;35 (April suppl):863–916.

[13] Moock PR, Leslie J. Childhood malnutrition and schooling in the Terai region of Nepal. Population and Human Resources Division Discussion Paper No. 82-14. Washington, DC: World Bank, 1982.

[14] Pollitt E. Malnutrition and infection in the classroom. Paris: UNESCO, 1990.

[15] Leslie J. Child malnutrition and diarrhea: a longitudinal study from Northeast Brazil. Doctor of Science Thesis, Johns Hopkins University School of Hygiene and Public Health, Baltimore, Md, USA, 1982.

[16] Scrimshaw NS, Taylor CE, Gordon JE. Interactions of nutrition and infection. Geneva: World Health Organization, 1968.

[17] Tomkins A, Watson F. Malnutrition and infection—a review. Nutrition Policy Discussion Paper No. 5. New York: United Nations Agency Coordinating Committee, Sub-Committee on Nutrition, 1989.

[18] Keusch GT. Nutrition-infection interactions. In: Geurrant RL, Walker DH, Weller PF. Tropical infectious diseases: principles, pathogens and practice. Vol 2. Philadelphia, Pa, USA: Churchill Livingstone, 1999:62–75.

[19] Powanda MC, Beisel WR. Metabolic effects of infection on protein and energy status. J Nutr 2003;133: 322S–7S.

[20] Scrimshaw NS, Bistrian BR, Brunser O, Elia M, Jackson AA, Jian Z-M, Kinney JM, Rosenberg IH, Wolf RR. Effect of disease on desirable protein energy rations. 385–398 In: Scrimshaw NS, Schurch B, eds. Proteinenergy interactions. Lausanne, Switzerland: Nestlé Foundation, 1991.

[21] Chen C, for Research Group. Research on the physical characteristics, fitness, and vital indicators of Chinese children and young adults. Beijing: Science and Technical Papers Publishing House, 1982.

[22] Jamison DT, Trowbridge FL. The nutritional status of children in China: a review of the anthropometric evidence. Population, Health and Nutrition Department Technical Note GEN-17. Washington, DC: World Bank, 1983.

[23] Jamison DT, Evans JR, King T, Porter I, Prescott N, Prost A. China: the health sector. Country Study Series. Washington, DC: World Bank, 1984.

[24] State Statistical Bureau. China statistical yearbook. Beijing: State Statistical Bureau, 1982.
[25] Piazza A. Food consumption and nutritional status in the PRC. Westview Special Studies on China. Boulder, Colo, USA: Westview Press, 1986.
[26] World Bank. World development report. Washington, DC: World Bank, 1979.
[27] World Bank. Social indicators data sheet. Washington, DC: World Bank, 1976.
[28] Graham GG, Creed HM, MacLean WC Jr, Kallman CH, Rabold J, Mellitis ED. Determinants of growth among poor children: nutrient intake-achieved growth relationships. Am J Clin Nutr 1981;34:539–54.
[29] Becker S, Black RE, Brown KH. Relative effects of diarrhea, fever, and dietary energy intake on weight gain in rural Bangladeshi children. Am J Clin Nutr 1991;53: 1499–1503.
[30] Chernichovsky D. The economic theory of the household and impact measurement of nutrition and related health programs. World Bank Staff Working Paper No. 302. Washington, DC: World Bank, 1978.
[31] Bhargava A. Modelling the health of Filipino children. J R Statist Soc, Ser A, 1994;157:417–32.
[32] Sokoloff KL, Villaflor GC. The early achievement of modern stature in America. Soc Sci Hist 1982;6: 453–81.
[33] Komlos J. Preface. In: Komlos J, ed. Stature, living standards and economic development. Chicago, Ill, USA: University of Chicago Press, 1994:ix–xv.
[34] Sokoloff KL. The heights of Americans in three centuries: some economic and demographic implications. In: Komlos J, ed. The biological standard of living on three continents. Boulder, Colo, USA: Westview Press, 1995: 133–50.
[35] Steckel RH, Prince JM. Tallest in the world: Native Americans of the Great Plains in the nineteenth century. Am Econ Rev 2001;91:287–94.
[36] Golden MHN. The nature of nutritional deficiency in relation to growth failure and poverty. Acta Paed Scand Suppl 1991;374:95–110.
[37] Hutchinson J. British aid and the relief of malnutrition. Overseas Development Paper No. 2. London: Her Majesty's Stationery Office, 1975.
[38] Meredith HB. Findings from Asia, Australia, Europe, and North America on secular changes in mean height of children, youths, and young adults. Am J Phys Anthrop 1976;44:315–26.
[39] Fogel RW. Economic growth, population theory, and physiology: the bearing of long-term processes on the making of economic policy. Am Econ Rev 1994;84: 369–95.
[40] Brown ML, ed. Present knowledge in nutrition. Washington, DC: International Life Sciences Institute Nutrition Foundation, 1990.
[41] Jamison DT, Lau LJ. Farmer education and farm efficiency. Baltimore, Md, USA: Johns Hopkins University Press, 1982.
[42] Stoker TM. Empirical approaches to the problem of aggregation over individuals. J Econ Lit 1993;31 (December):1827–74.

[43] King G. A solution to the ecological inference problem: reconstructing individual behavior from aggregate data. Princeton, NJ, USA: Princeton University Press, 1997.

[44] Scrimshaw NS. Through a glass darkly: discerning the practical implications of human dietary protein-energy interrelationships. Nutr Rev 1977;35:321-37.

[45] Martorell R, Leslie J, Moock PR. Characteristics and determinants of child nutritional status in Nepal. Population and Human Resources Division Discussion Paper No. 82-15. Washington, DC: World Bank, 1982.

[46] Martorell R, Yarbrough C, Lechtig A, Delgado H, Klein RE. Upper arm anthropometric indicators of nutritional status. Am J Clin Nutr 1976;29:46-53.

[47] Steckel RH. Heights and health in the United States, 1710-1950. In: Komlos J, ed. Stature, living standards and economic development. Chicago, Ill, USA: University of Chicago Press, 1994:153-70.

[48] Thomas D, Strauss, J. Health and wages: evidence on men and women in urban Brazil. J Econometrics 1997;77:159-185.

[49] Svedberg P. Malnutrition and poverty. Oxford, UK: Oxford University Press, 2002.

[50] Deolalikar AB, Behrman JR, Lavy V. Child growth in rural south India: economic and biological determinants. Unpublished paper, Department of Economics, University of Pennsylvania, Philadelphia, Pa, USA, 1992.

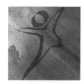

CHAPTER 18

Family Health Care Spending in Latin America

Acknowledgments

I acknowledge with thanks the help of Louise Fox and William McGreevey of the World Bank in obtaining the Brazilian data used in the analysis, and that of Mark Crowley of the Pan American Health Organization in estimating the regressions reported in Table 18.4.

Introduction

Expenditures by consumers on health care are in many respects like any other kind of expenditure; they are directed toward particular goods and services in order to satisfy wants for a more general good ('health'), and the process by which health is built up by investment or lost by depreciation or accident can be described by models of utility maximization under a variety of constraints and suppositions [Grossman (1982), Rapaport et al. (1982)]. In other respects, spending on health care is different from any other element of the consumer budget, because a large share of it is provided publicly although it is neither entirely a public good nor is it something required by law (such as education). In consequence, in order to understand how much health care households demand and buy, one needs to analyze the determinants of total health care expenditure and also the interaction between public and private spending.

Reprinted from *Journal of Health Economics 2*, Copyright 1983, with permission from Elsevier Science.

Previous analyses [Kleiman (1974), Newhouse (1977), Maxwell (1981)] have typically relied on highly aggregated data, and have concentrated on understanding total health spending. They indicate that health care is relatively elastic with respect to income across countries, with the elasticity declining toward one as income rises; that income and spending are much less related within countries; and that inter-country differences depend not only on income but on relative costs of particular medical services, the age structure and health problems of the population, the mechanisms of payment and other factors. Private expenditure, as a share of the total, depends not only on the factors determining demand for health care but on the availability and cost of public services and on the coverage and operation of private insurance.

Most of the analyses cited above have been limited to high-income countries, in part because of the limitations of data, especially data on private spending and its determinants. Studies of health care financing in poor countries have been based almost exclusively on a national accounts estimates [Pan American Health Organization (1982), Zschock (1978)] which give little more than a disaggregation of public financing by major source and a rough estimate of total private spending. More detailed studies, as for example of the social security system [Mesa-Lago (1978), Zschock (1983)] make use of the disaggregated information collected by public institutions, but still provide very little analysis of out-of-pocket spending by consumers. This situation is beginning to change, as surveys are undertaken with the specific objectives of measuring private expenditures and their causes [World Bank (1982)] or the use by consumers of the public health system [Selowsky (1979)]. Data of this type are still limited to very few countries and have so far been subject to relatively little analysis.

Meanwhile, given the preponderance of public sector data and of aggregated estimates, it may be valuable to make use of standard household income and expenditure surveys to study private health care spending. Data of this sort are also relatively rare in Latin America, but not nearly so rare as information collected specifically to study how health care is demanded and financed. Without adjustments for subsidies and transfers, such data are also likely to give biased measures of net expenditure and of the amount of medical care actually obtained; this problem is discussed further below. However, family budget data have the great advantage of covering a wide range of incomes and of other relevant variables, including detailed geographic and demographic information. In the long run, there may be no reason to expect much association between income and health care spending, or between the latter and actual health status, because of the great changes in medical technology and in living conditions generally [Fuchs (1979)], but in a cross-section at a given time it may be possible to measure a definite income elasticity. This is all the more likely if private spending only is studied, since the choice between private and public care may be highly income-dependent once public care is available to a consumer. This reasoning suggests that a family's income and its access to publicly-provided services—perhaps indicated by where it lives—should be worth studying in household budget data, even if other features which influence the need for health care and which belong in a full model of family decision-making are not considered.

This paper used such data from several household surveys in six Latin American countries between 1966 and 1975, primarily to estimate income elasticities and—for the one survey with substantial geographic variation—to investigate how the availability of public services and the way they are provided and paid for appear to affect family expenditures. Other sources are used to provide some information on these public services, but it should be emphasized that these data are not available in the same detail as private expenditures; some of the findings, while plausible and perhaps easy to confirm with more disaggregated public sector data, should therefore be regarded more as hypotheses than as conclusions until more thorough research is conducted.

In a previous study of household incomes and expenditures based on data from ten South American cities in five countries [Musgrove (1978a)], I estimated expenditure elasticities for total family health care spending and also for spending on insurance other than social security contributions, of which health insurance is a component. The results, show below, give fairly precise estimates of the health spending elasticity, which however differ among countries by more than 50 percent (from 0.81 to 1.34). Much of this variation may be due to differences in the cost and availability of public services, on which the surveys contained no information. Health and other insurance elasticities vary even more and are less precise. In the case of Chile, there is some evidence that the health care elasticity converges toward one as income rises, but the errors of estimate are quite large. The regressions from which these elasticities come also show health care spending to be influenced by family size, age of head of household, and employment of spouse, but these variables do not have consistent effects across countries. See Table 18.1.

In the case of spending on education—which like health care includes a great many zero values, and much variation due to factors besides income—elasticities estimated from the individual observations appear to be understated. When I used as observations the means of spending on education and of total spending by income quartiles, eliminating any transitory income effects within quartiles, the elasticities rose from about 1.0 to nearly

Table 18.1 Elasticities with Respect to Total Expenditure (Standard Errors in Parentheses)

CHILE (SANTIAGO)	COLOMBIA (4 CITIES)	ECUADOR (2 CITIES)	PERU (LIMA)	VENEZUELA (2 CITIES)
Total health care spending, except private health insurance				
0.844 (0.052)	1.171 (0.040)	0.904 (0.050)	0.808 (0.055)	1.341 (0.063)
Total insurance, including health insurance, excluding social security				
NA	1.116 (0.204)	1.205 (0.383)	0.756 (0.033)	1.253 (0.090)
Chile, total health care spending, elasticity by stratum				
Low 1.283 (0.709) High 1.071 (0.166)				

2.0 [Musgrove (1978b)]. I have therefore applied the same procedure to the data on health spending, combining observations for all ten cities. The results appear in Table 18.2, quartiles being defined by income per person in households and compared in dollars of equal purchasing power. The data are also shown in Figure 18.1, yielding an estimated elasticity of 1.5, higher than any of the individual countries' values for disaggregated data. In one city (Caracas) a second survey was taken nine years later, permitting an analysis of how spending changed as real income rose. I have calculated quartile-specific price indexes and used them to compare incomes and expenditures in real terms in the two years [Musgrove (1981)]; the results for health care spending also appear in Table 18.2. In the top three quartiles, the shifts imply an elasticity of about 0.9, but in the poorest quartile family health care spending declined, the implicit elasticity being about –0.5. It is not clear whether this is due to expansion of free public services, which would have reduced the need for private spending, or whether it reflects other factors such as better nutrition and sanitation, which would have improved the health of the poorest families.

The largest household expenditure survey yet taken in Latin America was conducted in Brazil in 1974–75 [FIBGE (1978)]. Published tables show means of total family spending (on several slightly different definitions) and of spending in total on health care and on several components such as doctors, hospitalization and surgery, drugs and medicines, etc., by region of the country, metropolitan/other urban/rural location, and class of total expenditure (nine classes are distinguished for most regions and locations). The Brazilian public health care system has recently been extensively analyzed

Table 18.2 Estimated Total Family Expenditure per Person and Private Health Care Expenditure, by Quartile 1 (low) to 4 (high) of Total Spending per Person, in Ten South American Cities (1968 Dollars per Year)[a]

	QUARTILE 1		2		3		4	
CITY	TOTAL	HEALTH	TOTAL	HEALTH	TOTAL	HEALTH	TOTAL	HEALTH
Cali	174	0.96	293	2.81	531	8.87	961	20.66
Barranquilla	201	2.77	339	5.93	504	12.55	924	36.87
Medellín	146	1.02	247	3.80	421	6.69	915	29.19
Quito	156	3.67	320	11.10	586	17.76	1236	35.97
Guayaquil	160	2.18	266	5.83	512	9.42	1044	27.14
Maracaibo	192	1.31	330	2.81	494	5.04	924	20.70
Santiago	220	1.96	421	5.14	714	9.00	1483	27.58
Bogota	229	2.89	384	3.80	586	11.25	1227	40.73
Lima	220	4.36	394	6.54	631	13.88	1290	34.06
Caracas	320	4.64	677	19.84	1162	45.32	2050	129.56

Caracas, Venezuela, only, in 1966 and 1975 (expenditures in bolivars per person per month; 1966 bolivars, 1975 deflated by a variable index)

	TOTAL	HEALTH	TOTAL	HEALTH	TOTAL	HEALTH	TOTAL	HEALTH
1966	122	3.57	217	8.10	384	26.46	835	51.60
1975: Nominal	126	2.32	265	8.88	505	28.91	1114	59.46
Real		2.72		9.99		31.84		62.75

[a]Cities are ordered by ascending median family income, in 1968 dollars, at purchasing-power-parity exchange rates. Values of total spending are medians within quartiles (12.5, 37.5, 62.5 and 87.5 percent of the cumulative distribution). 1975 real health spending in Caracas includes an adjustment for differential inflation of medical prices.

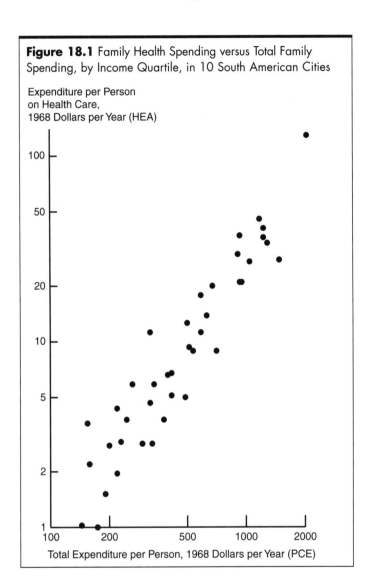

Figure 18.1 Family Health Spending versus Total Family Spending, by Income Quartile, in 10 South American Cities

Expenditure per Person on Health Care, 1968 Dollars per Year (HEA)

Total Expenditure per Person, 1968 Dollars per Year (PCE)

[McGreevey (1982)], but there has been little if any previous analysis of spending by families although some such research is now planned [Programa de Investigação em Serviços de Saúde (1982)]. I have used the data on total health care spending, shown in Table 18.3 and Figure 18.2, for the same analysis as that discussed above, with one difference: the much greater number of observations makes it possible to estimate the effects of region and location as well as an elasticity with respect to total expenditure.

Table 18.3 Mean Values of Total Family Expenditure (PCE) and Private Health Care Spending (HEA), within Each of Nine Classes of Total Family Expenditure, by Urban and Rural Areas, in Four Regions of Brazil (Cruzeiros of August 1974 per Year). The classes of Total Expenditure are Defined by Successive Non-Overlapping Intervals of this Variable; Class 1 Starts at Zero Expenditure, and Class 9 is Open-Ended. The Boundaries of the Expenditure Classes Vary among Regions and between Urban and Rural Areas, so as to Reduce the Number of Empty Classes (only Four High-Income Classes in the Rural Areas of Two Regions are Empty)

	1.		2		3		4		5		6.		7.		8		9	
	PCE	HEA	PCE	HEA	PCE	HEA	PCE	HEA	PCE	HEA	PCE	HEA	PCE	HEA	PCE	HEA	PCE	HEA
Metropolitan Areas																		
Rio de Janeiro (Region 1)	3256	92	7103	168	12569	335	18993	548	26684	803	37698	1300	54682	2052	93196	4467	212233	11172
Curitiba (Region 3)	3309	156	7229	178	12423	272	19064	563	26738	885	37389	1184	56119	2466	93965	3677	208811	12827
Porto Alegre (Region 3)	3403	77	7287	234	12616	357	19241	643	26723	899	37289	1148	55635	1741	94170	3701	173224	4902
Belo Horizonte (Region 4)	3207	115	6997	211	10197	284	13462	363	18967	619	26717	880	37512	1748	54345	2039	137471	6521
Fortaleza (Region 5)	3103	54	5730	111	7895	139	10211	230	12466	258	14690	334	18841	547	26526	765	56977	2243
Recife (Region 5)	3172	84	5712	140	7897	193	10072	272	12454	348	14738	411	18785	519	26978	767	61722	2274
Salvador (Region 5)	3196	96	5672	113	7909	135	10118	200	12422	264	14685	319	18784	387	26575	595	74222	2656
Other Urban Areas																		
Region 1	3270	72	7101	212	12319	406	18992	778	26485	1071	37386	1488	53161	2490	88696	6064	197940	6790
Region 3	3465	137	7026	264	12375	491	19053	805	26775	1206	37467	1785	54110	2984	88782	3707	192455	12050
Region 4	2849	104	6806	289	10101	441	13502	620	18802	926	26497	1248	36973	2073	54838	3317	95043	5406
Region 5	3023	88	5614	137	7891	229	10096	295	12391	329	14702	429	18853	569	26772	942	54202	2350
Rural Areas																		
Region 1	3171	91	6784	197	11191	392	18552	793	26376	1095	36628	1687	—	—	—	—	—	—
Region 3	3329	89	6876	336	12100	739	18841	1325	26654	1745	36647	2787	52685	4104	88451	5586	—	—
Region 4	1591	35	2864	71	3962	143	5614	215	7870	350	11832	617	18688	1322	26445	1792	55040	4650
Region 5	1638	35	2896	60	3943	94	5032	140	6189	173	7340	224	8453	269	12755	458	35950	1504

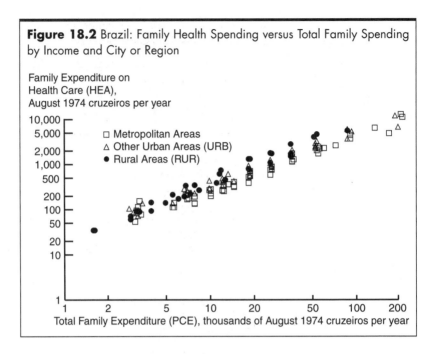

Figure 18.2 Brazil: Family Health Spending versus Total Family Spending by Income and City or Region

Family Expenditure on Health Care (HEA), August 1974 cruzeiros per year

□ Metropolitan Areas
△ Other Urban Areas (URB)
● Rural Areas (RUR)

Total Family Expenditure (PCE), thousands of August 1974 cruzeiros per year

As Figure 18.2 makes clear, the relation of household income to private health spending shows approximately constant elasticity. Moreover, at any level of total spending, rural families spend the most on health care, families in small and medium-sized cities spend less and households in the largest urban areas (seven of which are distinguished in the four regions studied) spend the least. These relations are tested by regression analysis, the results of which appear in Table 18.4. Regional differences as a whole are significant, because spending is higher in Region 5 than in Region 4, but most pairs of regions do not differ. The metropolitan/other urban/rural differences are significant and of the order of 30 percent (urban) and 50 percent (rural) with respect to metropolitan areas. The estimated income elasticity is 1.17, and differs insignificantly among the four specifications tested. There is no evidence, in the range of total expenditure studied, either of saturation at high incomes or of a threshold below which families show a much higher elasticity.

All three of these results—the high income elasticity, the regional differences and the differences by location—are consistent with the following simple model: total health care spending is a normal good, with an income elasticity declining toward one [Newhouse (1977)], but private care is a

Table 18.4 Brazil, 1974: Private Family Health Care Spending as a Function of Total Family Expenditure, Region and Metropolitan/Other Urban/Rural Differences.

Variables:	HEA	$= \log_{10}$ health care expenditure
	PCE	$= \log_{10}$ total expenditure
	URB	= non-metropolitan urban area
	RUR	= rural area
	REG 1, 3, 4, 5	= region (Rio de Janeiro; Parana, Santa Catarina, Rio Grande do Sul; Minas Gerais and Espirito Santo; nine northeastern states)

Regression results (coefficient standard errors in parentheses)

(1) $HEA = 1.1728 \, PCE - 2.2745 \, REG \, 1 - 2.2149 \, REG \, 3 - 2.1873 \, REG \, 4$
    (0.0162)   (0.0740)   (0.0738)   (0.0715)
    $-2.3339 \, REG \, 5 + 0.1100 \, URB + 0.1633 \, RUR, \; R^2 = 0.9992, \, F = 21499$
    (0.0678)   (0.0177)   (0.0188)

(2) $HEA = 1.1446 \, PCE - 2.0700 \, REG \, 1 - 2.0255 \, REG \, 3 - 1.9787 \, REG \, 4$
    (0.0203)   (0.0908)   (0.0910)   (0.0870)
    $-2.1653 \, REG \, 5, \; R^2 = 0.9986, \, F = 17996$
    (0.0836)

(3) $HEA = -2.2841 + 1.1994 \, PCE + 0.1270 \, URB + 0.1885 \, RUR, \; R^2 = 0.9711, \, F = 1422$
    (0.0805)   (0.0186)   (0.0210)   (0.0223)

(4) $HEA = -2.1945 + 1.1736 \, PCE, \; R^2 = 0.9522, \, F = 2572$
    (0.0982)   (0.0231)

Marginal F-tests: Adding all binary variables to (4) $F = 1414$
                 Adding regional variables to (3) $F = 1057$
                 Adding URB and RUR to (2) $F = 43$

$N = 131$ observations

luxury relative to publicly-provided free or subsidized services. Therefore private health care spending can have an elasticity above one even at very high incomes, because as household incomes rise, private services replace public services; and at a given level of income private spending will be higher where fewer public services are available. In Brazil, most public health care is provided through the Instituto Nacional de Assistência Médica da Previdência Social (INAMPS), which is part of the social security system. Expenditures by INAMPS are high relative to government tax revenues (including the payroll taxes which finance much of the system) in the poorer regions of the country [McGreevey (1982, p. 54)] so that there is some net transfer from richer to poorer regions; but expenditures per capita are still lower in the poorer regions [McGreevey (1982, Tables 8 and V.14)]. Private expenditure is higher in Region 4 (Center-West), where INAMPS spending per head of population is 95 percent of the national average, than in Regions 1 and 3 (South and Southeast), where INAMPS spending runs 20 percent above the average. This relation breaks down, however, for Region 5 (Northeast, the poorest part of the country), where INAMPS spending is only half the national average and private spending is also lowest; in this comparison, private and public spending appear to be complements rather than substitutes, perhaps because the relative importance of different components of medical care changes. (This point is considered further, below.)

As for the metropolitan/other urban/rural differences, coverage of the population by INAMPS is more complete in urban areas, although Brazil is one of the relatively few Latin American countries in which there is substantial rural coverage [Zschock (1983, pp. 35–37)]. Much of the urban/rural difference might be due to the difficulties of providing public health care to agricultural workers, so I repeated the analysis in Table 18.3 using an agricultural/non-agricultural classification. Private expenditure is higher, for a given total expenditure, in the agricultural sector, as expected; there is also no significant difference among the three agricultural occupations distinguished in the survey, or among the eight non-agricultural occupations. However, the way in which INAMPS provides care probably exaggerates the real difference in private spending by location: in the metropolitan areas, most health care is provided directly, with little or no out-of-pocket cost to the consumer, whereas in smaller cities and rural areas INAMPS often reimburses consumers for private expenditures, as well as paying other public-sector institutions for services provided. Since the household budget data do not show medical spending net of reimbursements, private costs are somewhat overstated in non-metropolitan areas [Zschock (1983, p. 6)]. Data do not seem to have been assembled showing the distinction between direct provision and reimbursements for urban and rural areas; but 'complementary services paid by INAMPS', which include reimbursements, are available by state and region [McGreevey (1982, p. 116)]; these are a slightly higher share of total outlays in the more rural Northeast, and a notably low share in the more urban South of the country.

The simple constant-elasticity relation characterizing total private health spending does not apply to all components; regional and locational differences in spending also vary according to which component is studied. Table 18.5 shows mean expenditures on the two items which diverge most from the pattern for the total—drugs and medicines, and hospitalization and surgery. The data for the former are also displayed in Figure 18.3, which shows that expenditure on drugs tends toward saturation, irrespective of region and

Table 18.5 Mean Values of Private Family Expenditure on Drugs and Medicines and on Hospitalization and Surgery, within Each of Nine Classes of Total Family Expenditure, by Urban and Rural Areas, in Four Regions of Brazil (Cruzeiros of August 1974 per Year). The Limits of the Classes of Total Family Expenditure (PCE), and the Means of Total Spending in the Classes, are the Same as in Table18.3 and are Not Repeated Here

	DRUGS AND MEDICINES									HOSPITALIZATION AND SURGERY								
	1	2	3	4	5	6	7	8	9	1	2	3	4	5	6	7	8	9
Metropolitan Areas																		
Rio de Janeiro	75	134	233	336	452	594	659	1059	1350	0	2	18	37	91	142	382	984	2356
Curitiba	125	101	182	325	381	386	575	593	830	0	28	18	70	133	262	796	1104	5903
Porto Alegre	70	180	250	428	499	630	557	679	966	0	5	5	19	68	84	268	929	234
Belo Horizonte	104	176	228	261	362	458	619	589	1040	1	6	16	19	76	106	139	249	901
Fortaleza	42	95	112	184	220	246	391	447	771	1	1	2	12	7	7	46	70	460
Recife	77	120	169	236	296	324	385	483	742	0	2	5	2	9	10	16	55	511
Salvador	88	102	116	158	188	253	294	395	670	1	0	0	2	24	1	7	18	527
Other Urban Areas																		
Region 1	67	175	305	525	651	770	921	1779	1293	4	1	14	68	88	97	350	818	1330
Region 3	90	181	317	420	604	598	935	888	1212	17	37	77	146	193	447	934	731	6182
Region 4	88	233	307	446	534	632	860	1195	1414	0	5	22	36	95	106	263	702	1351
Region 5	71	105	175	220	248	330	383	562	740	2	7	12	15	29	17	49	120	716
Rural Areas																		
Region 1	76	161	290	618	664	715	—	—	—	2	4	13	10	66	255	—	—	—
Region 3	58	160	307	471	569	818	1080	1109	—	18	93	242	503	631	1111	2088	3809	—
Region 4	33	61	111	152	253	396	707	771	1707	0	0	6	11	30	61	271	393	1629
Region 5	28	47	72	113	130	170	205	304	603	0	2	3	6	9	16	17	53	364

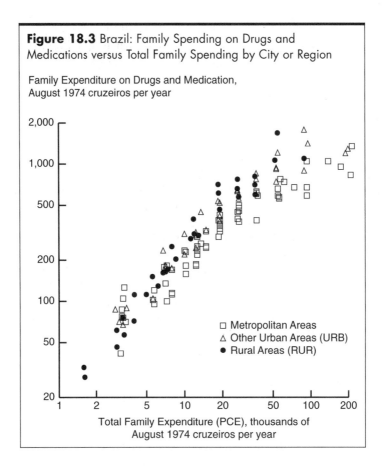

Figure 18.3 Brazil: Family Spending on Drugs and Medications versus Total Family Spending by City or Region

location. Rural spending is higher than in metropolitan or other urban areas at high levels of total household spending, but at low levels, rural families appear to spend less on drugs and medicines; this may reflect a distribution of the poorest rural families in areas where even pharmacies are rare, so that the explanation again turns on the availability of the goods and services.

Hospitalization and surgery, in contrast, shows an explosive growth with increasing income; this is undoubtedly the category for which private care is most clearly a luxury compared to public hospital services, so that the poorest families spend essentially nothing in this category. Metropolitan/other urban/rural differences do not seem to be stable across regions, but there are pronounced regional differences, with especially high expenditure in Region 3 (South) in all three locations. Brazil is unusual among Latin American countries in having a high share of private hospital beds [Zschock (1983,

Table 2)], which may be concentrated in the relatively urban, high-income South of the country. Of course, to the extent that private hospital care is reimbursed to consumers, net expenditures may be exaggerated much more than net total private health care spending.

References

Fuchs, Victor, 1979, Economics, health and post-industrial society, Milbank Memorial Fund Quarterly / Health and Society 57, 153–182.

Fundação Instituto Brasileiro de Geografia e Estatística, 1978. Estudo nacional de despesa familiar, Dados preliminares: Despesas das famílias, Regiões I, III, IV, V, VI, VII (FIBGE, Rio de Janeiro).

Grossman, Michael, 1982, The demand for health after a decade, Journal of Health Economics 1, 1–3.

Kleiman, Ephraim, 1974, The determinants of national outlay on health, in: Mark Perlman, ed., The economics of health and medical care (Wiley, New York).

Maxwell, Robert J., 1981, Health and wealth (Heath, Boston, MA).

McGreevey, William, 1982, Brazilian health care financing and health policy; An international perspective (World Bank, Population, Health and Nutrition Department, Washington, DC).

Mesa-Lago, Carmelo, 1978, Social security in Latin America (University of Pittsburgh Press, Pittsburgh, PA).

Musgrove, Philip, 1978a, Consumer behavior in Latin America (Brookings Institution, Washington, DC).

Musgrove Philip, 1978b, La contribución familiar al financiamiento de la educación en América Latina, in: Mario Brodersohn and María Ester Sanjurjo, eds., Financiamiento de la educación en América latina (Fondo de Cultura Económica, México).

Musgrove, Philip, 1981, The oil price increase and the alleviation of poverty; Income distribution in Caracas, Venezuela, in 1966 and 1975, Journal of Development Economics 9, 229–250.

Newhouse, Joseph, 1977, Medical-care expenditure: A cross-national survey, Journal of Human Resources 12, 115–124.

Pan American Health Organization, XXI Sanitary Conference, 1982, Plan de acción para la instrumentación de las estrategias de salud para todos en el año 2000: Implicaciones financieras y presupuestarias, Document CSP 21/21 (PAHO, Washington, DC).

Programa de Investigação em Serviços de Saúde, 1982, Acordo MEC/MS/MPAS/OPAS, Termos de Referencia (Brasília).

Rapaport, John, Robert L. Roberton and Bruce Stuart, 1982, Understanding health economics (Aspen, Rockville, MD).

Selowsky, Marcelo, 1979, Who benefits from public expenditure? A case study of Colombia (Johns Hopkins, Baltimore, MD).

World Bank, 1982, Colombia: Health sector review (World Bank, Population, Health and Nutrition Department, Washington, DC).

Zschock, Dieter, 1978, Health care financing in developing countries (American Public Health Association, Washington, DC).

Zschock, Dieter, 1983, Medical care under social insurance in Latin America: Review and analysis (Stony Brook, NY) (*date unknown*).

CHAPTER 19

Basic Patterns in National Health Expenditure

Scope of the Analysis

We describe what WHO's 191 Member States spend on health and how it is financed from out-of-pocket spending and prepayments, including social health insurance contributions, government "general revenue," and voluntary and employment-related insurance. To analyze the adequacy of spending, and the distribution of financial burden among sources of finance and households, we used simple comparisons and linear regression analyses. Most of the analyses consider all the Member States, to maximize the number of observations, and cover a wide range of incomes. Some analyses were also conducted on a regional basis, the results of which are sometimes reported, but not shown in detail.

The principal source of our data is the set of national health accounts estimates prepared by WHO, with revisions up to 31 May 2001. Because of subsequent revisions, the numbers do not always match those that have been published previously (1). The estimates refer to 1997, although they may be based on data for earlier years as well. We do not discuss the primary data sources or estimation methods here, since they have been described elsewhere (2). The quality of the information varies considerably among countries, so that initial estimates for 1997 were classified as follows: "complete data with high reliability", "incomplete data with high-to-medium reliability", or "incomplete data with low reliability". Originally, there were only 15 countries in the last category. The classification has not been

Co-authored with Riadh Zeramdini and Guy Carrin. Reprinted, with permission, from *Bulletin of the World Health Organization* 80(2), February 2002.

modified as improved data have been obtained, so the data for a country are at least as good as the categorization shown here. We do not expect that revisions to the data used here will significantly modify the patterns found.

The three data categories are always distinguished in the graphical presentations which follow, and in the statistical analyses. Table 19.1 shows WHO estimates {of three absolute expenditures in international dollars per capita, and of nine percentage shares}, and Table 19.2 classifies countries according to WHO region and per capita income level, distinguished as follows: very low income (<US$ 1000), low (US$ 1000–2200), middle (US$ 2200–7000), and high-income (>US$ 7000). Although WHO regions are further divided into strata according to estimated adult and child mortality levels (3), as indicated in Table 19.2, we did not analyze the data according to the strata because sometimes there were very few countries in a region/mortality cell.

The analysis begins with total health spending relative to gross domestic product (GDP), as a function of GDP per capita (GDPC). To visualize relations to income, we took natural logarithms of all money amounts. Fig. 19.1 shows the share of total health expenditures in GDP as a percentage of GDP (THE%GDP), as a function of Ln (GDPC), over the income range 6–11 (ca. US$ 400–60,000). Figs. 19.2 to 19.4 refer to the same income range. All graphical, and most statistical, analyses refer to percentage shares, relative to total health expenditure, government revenues, or total public or central government expenditure. Comparisons to the need for health spending, however, require amounts in US$, so per capita levels of total health expenditure, out-of-pocket spending, and total public spending are compared to per capita income in purchasing power parity dollars (PPP$).

What Do Countries Spend on Health?

The THE%GDP rises from 2% to 9% as income increases (Fig. 19.1). Regression analysis shows that health spending is (slightly) a luxury good: the regression coefficient on income for all countries together is 0.0109, and 0.0137 for the set of 72 countries with high-quality national expenditure data. The complete regression statistics for all three country groups according to data quality, and for all 191 countries together, are shown in Table 19.3. In this and all other regressions, the absolute value of the coefficient is greater for the high-quality data, but the difference between the estimated coefficients for all countries and for the high-reliability group is

Table 19.1 National Health Accounts Estimates for 191 WHO Member States for 1997, Revised Data as of 31 May 2001[a]

COUNTRY	THE/ GDP	PHE/ THE	PvHE/ THE	PHE/ GGE	SocSec/ THE	GenRev/ PHE	ExtRes/ PHE	PvIns/ PvHE	OOPS/ PvHE	THE	PHE	OOPS
					% SHARES[b]					PER CAPITA EXPENDITURES IN PPP $[c]		
Afghanistan (L)	1.4	52.6	47.4	3.6	0.0	92.5	7.5	0.0	100.0	7	4	4
Albania (M)	3.8	71.5	28.5	9.5	17.5	81.6	0.9	46.0	54.1	107	76	16
Algeria (H)	4.0	79.8	20.2	11.3	66.7	33.3	0.0	0.0	100.0	195	155	39
Andorra (L)	9.3	86.6	13.4	22.1	84.8	15.3	0.0	0.0	100.0	1557	1348	209
Angola (M)	4.1	47.9	52.1	6.1	0.0	89.1	10.9	0.0	100.0	62	30	32
Antigua and Barbuda (M)	5.5	62.9	37.1	15.0	0.0	100.0	0.0	0.0	100.0	508	320	188
Argentina (H)	8.0	55.2	44.8	20.1	60.2	39.7	0.2	24.8	75.3	953	526	322
Armenia (M)	7.8	41.5	58.5	12.2	0.0	92.1	7.9	0.0	100.0	160	67	94
Australia (H)	8.4	68.3	31.8	16.2	0.0	100.0	0.0	29.6	50.7	1917	1309	309
Austria (H)	8.0	71.4	28.6	11.2	59.5	40.5	0.0	27.0	58.8	1819	1299	306
Azerbaijan (M)	2.9	79.3	20.7	10.6	0.0	94.4	5.6	0.0	100.0	58	46	12
Bahamas (M)	6.5	53.7	46.3	13.7	0.0	100.0	0.0	0.0	92.6	785	421	337
Bahrain (M)	5.0	58.5	41.5	8.7	0.0	100.0	0.0	0.0	90.9	706	413	267
Bangladesh (H)	4.5	45.4	54.6	9.1	0.0	92.0	8.0	0.0	95.0	50	23	26
Barbados (M)	7.0	71.0	29.0	15.1	0.0	100.0	0.0	0.0	100.0	901	640	262
Belarus (M)	5.9	82.6	17.4	10.5	0.0	99.9	0.1	0.0	100.0	344	285	60
Belgium (M)	8.6	71.0	29.0	12.2	88.0	12.0	0.0	6.8	46.7	1995	1416	271
Belize (M)	4.7	51.0	49.0	8.2	0.0	95.5	4.5	0.0	100.0	226	115	111
Benin (M)	3.1	48.5	51.5	6.0	0.0	85.8	14.2	0.0	100.0	27	13	14
Bhutan (M)	4.7	72.2	27.8	10.1	0.0	70.3	29.7	0.0	100.0	27	19	7

a Countries are classified according to whether their data are judged by WHO to be complete and of high reliability (H), incomplete and of medium to high reliability (M), or incomplete and of low reliability (L).

b Abbreviations HE = health expenditure; T = total; P = public; Pvt = private; GGE = general government expenditure; SocSec = social security; GenRev = general revenue (tax funded); ExtRes = external resources; Ins = insurance; OOPS = out-of-pocket spending.

c PPP = purchasing power parity.

Table 19.1 (continued)

COUNTRY	THE/GDP	PHE/THE	PVTHE/THE	PHE/GGE	SocSec/THE	GenRev/PHE	ExtRes/PHE	Pvths/PvHE	OOPS/PvHE	PER CAPITA EXPENDITURES IN PPP $[c]		
										THE	PHE	OOPS
Bolivia (H)	4.7	63.9	36.1	9.1	65.3	24.9	9.8	7.8	85.7	104	66	32
Bosnia and Herzegovina (M)	4.0	55.4	44.6	6.2	0.0	69.1	30.9	0.0	100.0	20	11	9
Botswana (M)	3.4	70.5	29.5	5.9	0.0	98.5	1.6	52.9	37.1	220	155	24
Brazil (M)	6.5	40.4	59.7	9.7	0.0	100.0	0.0	48.1	52.0	438	177	136
Brunei Darussalam (M)	5.4	40.6	59.4	4.5	0.0	100.0	0.0	0.0	100.0	939	381	557
Bulgaria (H)	4.4	80.0	20.0	8.9	10.5	89.5	0.0	0.0	93.5	209	167	39
Burkina Faso (M)	4.0	67.6	32.4	11.3	0.0	76.4	23.6	0.0	100.0	32	22	10
Burundi (M)	2.1	42.2	57.8	4.0	0.0	69.4	30.6	0.0	100.0	12	5	7
Cambodia (M)	7.2	9.4	90.6	7.0	0.0	49.0	51.0	0.0	100.0	87	8	79
Cameroon (M)	3.0	34.2	65.8	7.2	0.0	71.0	29.0	0.0	81.6	44	15	23
Canada (H)	9.0	69.9	30.1	15.4	1.6	98.4	0.0	36.1	56.9	2181	1524	374
Cape Verde (M)	2.6	71.8	28.2	4.7	0.0	75.8	24.2	0.0	100.0	87	62	24
Central African Republic (M)	2.4	51.4	48.6	4.0	0.0	75.7	24.3	0.0	77.3	25	13	9
Chad (M)	3.1	79.3	20.7	13.2	0.0	78.0	22.0	0.0	100.0	25	20	5
Chile (H)	7.0	36.3	63.7	10.8	89.3	10.3	0.4	33.7	66.3	609	221	257
China (H)	4.2	39.4	60.6	13.6	87.0	12.6	0.4	0.0	78.9	125	49	60
Colombia (H)	9.3	57.6	42.4	18.2	40.3	59.5	0.2	38.9	61.1	569	328	147
Comoros (M)	4.5	68.2	31.8	8.7	0.0	75.8	24.2	0.0	100.0	53	36	17
Congo, Republic of (H)	2.8	64.6	35.4	4.8	0.0	84.5	15.5	0.0	100.0	28	18	10
Cook Islands (M)	5.3	67.1	32.9	10.3	0.0	99.8	0.2	0.0	100.0	319	214	105
Costa Rica (H)	7.0	78.3	21.7	21.6	84.9	14.5	0.6	3.0	97.0	498	390	105
Côte d'Ivoire (M)	3.0	46.0	54.0	5.7	0.0	81.6	18.4	14.9	85.1	46	21	21
Croatia (H)	8.2	80.5	19.5	13.2	92.6	7.4	0.0	0.0	100.0	530	427	103
Cuba (M)	6.3	87.5	12.5	10.0	20.9	79.0	0.1	0.0	100.0	87	76	11
Cyprus (H)	6.4	36.3	63.7	6.3	80.9	19.1	0.0	0.0	97.9	1085	394	677
Czech Republic (M)	7.1	91.7	8.3	14.7	89.5	10.5	0.0	0.0	100.0	910	835	76
Democratic People's Republic of Korea (L)	3.0	83.5	16.5	5.6	0.0	99.0	1.0	0.0	100.0	31	25	5

	1.6	74.1	25.9	12.3	0.0	90.5	9.5	0.0	100.0	15	11	4
Democratic Republic of the Congo (M)												
Denmark (H)	8.2	82.3	17.7	12.9	0.0	100.0	0.0	7.9	92.1	1969	1620	322
Djibouti (M)	4.6	44.4	55.6	5.7	0.0	96.7	3.3	0.0	29.8	62	27	10
Dominica (M)	5.9	69.6	30.4	11.0	0.0	97.5	2.5	17.7	82.4	309	215	77
Dominican Republic (M)	6.4	29.1	70.9	10.5	22.3	75.4	2.3	13.2	77.0	291	85	159
Ecuador (H)	3.7	50.8	49.2	7.0	48.8	49.1	2.1	10.6	65.4	120	61	39
Egypt (H)	4.3	31.8	68.2	4.5	39.6	56.1	4.3	0.4	93.2	123	39	78
El Salvador (H)	8.1	38.7	61.3	22.6	43.3	53.6	3.1	2.7	97.1	328	127	195
Equatorial Guinea (M)	3.6	56.0	44.0	7.9	0.0	85.9	14.1	0.0	100.0	59	33	26
Eritrea (L)	4.4	65.8	34.2	5.3	0.0	83.1	16.9	0.0	100.0	42	28	14
Estonia (H)	6.4	78.9	21.2	13.6	0.0	99.9	0.1	0.0	46.1	481	379	47
Ethiopia (M)	4.7	41.4	58.6	8.1	0.0	85.9	14.1	0.0	87.6	29	12	15
Fiji (H)	4.0	66.7	33.3	7.4	0.0	99.2	0.8	0.0	100.0	179	119	60
Finland (H)	7.3	76.1	23.9	10.7	19.6	80.4	0.0	10.4	83.0	1517	1154	301
France (H)	9.4	77.7	22.3	13.3	100.0	3.2	0.0	55.4	47.1	1994	1550	209
Gabon (M)	3.1	66.5	33.5	6.2	0.0	92.6	7.4	0.0	100.0	197	131	66
Gambia (M)	3.0	78.7	21.3	11.5	0.0	86.2	13.8	0.0	100.0	45	36	10
Georgia (H)	4.4	8.6	91.4	2.6	0.0	91.6	8.4	0.0	100.0	222	19	203
Germany (H)	10.5	76.6	23.4	14.5	90.7	9.3	0.0	29.5	66.0	2336	1789	361
Ghana (M)	3.6	55.1	44.9	9.6	0.0	72.1	27.9	0.0	100.0	63	35	28
Greece (H)	8.5	57.7	42.3	11.9	37.2	62.8	0.0	5.3	89.4	1177	679	445
Grenada (M)	4.6	65.7	34.3	10.4	0.0	98.2	1.8	0.0	100.0	265	174	91
Guatemala (M)	4.3	44.9	55.1	15.5	57.7	36.3	6.1	3.8	92.3	149	67	76
Guinea (M)	3.6	57.2	42.8	9.7	0.0	73.9	26.1	0.0	100.0	58	33	25
Guinea-Bissau (M)	3.9	64.0	36.0	2.2	0.0	79.2	20.8	0.0	100.0	34	22	12
Guyana (M)	4.6	81.5	18.5	8.6	0.0	99.4	0.6	0.0	93.9	180	147	31
Haiti (M)	3.6	33.5	66.5	10.2	0.0	63.4	36.6	0.0	43.2	45	15	13
Honduras (M)	6.4	55.4	44.6	17.0	9.7	84.9	5.3	0.1	91.4	158	88	64
Hungary (H)	6.8	75.3	24.7	10.4	35.5	64.5	0.0	0.0	46.9	677	510	78
Iceland (H)	8.0	83.7	16.3	18.9	31.5	68.5	0.0	0.0	100.0	1951	1633	318
India (H)	5.5	15.3	84.7	4.7	0.0	96.0	4.1	0.0	97.3	109	17	90
Indonesia (H)	2.7	22.9	77.1	3.0	69.5	23.0	7.5	16.0	84.0	82	19	53

Table 19.1 (continued)

COUNTRY	THE/GDP	PHE/THE	PVTHE/THE	PHE/GGE	SocSec/THE	GenRev/PHE	ExtRes/PHE	Pvhs/PvtHE	OOPS/PvtHE	THE	PHE	OOPS
					% SHARES[b]					PER CAPITA EXPENDITURES IN PPP $[c]		
Iran, Islamic Republic of (H)	5.9	46.4	53.6	10.4	25.7	74.3	0.0	0.0	100.0	275	128	148
Iraq (M)	4.2	58.9	41.1	12.5	0.0	100.0	0.0	0.0	100.0	136	80	56
Ireland (H)	7.0	75.6	24.4	16.3	8.3	91.7	0.0	32.9	54.7	1453	1099	193
Israel (H)	8.6	70.3	29.8	12.5	0.0	100.0	0.0	0.0	90.2	1553	1091	417
Italy (H)	8.3	67.5	32.5	11.2	0.4	99.6	0.0	3.9	72.5	1742	1176	410
Jamaica (M)	5.4	56.0	44.0	8.7	0.0	97.3	2.7	26.4	53.5	210	118	50
Japan (H)	7.4	79.5	20.5	16.7	89.0	11.0	0.0	0.0	78.9	1810	1439	293
Jordan (M)	7.1	70.3	29.7	13.4	0.0	97.8	2.2	0.0	73.7	285	200	62
Kazakhstan (M)	3.3	65.5	34.5	10.1	47.0	52.5	0.5	0.0	100.0	172	113	59
Kenya (M)	7.6	28.2	71.8	7.9	13.5	60.1	26.3	4.7	73.9	76	21	40
Kiribati (M)	8.9	99.2	0.9	12.9	0.0	98.5	1.5	0.0	100.0	175	174	1
Kuwait (M)	3.3	87.4	12.6	8.4	0.0	100.0	0.0	0.0	100.0	628	549	79
Kyrgyzstan (M)	4.0	69.4	30.6	10.4	0.8	94.0	5.2	0.0	100.0	90	62	27
Lao People's Democratic Republic (M)	4.3	36.8	63.2	6.0	0.6	86.3	13.1	0.0	100.0	74	27	47
Latvia (H)	6.0	60.6	39.4	9.6	52.5	47.4	0.1	0.0	100.0	338	205	133
Lebanon (H)	9.8	29.6	70.4	6.8	26.9	72.6	0.5	23.7	76.3	501	148	269
Lesotho (H)	5.3	76.0	24.0	12.4	0.0	79.5	20.5	0.0	100.0	96	73	23
Liberia (L)	2.5	66.7	33.3	6.7	0.0	88.8	11.2	0.0	100.0	94	62	31
Libyan Arab Jamahirya (L)	3.7	47.6	52.4	2.6	0.0	100.0	0.0	0.0	90.9	260	124	124
Lithuania (H)	6.6	73.9	26.1	14.4	68.6	31.4	0.0	0.0	90.9	280	207	66
Luxembourg (H)	5.9	92.5	7.5	12.7	86.0	14.0	0.0	19.5	99.2	2076	1920	155
Madagascar (M)	2.3	57.2	42.8	7.6	0.0	87.1	12.9	0.0	100.0	17	10	7
Malawi (M)	7.3	50.6	49.4	14.6	0.0	61.3	38.7	1.6	35.4	41	21	7
Malaysia (H)	2.3	57.6	42.4	5.6	0.0	98.8	1.2	0.0	100.0	214	123	91
Maldives (M)	7.1	74.5	25.5	10.9	0.0	91.6	8.4	0.0	100.0	274	204	70
Mali (M)	4.2	45.8	54.2	7.9	0.0	74.9	25.1	0.0	89.9	28	13	14
Malta (H)	6.3	58.9	41.1	8.9	98.5	1.5	0.0	0.0	92.6	873	514	332

Marshall Islands (L)	9.2	61.9	38.1	14.1	0.0	61.5	38.5	0.0	100.0	141	87	54
Mauritania (M)	2.9	69.7	30.3	7.8	0.0	84.8	15.2	0.0	100.0	44	31	13
Mauritius (M)	3.4	51.1	48.9	7.1	0.0	79.1	20.9	0.0	100.0	277	141	135
Mexico (H)	5.3	43.3	56.7	6.0	73.6	27.6	0.0	2.7	93.7	406	176	216
Micronesia, Federated States of (L)	7.6	79.7	20.3	11.3	0.0	100.0	0.0	0.0	100.0	164	131	33
Monaco (L)	7.0	50.0	50.0	17.8	93.8	6.3	0.0	0.0	100.0	1549	775	775
Mongolia (H)	5.5	62.7	37.3	13.4	12.2	76.5	11.4	0.0	73.3	88	55	24
Morocco (M)	4.6	28.6	71.4	3.9	8.4	89.8	1.8	23.1	76.9	142	41	78
Mozambique (H)	3.9	56.2	43.8	11.2	0.0	39.8	60.2	0.0	41.2	28	16	5
Myanmar (M)	2.3	18.6	81.4	4.4	0.0	99.9	0.1	0.0	100.0	26	5	21
Namibia (M)	7.9	54.3	45.7	11.1	0.0	91.6	8.4	91.3	3.0	411	223	6
Nauru (L)	4.9	97.4	2.6	9.6	0.0	100.0	0.0	0.0	100.0	213	208	6
Nepal (M)	4.7	20.6	79.5	5.3	0.0	67.1	32.9	0.0	73.5	58	12	34
Netherlands (H)	8.7	68.9	31.1	12.6	93.8	6.2	0.0	57.5	23.2	1960	1350	142
New Zealand (H)	7.6	77.3	22.7	12.7	0.0	100.0	0.0	29.8	68.9	1381	1068	216
Nicaragua (M)	7.3	49.5	50.5	22.1	18.7	61.2	20.1	0.0	100.0	318	157	161
Niger (M)	3.0	51.1	48.9	6.0	0.0	61.0	39.1	0.0	81.4	19	10	8
Nigeria (M)	1.9	27.0	73.0	3.5	0.0	53.8	46.2	0.0	100.0	14	4	10
Niue (L)	7.6	97.3	2.7	13.0	0.0	100.0	0.0	0.0	100.0	774	753	21
Norway (H)	8.1	83.0	17.0	15.2	0.0	100.0	0.0	0.0	88.9	2152	1785	326
Oman (H)	3.2	82.1	17.9	6.9	0.0	100.0	0.0	0.0	49.9	319	262	28
Pakistan (M)	4.0	22.9	77.1	2.9	55.1	42.0	2.9	0.0	100.0	66	15	51
Palau (L)	6.1	87.5	12.5	8.9	0.0	100.0	0.0	0.0	100.0	520	455	65
Panama (H)	7.6	66.7	33.3	18.7	60.6	38.8	0.6	16.8	76.8	396	264	101
Papua New Guinea (M)	3.3	90.6	9.5	9.6	0.0	83.5	16.5	0.0	100.0	78	71	7
Paraguay (M)	7.5	33.1	66.9	13.6	47.8	48.8	3.5	20.8	69.2	338	112	156
Peru (H)	3.5	57.3	42.7	11.8	61.1	36.3	2.6	7.1	86.4	160	91	59
Philippines (H)	3.5	48.5	51.5	7.2	30.9	67.6	1.5	4.6	95.4	132	64	65
Poland (H)	6.1	72.0	28.0	10.1	0.0	100.0	0.0	0.0	100.0	456	328	128
Portugal (H)	10.7	55.6	44.4	14.2	6.3	93.7	0.0	2.7	90.6	1619	900	652
Qatar (M)	5.3	57.5	42.5	7.6	0.0	100.0	0.0	0.0	100.0	1433	824	609
Republic of Korea (H)	5.0	41.0	59.0	10.1	71.9	28.1	0.0	11.3	78.2	743	305	342
Republic of Moldova (H)	8.0	75.4	24.6	11.9	0.0	97.6	2.4	0.0	100.0	173	130	42

Table 19.1 (continued)

COUNTRY	THE/ GDP	PHE/ THE	PVTHE/ THE	PHE/ GGE	% SHARES[b]					PER CAPITA EXPENDITURES IN PPP $[c]		
					SocSec/ THE	GenRev/ PHE	ExtRes/ PHE	Pvhs/ PvHE	OOPS/ PvHE	THE	PHE	OOPS
Romania (H)	4.1	62.9	37.1	7.5	18.7	80.3	1.0	0.0	100.0	253	159	94
Russian Federation (H)	5.2	76.8	23.2	10.6	83.8	15.7	0.5	0.0	100.0	376	289	87
Rwanda (M)	5.2	34.1	65.9	8.7	0.9	28.5	70.6	0.2	62.4	35	12	14
Saint Kitts and Nevis (M)	4.7	68.4	31.6	10.9	0.0	92.5	7.5	0.0	100.0	498	340	157
Saint Lucia (M)	4.1	62.3	37.3	9.0	0.0	97.0	3.0	0.0	100.0	226	141	85
Saint Vincent and the Grenadines (M)	6.3	63.8	36.2	9.8	0.0	99.9	0.1	0.0	100.0	286	182	103
Samoa (M)	3.5	71.4	28.6	12.5	0.0	97.8	2.2	0.0	100.0	176	126	50
San Marino (L)	7.6	85.2	14.8	9.9	93.6	6.4	0.0	0.0	100.0	2350	2002	348
Sao Tome and Principe (M)	3.0	66.7	33.3	2.9	0.0	78.8	21.3	0.0	100.0	45	30	15
Saudi Arabia (M)	4.0	80.2	19.8	9.4	0.0	100.0	0.0	10.5	31.9	444	356	28
Senegal (M)	4.5	55.7	44.3	13.2	0.0	83.6	16.4	0.0	100.0	61	34	27
Seychelles (M)	6.4	77.1	22.9	8.8	0.0	78.0	22.0	0.0	100.0	736	568	169
Sierra Leone (M)	3.0	41.4	58.6	7.2	0.0	73.2	26.8	0.0	100.0	17	7	10
Singapore (H)	3.2	35.8	64.2	5.5	23.2	76.8	0.0	0.0	100.0	663	237	425
Slovakia (H)	7.8	79.8	20.2	12.4	92.8	7.2	0.0	0.0	100.0	736	587	149
Slovenia (H)	8.9	79.3	20.7	16.3	96.3	3.7	0.0	48.1	51.9	1236	981	133
Solomon Islands (M)	3.5	95.3	4.7	11.4	0.0	85.3	14.8	0.0	6.7	102	98	0
Somalia (M)	2.4	62.5	37.5	5.6	0.0	92.6	7.4	0.0	100.0	11	7	4
South Africa (H)	10.3	47.3	52.7	12.7	0.0	99.8	0.2	77.8	20.2	770	364	82
Spain (H)	7.0	77.2	23.5	13.5	10.9	89.1	0.0	23.4	76.6	1162	897	210
Sri Lanka (H)	3.2	49.5	50.5	6.0	0.0	95.8	4.2	1.0	99.0	94	47	47
Sudan (M)	4.4	20.9	79.1	3.4	0.0	100.0	0.0	0.0	100.0	46	10	36
Suriname (M)	6.2	62.1	37.9	19.9	44.7	22.8	32.5	0.0	100.0	191	119	72
Swaziland (M)	3.4	72.3	27.7	8.2	0.0	79.3	20.7	0.0	100.0	148	107	41
Sweden (H)	8.1	84.3	15.8	11.5	0.0	100.0	0.0	0.0	100.0	1743	1469	275

Country											
Switzerland (H)	10.2	74.1	26.8	14.5	79.3	20.7	0.0	41.7	16.6	2598	1924	116
Syrian Arab Republic (M)	2.5	33.6	66.4	2.9	0.0	99.5	0.5	0.0	100.0	74	25	49
Tajikistan (M)	3.0	66.0	34.0	9.4	0.0	96.6	3.5	0.0	100.0	22	14	7
Thailand (H)	3.7	56.9	43.1	8.5	8.4	91.5	0.1	13.6	86.2	234	133	87
The former Yugoslav Republic of Macedonia (L)	6.5	84.8	15.2	15.6	89.6	9.9	0.5	0.0	100.0	276	234	42
Togo (M)	2.8	42.8	57.2	4.3	0.0	84.7	15.3	0.0	100.0	40	17	23
Tonga (M)	7.9	46.8	53.2	13.1	0.0	90.7	9.3	0.0	100.0	342	160	182
Trinidad and Tobago (M)	5.0	43.6	56.4	7.6	0.0	100.0	0.0	5.9	88.0	373	162	185
Tunisia (M)	5.3	40.4	59.6	6.7	42.7	57.2	0.1	0.0	90.9	281	114	152
Turkey (M)	4.2	71.6	28.4	10.1	33.2	66.8	0.0	0.2	99.6	265	190	75
Turkmenistan (M)	3.9	74.5	25.5	11.7	9.9	87.7	2.4	0.0	100.0	110	82	28
Tuvalu (M)	8.9	71.4	28.6	7.7	0.0	94.2	5.8	0.0	100.0	151	108	43
Uganda (M)	3.7	50.7	49.3	11.5	0.0	38.2	61.8	0.6	59.1	42	21	12
Ukraine (M)	5.4	75.0	25.0	9.3	0.0	99.2	0.8	0.0	100.0	177	133	44
United Arab Emirates (M)	3.7	79.3	20.7	26.9	0.0	100.0	0.0	19.1	65.9	771	611	105
United Kingdom (H)	6.7	83.7	16.3	14.3	11.6	88.4	0.0	21.3	67.1	1399	1171	153
United Republic of Tanzania (M)	5.1	47.1	52.9	14.8	0.0	63.3	36.7	0.0	85.9	21	10	10
United States of America (H)	13.0	45.5	54.6	18.0	31.9	68.1	0.0	60.6	28.2	3915	1780	603
Uruguay (H)	10.0	45.9	54.1	13.7	51.7	47.7	0.6	63.6	36.7	922	424	183
Uzbekistan (M)	4.6	82.9	17.1	11.6	0.0	99.4	0.6	0.0	100.0	94	78	16
Vanuatu (M)	3.3	64.3	35.8	9.6	0.0	51.6	48.4	0.0	100.0	104	67	37
Venezuela, Bolivarian Republic of (H)	4.1	64.1	35.9	10.5	33.4	66.6	0.0	4.7	86.6	247	159	77
Viet Nam (M)	4.5	20.3	79.7	4.0	0.0	93.3	6.7	0.0	100.0	71	14	56
Yemen (M)	2.9	37.9	62.1	3.3	0.0	90.1	9.9	0.0	100.0	22	8	14
Yugoslavia (M)	7.8	58.7	41.4	13.8	0.0	100.0	0.0	0.0	100.0	170	100	70
Zambia (M)	6.0	56.5	43.5	13.4	0.0	60.7	39.3	0.0	73.3	45	25	14
Zimbabwe (H)	9.5	59.1	40.9	15.4	0.0	61.9	38.1	21.0	67.0	242	143	66

Table 19.2 Countries Grouped by WHO Region, Mortality Stratum, and GDP per Capita

WHO REGION[a]	MORTALITY STRATUM (CHILD/ADULT)	PPP INCOME CLASS (GDP PER CAPITA)			
		VERY LOW (<US$ 1000)	LOW (US$ 1000–2200)	MIDDLE (US$ 2200–7000)	HIGH (>US$7000)
AFRO	Both high	Benin, Burkina Faso, Chad, Guinea-Bissau, Madagascar, Mali, Niger, Nigeria, Sierra Leone	Angola, Cameroon, Cape Verde, Comoros, Equatorial Guinea, Gambia, Ghana, Guinea, Mauritania, Sao Tome and Principe, Senegal, Togo,	Algeria, Gabon, Liberia	Mauritius, Seychelles
	High/very high	Burundi, Congo, Democratic Republic of the Congo, Eritrea, Ethiopia, Kenya, Malawi, Mozambique, Rwanda, United Republic of Tanzania, Zambia	Central African Republic, Côte d'Ivoire, Lesotho, Uganda	Botswana, Namibia, Swaziland, Zimbabwe	South Africa
AMRO	Both very low				Canada, USA
	Both low		Cuba	Belize, Brazil, Colombia, Dominica, Dominican Republic, El Salvador, Grenada, Guyana, Honduras, Jamaica, Panama, Paraguay, St Lucia, St Vincent, Venezuela	Antigua and Barbuda, Argentina, Bahamas, Barbados, Chile, Costa Rica, Mexico, St Kitts and Nevis, Suriname, Trinidad and Tobago, Uruguay
	Both high		Haiti	Bolivia, Ecuador, Guatemala, Nicaragua, Peru	
EMRO	Both low			Islamic Republic of Iran, Jordan, Lebanon, Syria, Tunisia	Bahrain, Cyprus, Kuwait, Libyan Arab Jamahiriya, Oman, Qatar, Saudi Arabia, United Arab Emirates
	Both high	Afghanistan, Somalia, Yemen	Djibouti, Pakistan, Sudan	Egypt, Iraq, Morocco	

Region	Mortality stratum				
EURO	Both very low			Croatia	Andorra, Austria, Belgium, Czech Republic, Denmark, Finland, France, Germany, Greece, Iceland, Ireland, Israel, Italy, Luxembourg, Malta, Monaco, Netherlands, Norway, Poland, Portugal, San Marino, Slovak Republic, Slovenia, Spain, Sweden, Switzerland, United Kingdom
	Both low	Bosnia and Herzegovina	Armenia, Azerbaijan, Tajikistan, Uzbekistan	Albania, Bulgaria, Georgia, Kyrgyz Republic, Macedonia, Romania, Turkey, Turkmenistan, Yugoslavia, Belarus, Kazakhstan, Latvia, Lithuania, Ukraine	
	Low/high	Moldova			Estonia, Hungary, Russian Federation
SEARO	Both low			Indonesia, Sri Lanka, Thailand	
	Both high	Bhutan, Myanmar	Bangladesh, Democratic People's Republic of Korea, India, Nepal	Maldives	
WPRO	Both very low				Australia, Brunei Darussalam, Japan, New Zealand, Singapore
	Both low		Cambodia, Kiribati, Lao People's Democratic Republic, Marshall Islands, Micronesia, Mongolia, Tuvalu, Vietnam	China, Cook Islands, Fiji, Nauru, Papua New Guinea, Philippines, Samoa, Solomon Islands, Tonga, Vanuatu	Malaysia, Niue, Palau, Republic of Korea

a AFRO = WHO Regional Office for Africa; AMRO = WHO Regional Office for the Americas; EMRO = WHO Regional Office for the Eastern Mediterranean; EURO = WHO Regional Office for Europe; SEARO = WHO Regional Office for South-East Asia.

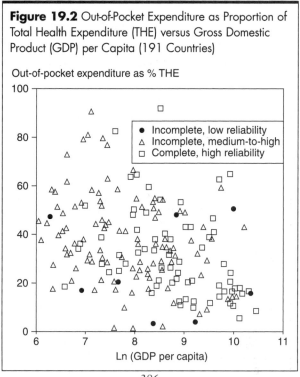

Figure 19.1 Total Health Expenditure as % of Gross Domestic Product (GDP) versus GDP per Capita (191 Countries)

Total health expenditure as % GDP
15
10
5
0
Incomplete, low reliability
Incomplete, medium-to-high
Complete, high reliability
6
7
8
9
10
11
Ln (GDP per capita)

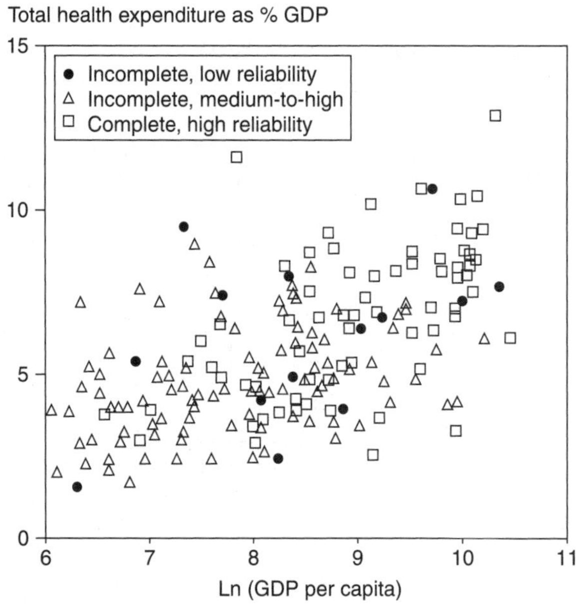

Figure 19.2 Out-of-Pocket Expenditure as Proportion of Total Health Expenditure (THE) versus Gross Domestic Product (GDP) per Capita (191 Countries)

Out-of-pocket expenditure as % THE
100
80
60
40
20
0
Incomplete, low reliability
Incomplete, medium-to-high
Complete, high reliability
6
7
8
9
10
11
Ln (GDP per capita)

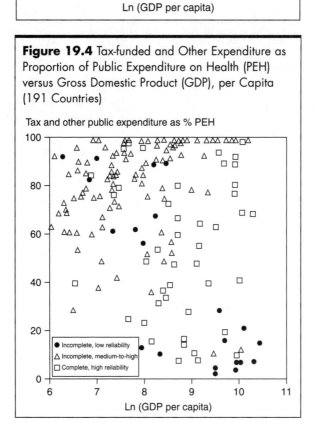

Figure 19.3 Public Expenditure as Proportion of Total Health Expenditure (THE) versus Gross Domestic Product (GDP), per Capita (191 Countries)

Public health expenditure as % THE
100
80
60
40
20
0
6
7
8
9
10
11
Ln (GDP per capita)
● Incomplete, low reliability
△ Incomplete, medium-to-high
□ Complete, high reliability

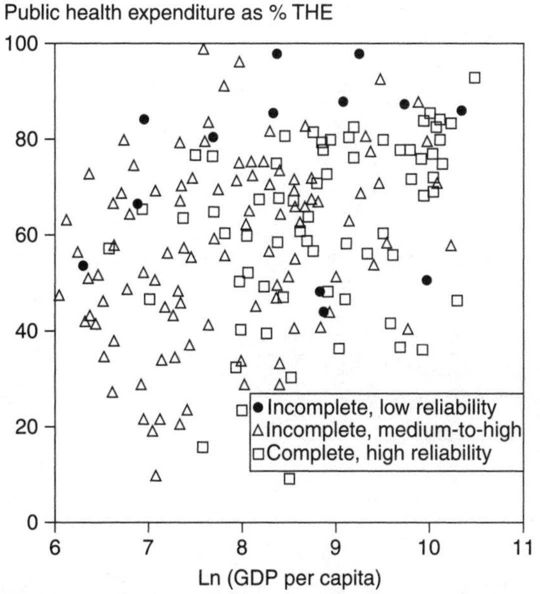

Figure 19.4 Tax-funded and Other Expenditure as Proportion of Public Expenditure on Health (PEH) versus Gross Domestic Product (GDP), per Capita (191 Countries)

Tax and other public expenditure as % PEH
100
80
60
40
20
0
6
7
8
9
10
11
Ln (GDP per capita)
● Incomplete, low reliability
△ Incomplete, medium-to-high
□ Complete, high reliability

Table 19.3 Regression Statistics for Health Expenditure as a Percentage of Gross Domestic Product

REGRESSION STATISTIC	DATA QUALITY			
	LOW	MEDIUM-TO-HIGH	HIGH	ALL DATA
Constant	−0.0328	−0.0020	−0.0567	−0.0353
Standard error	0.0437	0.0119	0.0220	0.0098
t-Statistic	−0.7484	−0.1702	−2.5090	−3.6092
Probability[a]	0.4675	0.8652	0.0144	0.0004
Coefficient of Ln (GDPC)	0.0110	0.0060	0.0137	0.0109
Standard error	0.0051	0.0015	0.0025	0.0012
t-Statistic	2.1218	4.1782	5.4798	9.3725
Probability[a]	0.0563	0.0001	0.0000	0.0000
R^2	0.2572	0.1461	0.3002	0.3173
Adjusted R^2	0.2000	0.1377	0.2902	0.3137
n	15	104	72	191

[a]Probability that the true value of the coefficient is zero.

never significant, and both coefficients always differ from zero. The fit of the regression line, adjusted for degrees of freedom, sometimes improves substantially when only the most reliable data are used. In summary, the inclusion of lower quality data introduces additional "noise", but does not appreciably change the slope of any relation.

A better comparison would be to use per capita income net of subsistence, rather than income without deduction for basic needs, but there is no common estimate of the concept. Many countries are so poor (28 have incomes under US$ 1000 per year; Table 19.2) that spending even 4% of total income on health is equivalent to a high share of non-subsistence income, comparable to that in richer countries. The share of health spending in total income varies greatly at all income levels: the standard deviation of the share is 0.014 for the very low income group, and 0.0198–0.021 for the three higher income groups.

The health share of GDP ranges from <3% to 6% among African countries at incomes under US$ 2500. This is as high as the 5–10% spread among the Americas at incomes of US$ 10 000–20 000, or the 3–6% range in the Eastern Mediterranean Region, for the same income interval. This counter-intuitive result—that countries which seem to have less scope for variation nonetheless vary as much as countries with more leeway for spending differences—shows up repeatedly in the analyses.

Shares of GDP translate into a wide range of US$ amounts per capita. All health expenditures are converted to US$ at the same PPP$ rates as incomes, because health-specific price indices are unavailable. Relative differences are largest in poor countries, as high as 5:1 at incomes under US$ 5000, but are about 2:1 among most countries at incomes of US$ 10 000–20 000. There are no marked regional differences in the shape or slope of the expenditure/income relation, so we do not show the results by region. There are bigger differences in how health is financed, but these do not systematically affect the total. In most countries, total health spending is low (less than US$ 45 per person per year in 25 countries with incomes below US$ 1000) and below US$ 110 in another 32 countries at incomes under US$ 2200.

Some countries spend less than the cost of a package of cost-effective services, estimated in 1993 to be US$ 12 per capita in very poor countries and US$ 22 in middle-income countries (4). This is not enough to assure availability of even a few highly justified services to the whole population, whether the justification is based on cost-effectiveness, protection from catastrophic expense, or other criteria. Inadequate spending in this sense is distinct from low health expenditure causing loss of potential economic growth (5).

Paying Beforehand or When Care is Needed

Because of its relation to financial risk, the crucial distinction in health spending is between prepayment in all forms, and payment out-of-pocket at time of service. Small out-of-pocket costs are harmless for all but the poorest users. High cost spending, however, should be covered via prepayment to avoid the risk of impoverishment, or of doing without needed care. Since the poorer a person is, the lower is the threshold for catastrophic expenses, the out-of-pocket share ought to be lower in poorer countries. However, exactly the opposite occurs: at low incomes, the average out-of-pocket share is high and extremely variable (20–80% of all health spending, Fig. 19.2).

With increasing income, the range also narrows: the standard deviation of the share drops 0.220–0.160 between the low- and high-income groups. Except for four or five countries with highly reliable data, there is a sharp frontier of maximal out-of-pocket spending in the total, visible as a downward-sloping diagonal in Fig. 19.2. This frontier also shows up separately in sub-Saharan Africa, the Americas and the Eastern Mediterranean and North Africa, but not in Europe, where the out-of-pocket share is nearly always below 40%. Regression analysis gives an income coefficient of

–0.0635 for the share of out-of-pocket expenditure as a percentage of total health expenditure (OOP%THE) for all countries together, and –0.0862 for countries with high-quality data. Both coefficients are significantly negative (Table 19.4). The declining share of out-of-pocket spending does not offset the rise in total spending on health, so the dollar amount spent out of pocket climbs rapidly but not quite proportionately as income and total spending increase. Absolute spending amounts are analyzed below.

A given overall share of out-of-pocket financing represents little financial risk to households when it is low and distributed in proportion to capacity to pay. Everyone then buys those, and only those, health goods and services that are individually affordable. In other cases, important financial risk is indicated by the percentage of households whose estimated health costs exceeded 50% of their income net of food expenditures, a measure of catastrophic spending. In household surveys in 21 countries, this proportion is usually below 5% of all households, but in a few cases the share exceeds 10% (6). There is no relation between this share and the level of income. The sample is rather small and includes no high-income countries; and there is no clear connection between the level of out-of-pocket spending and the fraction of households with very high levels of such spending. Preliminary WHO results from a larger sample of 44 countries, including some that are richer than the 21 countries considered here, seem to show this

Table 19.4 Regression Statistics for Out of Pocket Payments as a Percentage of Total Health Expenditure

REGRESSION STATISTIC	DATA QUALITY			
	LOW	MEDIUM-TO-HIGH	HIGH	ALL DATA
Constant	0.5735	0.8066	1.0781	0.8664
Standard error	0.3090	0.1355	0.1938	0.0926
t-Statistic	1.8559	5.9530	5.5627	9.3600
Probability[a]	0.0863	0.0000	0.0000	0.0000
Coefficient of Ln (GDPC)	−0.0375	−0.0555	−0.0862	−0.0635
Standard error	0.0366	0.0171	0.0214	0.0110
t-Statistic	−1.0246	−3.2059	−4.0220	−5.7494
Probability[a]	0.3242	0.0018	0.0001	0.0000
R^2	0.0747	0.0915	0.1878	0.1488
Adjusted R^2	0.0035	0.0826	0.1761	0.1444
n	15	104	72	191

[a]See footnote a, table 19.3

effect: the share of households with catastrophic spending, and the share of catastrophic spending in the total, both fall somewhat with rising income.

Household survey data usually do not indicate how families financed such catastrophic expenditures, but in India health needs often push families into selling assets or borrowing cash, even in the upper-income quintiles. Only about one-half of all families can afford a medical emergency out of current income or savings, and the loss of savings leaves them exposed to other risks (7). Similar evidence comes from a survey in northern Viet Nam in 1995: only 30% of poor households could rely on savings to pay for health services, while close to 40% had to spend less on essential items (food or fuel), or borrow money, or sell livestock (8). Reduced risk of asset loss or impoverishment is the chief benefit from extending prepayment and confining out-of-pocket payment to easily affordable services.

How is Prepayment Financed?

Some mechanisms are not widely used and contribute little to total health spending, such as "health cards" bought in advance of need and which entitle purchasers to a restricted amount of care. This was the case in the Thai Health Card Program established in 1983. In 1992, the program was converted to a voluntary health insurance program with a broad benefit package (9). Aside from schemes like these, there are three basic ways to finance prepayment: private insurance (voluntary or employment-related), social health insurance contributions, and taxes (general revenue). All publicly financed health is prepaid; private spending is divided between insurance and out-of-pocket payments. When private insurance is negligible, which is the case in most countries and virtually all poor countries, the prepayment/out-of-pocket distinction coincides with that between public and private expenditure. Public spending is then the complement of out-of-pocket spending. Relative to total health spending, public spending shows a similar frontier, for the minimum rather than the maximum share (Fig. 19.3).

The share of public health expenditure as a percentage of total health expenditure (PHE%THE) rises with income, with a regression coefficient of 0.0573 for all countries together and 0.0758 for countries with the most reliable data (Table 19.5). Europe is the only region where the public share is always above 40% and nearly always above 60%, with little relation to income. Finally, the relative variation in public spending shrinks: the standard deviation decreases from 0.228 in the low-income group to 0.160

Table 19.5 Regression Statistics for Public Health Expenditure as a Percentage of Total Health Expenditure

REGRESSION STATISTIC	DATA QUALITY			ALL DATA
	LOW	MEDIUM-TO-HIGH	HIGH	
Constant	0.4329	0.1150	−0.0605	0.1288
Standard error	0.1397	0.1375	0.1940	0.0950
t-Statistic	1.3539	0.8368	−0.3123	1.3557
Probability[a]	0.1988	0.4047	0.7557	0.1768
Coefficient of Ln (GDPC)	0.0363	0.0586	0.0758	0.0573
Standard error	0.0379	0.0174	0.0214	0.0113
t-Statistic	0.9598	3.3611	3.5310	5.0524
Probability[a]	0.3546	0.0011	0.0007	0.0000
R^2	0.0662	0.0997	0.1511	0.1190
Adjusted R^2	−0.0056	0.0909	0.1390	0.1143
n	15	104	72	191

[a]See footnote a, table 19.3

at high incomes. This illustrates the same phenomenon as the reduced variation in the out-of-pocket share in total health spending. Public spending includes both social health insurance contributions (the "Bismarck" model) and general revenues or "tax-funded" expenditure (the "Beveridge" model). The latter is the predominant, often the only, mode in most countries (Fig. 19.4). Countries where social security is the principal mode of public spending are concentrated in Europe (10). In high-income countries, either model can achieve essentially universal financial protection and account for a large share of total health expenditure. In low-income countries often neither mode accounts for even half of total spending.

The social security/general revenue distinction shows no convergence as income rises. High-income countries rely chiefly on one model or the other, whereas at lower incomes part of the population is covered by social health insurance and another part is protected by Ministry of Health financing, chiefly from general revenue. Particularly in Latin America, there is a great variety of institutional arrangements, and the population nominally covered under one scheme often also uses services financed by a different mode (11). The lack of convergence and the variety of financing combinations arise for historical reasons, unrelated to income. There is considerable debate whether social health insurance or general taxation is better (12), but nothing can be concluded from financing data alone, especially when public expenditure of both kinds together is only a small share of the total.

The third main mode of prepayment, private insurance, is virtually non-existent in the majority of countries. In only 47 countries does it account for 5% of private health expenditure (only five of which are in Africa), and that may mean a share of total spending as low as 1–2%. Private insurance is even more of a luxury than public spending, being important at high incomes, mostly in a few countries of the Americas and Europe. This is not surprising, since so many countries are poor and many people cannot afford a meaningful degree of financial protection of this form. Unless they are protected by publicly-financed health care, including the possibility of public subsidies for private insurance, many people rely on out-of-pocket financing and face the risk of catastrophic costs (1). Even where it is affordable by a larger part of the population, private insurance is not widespread in most countries because of the efficiency problems inherent in the distribution of medical risk among people, and uncertainty both on their part and on that of insurers (13).

The shares of insurance in total health spending vary considerably, from a significant form of prepayment (as in South Africa and the USA), to a complement of publicly funded services (as in Canada and several European and Latin American countries). The importance of private insurance also depends on whether the well-off must purchase it and leave the public system (as in the Netherlands), or may direct their social security contributions to private insurers (in Chile). Employers purchasing for their employees account for a large share of insurance in Brazil and the USA, and for much of health financing in the formal sector in many other countries.

How Much of Public Spending Goes for Health?

Public expenditure on health can be low because of low total public expenditure, or because a low share of public expenditure is devoted to health, or both. The ratio of public spending on health to total general government expenditure (PHE%TPE) seldom exceeds 20% and is below 10% for most countries, including almost all of the African and the Eastern Mediterranean Regions. The share increases as income rises, approximately from 5% to 10%, with an income coefficient of 0.0159 for all countries together

Table 19.6 Regression Statistics for Public Health Expenditure as a Percentage of Total Public Expenditure

REGRESSION STATISTIC	DATA QUALITY			
	LOW	MEDIUM-TO-HIGH	HIGH	ALL DATA
Constant	−0.0952	−0.0019	−0.0291	−0.0283
Standard error	0.0904	0.0302	0.0471	0.0216
t-Statistic	−1.0535	−0.0630	−0.6183	−1.3111
Probability[a]	0.3113	0.9499	0.5384	0.1914
Coefficient of Ln (GDPC)	0.0240	0.0123	0.0161	0.0159
Standard error	0.0107	0.0038	0.0052	0.0026
t-Statistic	2.2427	3.1981	3.1064	6.1483
Probability[a]	0.0430	0.0018	0.0027	0.0000
R^2	0.2789	0.0911	0.1211	0.1667
Adjusted R^2	0.2235	0.0822	0.1085	0.1622
n	15	104	72	191

[a]See footnote a, table 19.3

and 0.0161 for countries with more reliable data (Table 19.6). Variation around the mean share stays fairly constant across the four income groups, the standard deviation varying from 0.038 to 0.045.

IMF estimates of this relationship calculate total central government expenditure relative to GDP, and the shares for health, education, defense and interest payments (14, 15). These estimates do not match the national health account numbers estimated by WHO, when much expenditure passes through subnational governments, as in Brazil, China, and India. The average share of GDP spent by central governments increases only slightly (from 24% to 29%) from very low- to middle-income countries, with a further increase to 32% among high-income countries. Within the lower income groups, and often within each mortality stratum, there is variation of as much as 3:1.

Failure to capture much of a country's income for public use does not generally explain low health spending in poor countries, but it helps account for the low shares that central governments spend for health in countries such as El Salvador, China, and the United Arab Emirates. Chinese spending is much higher when general rather than central government is included. At high incomes and low mortality, the shares converge somewhat for total spending, but less so for health expenditure. The relation between the two fractions of GDP fans out as central government accounts for more of the economy. This is consistent with the widening variation in the share of GDP spent on health.

Summary of findings

The analysis of national health accounts estimates does not lead to striking or unexpected conclusions, so far as shares are concerned. Analysis of absolute dollar amounts shows that out-of-pocket spending, total health expenditure and total public spending all rise with income. The respective double-logarithmic elasticities are 0.9733, 1.2052 and 1.1431, for all countries together (Tables 19.7 to 19.9). When only the highly reliable data are used, the corresponding estimated coefficients are 0.8839, 1.2223, and 1.1944. These elasticities mean that the share of out-of-pocket spending in GDP falls modestly as countries become richer, and that such spending takes a decreasing share of non-subsistence income and becomes less of a burden on average. In contrast, both total health expenditure and total public expenditure of all kinds rise with income.

The relationships between different health expenditure concepts fall into two groups: some do not converge toward a common pattern as income

Table 19.7 Regression Statistics for Out-of-Pocket Payments per Capita as a Function of Income per Capita

| REGRESSION STATISTIC | DATA QUALITY | | | |
	LOW	MEDIUM-TO-HIGH	HIGH	ALL DATA
Constant	−4.8996	−3.9062	−3.1264	−4.0405
Standard error	1.7530	0.5643	0.6495	0.3738
t-Statistic	−2.7950	−6.9213	−4.8129	−10.8094
Probability[a]	0.0152	0.0000	0.0000	0.0000
Coefficient Ln (GDPC)	1.0330	0.9529	0.8839	0.9733
Standard error	0.2078	0.0715	0.0718	0.0446
t-Statistic	4.9716	13.3135	12.2967	21.8270
Probability[a]	0.0003	0.0000	0.0000	0.0000
R^2	0.6553	0.6370	0.6835	0.7170
Adjusted R^2	0.6288	0.6334	0.6790	0.7155
n	15	103	72	190

[a]See footnote a, table 19.3

Table 19.8 Regression Statistics for Total Health Expenditure per Capita as a Function of Income per Capita

REGRESSION STATISTIC	DATA QUALITY			
	LOW	MEDIUM-TO-HIGH	HIGH	ALL DATA
Constant	−5.2843	−4.1739	−4.7881	−4.6958
Standard error	0.8546	0.2674	0.3860	0.1909
t-Statistic	−6.1832	−15.6077	−12.4014	−24.6026
Probability[a]	0.0000	0.0000	0.0000	0.0000
Coefficient of Ln (GDPC)	1.2748	1.1330	1.2223	1.2052
Standard error	0.1013	0.0339	0.0427	0.0228
t-Statistic	12.5839	33.4118	28.6098	52.9171
Probability[a]	0.0000	0.0000	0.0000	0.0000
R^2	0.9241	0.9162	0.9212	0.9368
Adjusted R^2	0.9182	0.9154	0.9200	0.9364
n	15	104	72	191

[a]See footnote a, table 19.3

rises, whereas others clearly do. The former group includes the share of GDP spent on health; the share of public spending financed by general revenue rather than by social security; and the share of health in total government spending. Countries show little or no regularity in these shares. As income rises there is a convergence in the average level of the shares of

Table 19.9 Regression Statistics for Total Public Expenditure per Capita as a Function of Income per Capita

REGRESSION STATISTIC	DATA QUALITY			
	LOW	MEDIUM-TO-HIGH	HIGH	ALL DATA
Constant	−1.4957	−2.1643	−2.8433	−2.3769
Standard error	0.8496	0.3189	0.3590	0.2081
t-Statistic	−1.7603	−6.7857	−7.9202	−11.4216
Probability[a]	0.1018	0.0000	0.0000	0.0000
Coefficient of Ln (GDPC)	1.0688	1.1115	1.1944	1.1431
Standard error	0.1007	0.0404	0.0397	0.0248
t-Statistic	10.6120	27.4823	30.0667	46.0341
Probability[a]	0.0000	0.0000	0.0000	0.0000
R^2	0.8965	0.8810	0.9281	0.9181
Adjusted R^2	0.8885	0.8798	0.9271	0.9177
n	15	104	72	191

[a]See footnote a, table 19.3

health spending represented by public expenditure (increasing) and by out-of-pocket spending (decreasing). There is an even more marked common pattern for the variation in those shares at a given income level. As income rises, the relative variation in health spending among countries narrows; the public share becomes more uniformly high; and that of out-of-pocket spending becomes more uniformly low. Increased prepayment, most of which is public, is what allows the out-of-pocket share to fall markedly. This reduces catastrophic financial risk for households, while avoiding the market failure that makes competitive, private health insurance inefficient, because those who need it most can least afford it, if insurers charge according to risks (15).

Several conclusions emerge, as outlined below:

- In many poor countries total health spending is very low, even compared to the cost of a package of highly justified interventions.

- Out-of-pocket spending is already catastrophic for several percent of households. Even if consumers were willing to pay more for better quality services, the poor could not pay much more and would require preferential treatment (16).

- Prepayment via health insurance is limited to the wealthy and those with formal employment. The poor could afford meaningful insurance coverage only with public subsidy.

These conclusions, and the need to provide public goods and services with large externalities (which private markets will not deliver adequately), make public expenditure on health particularly important in poor countries. However, these are the countries with the lowest relative public spending in health. What actually happens appears to be at odds with what is needed.

Needs Versus Actual Spending

Nothing here indicates how much a country should spend on health, because there is no consensus as to what services to finance for its citizens, and different packages of services have different costs. It is particularly difficult to specify appropriate voluntary private spending on health, since people differ not only in needs, but in their tastes and their degree of risk aversion. Nonetheless, a given package of services corresponds to a relatively well-defined minimum cost, if it is provided for the whole population.

If a country is to deliver that package, it should spend at least the corresponding minimum amount. (It might spend considerably more for the same package, because the way health is financed can greatly affect costs.)

The cost for a package will depend on several characteristics of the country, including its income. The package might cost more to provide in high-income countries than in low-income ones, because inputs are more expensive. But in poorer countries, it may instead be costlier to reach everyone because the population is widely dispersed. The low level of schooling and worse health status may also require more intensive intervention. Thus, the need for spending the services in the package may be constant, or declining with per capita income, at least at low incomes.

Whatever the relationship between income and total need relative to the package, the need for public expenditure on those services, as a share of the

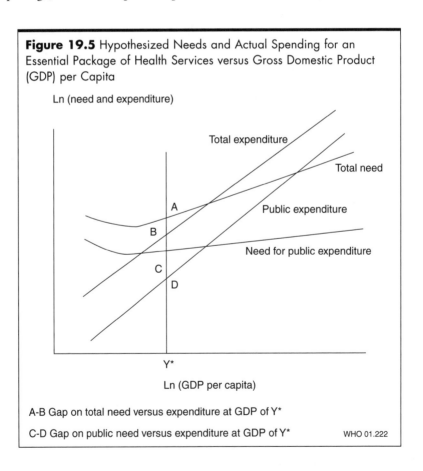

Figure 19.5 Hypothesized Needs and Actual Spending for an Essential Package of Health Services versus Gross Domestic Product (GDP) per Capita

Ln (need and expenditure)

Total expenditure

Total need

A

B

Public expenditure

Need for public expenditure

C

D

Y*

Ln (GDP per capita)

A-B Gap on total need versus expenditure at GDP of Y*

C-D Gap on public need versus expenditure at GDP of Y*

WHO 01.222

total need, almost surely declines with income. This can happen either by declining absolutely, or by rising more slowly the richer a country becomes. People can spend more privately, because out-of-pocket expenses are less onerous, or they can afford wider private insurance coverage. More public spending would simply crowd out some of that private expenditure.

The relation between actual total spending and actual public spending is just the opposite of that for needs: the difference between them narrows as income rises. Any gap between needs and actual expenditure is greater for the public component than for the total (Fig. 19.5). For a country with GDP per capita of Y*, spending is not enough to provide the package to everyone and there is a gap, A–B; the public gap, C–D, is much larger. Even if the total gap were closed, there might still be a shortfall of public spending. Part of the population would not benefit from the services, and the additional expenditure would buy other interventions and be distributed less equitably. These findings indicate that the challenge for poorer countries is not merely to spend more on health, but to spend more equitably by increasing prepayment, especially for potentially catastrophic expenses, and by public resources. Rich countries have not converged on a single health financing model or institutional arrangement, but they have converged on a high degree of protection from financial risk through prepayment.

References

[1] The world health report 2000—Health systems: improving performance. Geneva: World Health Organization; 2000.

[2] Poullier JP, Hernández P. Estimates of national health accounts (NHA) for 1997. Geneva: World Health Organization; 2000. WHO/EIP Discussion Paper No. 27.

[3] Lozano R. Mortality regionalization in the world. Geneva: World Health Organization, 2000 (unpublished note).

[4] World Bank. World development report 1993: investing in health. New York: Oxford University Press; 1993.

[5] Ruger JP, Jamison DT, Bloom DE. Health and the economy. In: Merson ME, Black RE, Mills AJ, eds. International public health. Gaithersburg (MD): Aspen; 2000. p. 617–66.

[6] Xu K, Murray CJL, Lydon P, Ortiz de Iturbide J. Estimates of the fairness of financial contribution. Geneva: World Health Organization. WHO/GPE Discussion Paper No. 26.

[7] India's future health system: issues and options. Washington (DC): World Bank, Health, Nutrition and Population Sector Unit, India; 2001.

[8] Ensor T, San PB. Access and payment for health care: the poor of Northern Vietnam. International Journal of Health Planning and Management 1996; 11:69–83.

[9] Supakankunti S. Future prospects of voluntary health insurance in Thailand. Health Policy and Planning 2000; 15:85–94.

[10] The reform of health systems: a review of seventeen OECD countries. Paris: Organisation for Economic Co-operation and Development; 1994.

[11] Londoño JL, Frenk J. Structured pluralism: towards an innovative model for health system reform in Latin America. Health Policy 1997; 41:1–39.

[12] Jönsson B, Musgrove P. Government financing of health care. In: Schieber GJ, editor. Innovations in health care financing. Proceedings of a World Bank conference, 10–11 March, 1997, Washington, DC. Washington (DC): World Bank, 1997.

[13] Arrow K. Uncertainty and the welfare economics of medical care. American Economic Review 1963; 53:941–73.

[14] International financial statistics. Washington (DC): International Monetary Fund; 2000.

[15] Government financial statistics. Washington (DC): International Monetary Fund; 2000.

[16] Newbrander W, Collins D, Wilson L. Ensuring equal access to health services: user fee systems and the poor. Boston (MA): Management Sciences for Health; 2000.

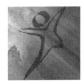

CHAPTER 20

Economic Crisis and Health Policy Response

Introduction: The Nature of the Question

"Health Policy" is something less well defined and much less quantitative than the phenomena demography normally deals with, so it seems appropriate to begin by explaining just what questions will be treated in what follows. This will also serve to make it clear that the approach of this paper is rather skeptical and conceptual, and has little new empirical information to offer.

Economic crisis versus structural adjustment

It is difficult to distinguish the demographic consequences of structural adjustment from the reactions to the economic crisis which provokes the need for adjustment, whether or not that adjustment is part of a formal program involving short-term foreign assistance and policy advice from institutions such as the World Bank. Thus it is not clear that whatever bad consequences for health occur should be attributed to the adjustment program (Cornia 1989) rather than to the economic mismanagement, sheer bad luck, or other factors causing the crisis. Focusing on the adjustment process may mean supposing that the alternative was not to adjust, rather than supposing that the only choice a country faced was how to get its macroeconomy back into balance, and *how soon* to start doing so. Whether adjustment looks like needlessly throwing the car into a skid and a possible collision, depends on whether the alternative looks like going over a cliff. The general question is whether the economic crisis, including such responses to it as a

©IUSSP 1997. Reprinted from *Demographic Responses to Economic Adjustment in Latin America*, edited by Georges Tapinos, Andrew Mason, and Jorge Bravo. (International Studies in Demography, 1997), by permission of Oxford University Press.

formal adjustment program, has had any systematic effect on health policy. Specific policy changes may be part of, or linked to, specific decisions on adjustment, but they need not be: they may be contemporaneous reactions to aspects of the crisis itself.

Connections to demographic phenomena

Ultimately, one wants to know what happened to births, deaths, age distributions, and other quantifiable demographic variables. This chapter does not carry the story that far, except for a brief discussion of previous empirical research on the health consequences of the crisis of the (early) 1980s. One of these sources (Grosh 1990) concentrated on expenditure on health care; the other (Musgrove 1988) also considered the output of services and the outcomes for health in the population. But since next to nothing was known about morbidity, the scant evidence available on health outcomes concerns mortality.

Here the emphasis is on what, if anything, happened to health policy. It is possible *a priori* that crisis or adjustment made for substantial changes in health policy, but without having much effect on anyone's health status. It is just as possible that there were large effects on morbidity and mortality, but that these had little to do with any official policy. To consider the likelihood of these and other possible outcomes, it will help first to think of the channels by which an economic downturn can affect health, and then to consider whether and how policy—particularly health policy—may be important in each of those channels.

Channels for health effects of economic crisis

Almost anything can affect one's health, and almost nothing in a modern economy is immune from the effects of economic contraction, so there is hardly any limit to the ways that economic crisis might affect the health of the population. Many of the possible channels are, however, likely to be quantitatively unimportant, affecting very few people or changing the incidence or prevalence of disease or other variables by insignificant amounts. Figure 20.1 (modified from Musgrove 1988) shows the principal ways by which an economic crisis could be expected to have significant effects on health. The diagram is incomplete in two demographically important respects: it does not show any of the mechanisms likely to affect birth rates, and because it has no spatial dimension it does not suggest impacts on migration.

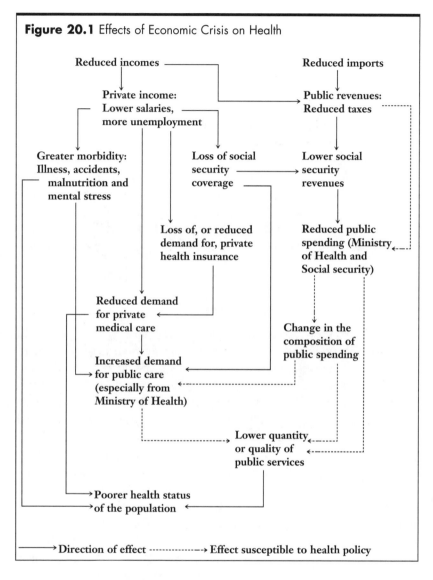

Figure 20.1 Effects of Economic Crisis on Health

Some of the channels portrayed are direct—that is, they modify the like-lihood of getting sick or hurt, or dying—while others are indirect, in that they pass through the health care system and would show no effect if the crisis did not affect that system. To the extent that publicly provided (or publicly subsidized) health care is free to users, it is particularly important what happens to the publicly-funded health sector. Health outcomes suffer most when the public health system shrinks in size or becomes less effective just when, because of lost employment, income, or insurance coverage, people's need for it increases. Whether the relation between need and demand for health care changes during an economic downturn is one of the major questions to which policy might be addressed.

In principle, one or more kinds of public policy are relevant to every channel of mediation between economic events and demographic outcomes, including health. Some of these, such as policies affecting prices, wages, and employment, are crucial to adjustment programs. Health policy can affect only some of the channels although, on a broad definition, these effects can reach far beyond the narrower decisions concerning the public provision of medical care. The diagram distinguishes those paths for which health policy is most relevant, in both the broad sense, including regulation and incentives, and in the narrow sense of spending public resources to buy or produce health care.

The reach and importance of health policy

Health policy is essentially unable to affect people's employment and income at the moment of a crisis, however much the provision of health care may overcome disabilities and raise people's productivities in the long run. The direct *economic* effects of economic downturn on health are therefore beyond the reach of health policy. Other direct effects, however, may be more amenable to control: health policy affecting the environment, and public health measures generally, are examples. Among the indirect effects, it is not only the public provision of care that responds to health policy; it may be just as important to determine who has access to social security medical care, or to regulate the private insurance market. In general, it can be expected that these indirect consequences of policy become more important as the economy, and the health sector, become more differentiated and complex. In a poor country where few people can afford private doctors and all hospital care is publicly provided, public policy affects health through fewer channels than in a richer country with a large private medical sector and substantial private insurance. Thus, apart from differences in the specific health policies of one and another country, there are differences in the *reach* of policy; this is reason enough to suspect that simple relations between policy and outcomes will be hard to find or nonexistent, that what is true of Nicaragua or Bolivia will not characterize Argentina or Brazil.

Health Policy: Definition, Ambiguity, and Attribution

Up to this point, the phrase "health policy" has been used as though it needed no definition and presented no ambiguity: it should be possible to tell what a policy is, whether and how it has changed, what caused any such change, and what effect that might be expected to have on health and demographic variables. On closer examination, all these assumptions appear questionable.

What do we mean by health policy?

Consider two extreme possible meanings for these words. One is that health policy is defined by the declarations of governments, in the broadest terms and at the highest political level. In that sense, every government that participated in the Alma Ata Conference in 1978 has a policy of giving priority to primary health care (World Health Organization 1978). Everything else—the definition of strategies for implementation, the decisions about investment, budget allocation, and regulation—would then be just the expression or working out of the policy. The limitations of this view are well known: what governments (and others) do, does not necessarily follow from what they say. In any case, what was said is often left so vague that it is hard even to tell whether a given action or decision is consistent with the supposed "policy".

At the other extreme, everything that a government does can be regarded as revealing or conforming to an implicit policy: "real" policy is the sum of actions. But this is no easier to interpret, because actions are so numerous, and so often apparently inconsistent, that policy may be too complex to mean anything more general. Policy itself may also be contradictory, which is hard to tell from the absence of policy. We are left with the puzzlement of Alice, listening to the White Knight explain the difference between the Thing, and the Name of the Thing, and What the Thing is Called, and What the Name of the Thing is Called (Carroll 1865, chapter 8). At the very least, it must be recognized that policy may be defined at different levels of generality, and bear different relations to what actually goes on in a health sector. Change in policy is therefore at least equally complicated, and different policies could change in inconsistent directions under the same, or simultaneous but unrelated, impulses.

How can we tell if policy has changed?

Clearly a change in rhetoric is a different thing from a change in activity, so whether a change in policy has occurred depends on whether one is concerned with words or deeds. But there is another dimension to policy change which is more subtle and probably more important than the distinction between saying and doing. That is the *conditional* reach of a policy, the period over which and the circumstances under which it is supposed to apply.

Consider a Ministry of Health whose budget has for several years been growing at 5 percent per annum, and which has routinely devoted 10 percent of the budget to capital investment. In the first year of an economic crisis—of unpredictable depth and duration—the budget is cut by 10 percent (the same as for the government budget generally), and all investment is stopped, leaving the recurrent budget the same as the year before. Was there a change of policy? If "policy" meant a constant share for investment, then clearly policy changed. But if it meant never reducing recurrent expenditure, then there was no change in policy, and the stoppage of investment was necessary to uphold the policy.

This simple example illustrates two important issues. First, it is neither easy nor fair to infer policies solely from certain actions. Criticizing the outcome is a different matter, and does not depend on what happened to policy along the way. Second, governments have competing objectives—to keep investing to expand services, but also to try never to cut existing services—and in general, *they do not really have a policy for reconciling those conflicts* when suddenly choices have to be made. Policies are seldom or never spelled out with all the "ifs" and "buts" that circumstances may impose, particularly if that would require a long planning horizon. As another example, there are good reasons why public expenditure on health care should be counter-cyclical, to cope with the fluctuation of needs mentioned earlier (Musgrove 1984), but no government in Latin America has such a policy. It would imply a privileged position for health in recessions (which every Minister of Health would endorse), but require reduced spending or at least reduced growth in boom times (which no Minister seems prepared to accept). It seems more nearly the case that there is one policy in good times and another in bad times, with no policy for getting from one situation to the other.

Attributing causes and effects

Much of the focus on the possible damage from recession and adjustment is on the issue of public spending, but the more interesting questions about health policy are not so narrow. Is there a shift among different kinds of interventions? Between one institution and another for delivery of care? Between hospital and ambulatory care? Does the government change its mind about user fees or internal prices and tariffs? Does it change the way staff are hired, assigned, or promoted? Does it change the way inputs other than staff are ordered and allocated, or the way they are paid for and the way they are combined with human inputs? Change in any of these dimensions may carry implications for the budget, but the impact may be very different from what the money amounts would suggest, and even run in the opposite direction.

An economic crisis is likely to have two kinds of adverse effects on health. It reduces people's incomes and therefore both exposes them to increased risk of getting sick and makes it harder for them to buy medical care if they need it; and it reduces government revenues and therefore makes it harder to provide or subsidize health services. Health policy cannot do anything about the loss of income, whether individual or public, but it can affect all three of the possible consequences just described.

A good health policy, or a good change in existing policy, would maintain the output of those services most essential to health, or even extend them, for the counter-cyclical reason mentioned earlier. It would reduce waste in the system both in the sense of technical inefficiency or lower than possible output for given inputs, and in the allocative sense of giving priority to those interventions which buy the greatest increase in health status per dollar spent (Jamison, Mosley, Measham. and Bobadilla 1993). Moreover, to the extent that economic hardship was regressive, policy would become offsettingly progressive, taking particular care to protect the poor. The latter aspect is usually described as "equity", although it is only one of the possible meanings of equity in a health care system (Musgrove 1986). Thus the opportunity for good change in policy is greater the worse policy was before the crisis. It is easier to fast, if one is too fat to start with, and it is easier to become more efficient or progressive if the system was initially wasteful or regressive. *Ceteris paribus*, we should expect improvements in health policy to be correlated negatively with the quality of prior policy.

Policy or policy change is bad if it reduces service coverage more than necessary, reduces it more than proportionally for the most valuable services, cuts back more on services to the neediest, or makes provision less efficient by (further) unbalancing the combination of inputs. The better a system was functioning before an economic shock, the greater the risk that it will become less effective or more regressive or inequitable. Because policy can be judged by four distinct criteria—total coverage, allocative efficiency, technical efficiency, and progressivity—it is obvious that many possible policy changes look good on one criterion and bad on another, with their total effect uncertain. Such ambiguous policies are particularly likely to have redistributional effects, benefiting or protecting some groups and worsening the situation of others. *A priori*, policies such as introducing or raising user fees fall into this category, with their outcome depending on what happens to demand, to net revenues, and to purchases of inputs.

What Happened in Latin America in the 1980s?

There were substantial changes in declared policy or actual public practice in many countries all over the world during the 1980s. In some cases these changes resulted from political upheaval rather than simply economic pressure; the formerly communist countries of eastern Europe, such as Romania (Fox 1992) or Poland (World Bank 1992), provide the most striking examples. In other cases, changes in the health sector have followed economic shock, as in Indonesia after the collapse of oil prices (World Bank 1991) or in Ghana, following an adjustment program that began in 1983 and led to substantial change in budgets and (temporarily) in real user fees (Berk 1992). These cases illustrate the diversity of causes leading to changes in health policy and the variety of possible responses and outcomes. The range of events in Latin America has been somewhat narrower, but it still shows the importance of political and ideological as well as economic factors in affecting health policy.

Declared policy change: words as policy

One approach to the question of how health policy responded to economic stress would be to review all the constitutional and legal changes affecting health over the decade in as many countries as possible. A study by Fuenzalida-Puelma and Scholle Connor (1989) limited the analysis of health policy to what is specified in national constitutions and certain major laws. Not surprisingly, these documents refer primarily to the right to health or health care, and sometimes to the duty of the state or government to guarantee or provide it. (The constitution of Guyana goes so far as to declare a right to a happy life, free of disease.) The degree to which rights and duties are spelled out depends very much on the age of the constitution, and on whether the country has a common law (formerly English) or civil law (formerly Spanish, Portuguese, or French) tradition. Nineteenth-century documents such as the constitutions of 1853 in Argentina or 1886 in Colombia (or 1787 in the United States), do not even mention health explicitly. Newer charters, particularly those adopted during the 1970s or 1980s in such countries as Brazil, Cuba, Ecuador, El Salvador, Guatemala, Guyana, Honduras, Nicaragua, Panama, and Peru are much more explicit, sometimes declaring it the duty of the state to provide care (Panama) or to provide it free to the indigent (El Salvador) or to everyone (Cuba).

Over the long run, the analysis of constitutional provisions shows a clear increase in the social importance of health and health care, and a steady expansion of "rights", generally in the direction of universal access. When budgets fall and services are curtailed or allowed to deteriorate in quality or equity, however, the disjunction between actual practice and the goals espoused in the law becomes temporarily wider. Certainly the law, at this level of generality, offers no guide to what will actually happen under economic pressure.

Evidence on spending: budgets as policy

What a government actually spends on health is commonly taken as a test of whether it has "put its money where its mouth is". If public expenditure on health care were to change substantially when nothing in the economic environment or in the burden of disease faced by society had changed, that would indeed be an indication that policy had changed, that health had acquired greater or lesser priority among claims on public resources. An economic crisis is obviously a poor time for that kind of test, since the economic environment changes abruptly, and that in turn may directly increase the burden of ill-health. It is still possible to ask the simpler question whether health expenditure was relatively protected or not, but even then there are at least three reasonable denominators to compare it to: population, total public spending, and gross domestic product. These three ratios do not necessarily move together, and even if they do, it is not clear what that indicates about policy.

Estimates of these ratios for thirteen countries, for 1980–5 or 1980–6, are shown in Table 20.1. The data refer to consolidated public sector spending, including sub-national governments, in four cases and to the central government only in the other nine. All data are shown as real, country-specific indexes, using 1982 as the base year. This was the year the debt

Table 20.1 Indices of Public Expenditures on Health (Central Government or Total Public Sector) in Thirteen Latin American and Caribbean Countries, 1980–86 (1982 = 100)

COUNTRY, CONCEPT AND COVERAGE	1980	1981	1982	1983	1984	1985	1986
Argentina (consolidated public sector)							
Per capita	149	127	100	148	47	53	64
As share of total public spending	121	111	100	125	42	47	55
As share of GDP	127	118	100	145	45	55	64
Bolivia (central government only)							
Per capita	219	134	100	91	88	85	60
As share of total public spending	124	103	100	103	94	73	70
As share of GDP	200	125	100	100	100	100	75
Brazil (central government only)							
Per capita	108	99	100	81	82	91	96
As share of total public spending	104	104	100	91	104	113	78
As share of GDP	94	96	100	85	87	89	89
Chile (consolidated public sector)							
Per capita	96	94	100	82	75	76	67
As share of total public spending	98	93	100	84	72	70	63
As share of GDP	94	79	100	84	74	74	63
Costa Rica (consolidated public sector)							
Per capita	205	136	100	109	108	106	110
As share of total public spending	142	114	100	94	89	91	91
As share of GDP	178	124	100	109	102	102	103
Dominican Republic (central government only)							
Per capita	99	110	100	102	89	77	85
As share of total public spending	83	93	100	93	99	84	82
As share of GDP	100	109	100	100	91	82	91
El Salvador (central government only)							
Per capita	132	114	100	94	95	76	69
As share of total public spending	131	105	100	107	83	89	72
As share of GDP	112	106	100	94	94	75	69
Ecuador (central government only)							
Per capita	84	108	100	89	87	88	
As share of total public spending	94	108	100	106	106	95	
As share of GDP	84	107	100	95	92	92	
Honduras (central government only)							
Per capita	103	98	100	100	95	93	105
As share of total public spending	105	114	100	94	78	76	95
As share of GDP	94	92	100	102	96	95	108
Jamaica (central government only)							
Per capita	91	95	100	90	71	64	57
As share of total public spending	88	93	100	92	90	91	86
As share of GDP	92	94	100	89	72	69	61
Mexico (central government only)							
Per capita	90[a]		100	93	94	95	83
As share of total public spending	100[b]		100	94	97	114	
As share of GDP			100	100	99	100	93

Uruguay (central government only)						
Per capita	91	104	100	91	91	93
As share of total public spending	120	119	100	111	113	131
As share of GDP	83	93	100	97	100	102
Venezuela (consolidated public sector)						
Per capita	92	100	100	131	108	115
As share of total public spending	94	92	100	157	147	155
As share of GDP	85	95	100	140	120	130

aCalculated from estimates to one digit only, in original source.
bFigures for 1979.
Sources: Argentina, Bolivia, Chile, Costa Rica, Dominican Republic, El Salvador, Jamaica and Venezuela: Grosh (1990), Tables A.II.R, A.II.9, A.II.19, A.II.24, A.II.29, A.II.34, A.II.39, A.II.44, A.III.5, and A.III.6; Brazil, Ecuador, Honduras, Mexico and Uruguay: Musgrove (1988), Cuadro [Table] 3-1. Gaps in table indicate data missing in original sources.

crisis began, and for many countries was therefore the last relatively normal budgetary year, with sharp retrenchment occurring in 1983 or 1984. (Costa Rica and El Salvador are notable exceptions, where spending declined substantially between 1980 and 1982.)

In every country except Honduras and Venezuela, public spending per person on health was lower, sometimes much lower, in the mid-1980s than it had been at the start of the decade. Whether expenditure could have been maintained more generally, despite failing incomes, is an open question: it would certainly have required a strong counter-cyclical commitment. The absence of any policy to give health more priority in times of hardship is also shown by the decline in the share of GDP which governments devoted to the sector: again, Honduras and Venezuela are exceptions.

It may be more reasonable to judge policy by comparing health spending with total public spending. This indicator also fell in most countries, often quite sharply, indicating that health lost in relative budgetary priority. The results are more varied both within and among countries, however. The share rose, at least temporarily, in Brazil, Ecuador, Mexico, and Uruguay—suggesting that there was no continuous policy but rather a year-to-year improvisation. Certainly these were not, in most countries, years in which conditions were favorable to defining and implementing stable, future-oriented policies.

Inputs and outputs: allocation and provision as policy

The expenditure estimates just presented have been purged, so far as possible, of general price inflation. It is, however, virtually impossible to standardize them for price changes specific to the health sector, or for changes in the mixture of inputs used or outputs produced: no one has made up the indices necessary for such deflation. Particularly during economic turmoil, it cannot be assumed that there is a stable relation between dollars spent and health gains produced. It is therefore natural to look specifically at some crude measures of sectoral output and at the absolute or relative amounts of different inputs used.

Given the magnitude of the decline in expenditure, it is surprising to find that public sector health output, in the form of ambulatory consultations and hospitalization, generally did not fall proportionately in the five countries where these measures were studied (Musgrove 1988: 40-53). There is a great deal of variation among countries and from year to year, but no evidence that output depended linearly on budgets. Four possible reasons may be suggested:

1. Investment was reduced very sharply, at least at the start of the crisis, so that recurrent expenditure was partly protected. This clearly happened in all countries.

2. Real salaries fell, so that although there was no reduction in public sector health staff, the cost of employing them declined. The tendency of employment to grow even during the crisis suggests that one of the few constant policies of most governments was to provide jobs for as many medical graduates as possible. The evidence on salaries is more mixed: these fell more often than not, however, indicating that medical personnel paid part of the cost of budget reductions. This is a reminder that "health policy" is not only policy about patients and their needs but also about staff and their demands, and that a major policy problem is to reconcile these two groups' claims.

3. Existing inefficiencies in the use of resources were reduced, by providing more ambulatory and less hospital care, or more preventive and less curative care, or by making better use of low-level staff relative to doctors, or by improving the balance among staff, drugs, and other inputs. Here the evidence is extremely mixed. Musgrove (1988) found almost no data by which to judge either allocative or technical efficiency. Hospital use increased in Honduras, largely because several new hospitals had been completed just before the recession began. It would have been a change of policy *not* to put them into operation, and consistent policy meant shortchanging ambulatory care. In Brazil,

there was a clear policy to hold down hospitalization and direct more resources to non-hospital care (Piola and Vianna 1991). Grosh (1990) found evidence of reductions in the already low ratios of nurses to doctors, suggesting that inefficiency actually increased in several countries during the 1980s. And in the case of social security medical care in Peru, Petrera (1989) found that expenditure on drugs was cut drastically while staff increased, clearly indicating a worsening of inefficiency.

4. Quality declined, so that consultations and hospitalizations made poorer contributions to health improvements than before. This idea is hard to distinguish from that of reduced efficiency, and there is almost no direct evidence bearing on it—no evidence, in particular, of lower gains in healthy life years or other outcome measures.

These four possible explanations refer to total output in the form of consultations and hospitalizations. It is a different question whether health outcomes varied in relation to sectoral output. Almost nothing systematic could be found out about allocation among different programs or health problems. However, immunization programs were generally protected and this probably helps account for the continued decline in infant mortality in several countries during the 1980s.

What do these fragments of evidence say about how health policy reacted to the budget reductions? The short answer has to be, not much: what evidence there is, is too incomplete and inconsistent, and often is based on very crude indicators. Nonetheless, two conclusions suggest themselves. One is that there is a cost to changing policy, even when changed circumstances require it. The choice may be between leaving new investments idle, and using them even though cheaper or more effective programs had to be cut back, as seems to have occurred in Honduras. Because investment in buildings and people takes a long time to mature, quick and substantial changes in input use are difficult and costly. Second, while it might be possible to define coherent policy change with respect to one objective, there is no easy way to take account of competing objectives. This is true not only when allocating resources to different treatments, which means making choices among patients, but also when sharing the burden of recession between patients and health sector workers. The burden seems to have been shared quite differently in different countries.

Improvisation, coping, and interest group struggles

The foregoing discussion suggests that not only has there been no uniform response to economic crisis and adjustment across countries in Latin America but that even within any one country, "policy change" has usually not been well defined or internally consistent. Implicit policy, indicated by how much is spent and on what, has of course changed, but in an often erratic fashion. Moreover, the explicit enunciation of policy, particularly when embodied in constitutions, laws, and statements for political public consumption, may have little to do with reality.

Significant, coherent shifts of policy can be debated and implemented. But that process is not automatic, takes more time than an abrupt economic crisis allows (at least in the first year or two), and is likely to respond to other, long-term factors independent of the crisis. Particularly in the short run, what happens is much more a matter of *coping* with the immediate financial pressures, *improvising* adjustments within the public health sector, and *struggles* between interest groups over who and what is to be protected, or sacrificed. These are messy processes, which helps explain both the year-to-year variation in expenditure and service production and the frequent inconsistency between what is said and what is done.

Coping is what administrators of clinics and programs have to do, when their budgets are cut or they face some other restrictions such as failure to deliver drugs and supplies. Traditionally, Latin American public health systems have been grossly over-centralized, so that administrators cannot reallocate budgets significantly, make their own personnel decisions, or otherwise respond effectively to resource shortage. This problem long antedates the economic crisis, and would need fixing even if no recession had occurred; the crisis has merely made more painfully evident the inefficiency such centralization imposes.

Improvising means trying to adjust policy in the short run, usually without an adequate conceptual basis. Particularly in the first years of a crisis, improvising is nearly all that can be done: there is too little experience from which to predict the consequences of policy changes, and the system usually starts so far from equilibrium that many different possible changes appear to make sense or at least to offer some good effects. Many improvisations are implicitly revealed in the budget, but as was argued above, it is hard to read any clear policy shift out of them. What is needed is detailed research on what actually happened at the level of programs and facilities, who took the relevant decisions, and what if any difference they made.

Some research exists, particularly in the case of Brazil (Piola and Vianna 1991; Couttolenc 1991), but in most countries rather little is known about the details of policy improvisation.

Struggling for resources and control goes on all the time within governments and among the interest groups affected by the crisis in health care finance, but it can be expected to intensify when funds are reduced. Ideally, policy means a decision about who is to bear the burden, who is to win and who is to lose. These decisions are seldom made clearly or enforced consistently, and the results often escape the control of those trying to make health policy. For example, doctors in Honduras secured most of the budget increases in the form of higher salaries for themselves, blocking any expansion of services (Musgrove 1988, Chapter 6). In Brazil, the largest struggle has been over the sharing of funds and responsibilities among the federal, state and municipal governments, with revenue-sharing determined outside the health sector and central health policy having to adjust to the new financing pattern (Piola and Vianna 1991).

Exogenous trends in policy

In the absence of economic crisis and adjustment the need to cope and the pressure to improvise would have been much less, and it would have been easier to accommodate the normal struggles between interest groups. But there would still have been some strong scientific and intellectual or ideological currents running in the Latin American health sector, and it is reasonable to suppose they would still have had some influence on health policy. Three such tendencies are those towards specific, cost-effective interventions, particularly those applied in "child survival" programs (Task Force for Child Survival 1990), towards privatization in the provision of services (Roth 1987; World Bank 1987); and towards "cost recovery" or user fees at public facilities (Jimenez 1987; Griffin 1988).

Each of these ideas has been sold on the grounds that governments' economic difficulties require them to concentrate on what works best and costs least—that faced with a crisis, they cannot afford the "luxury" of high-cost, ineffective care (usually identified with hospital care), or of inefficient public provision, or of free care for everyone in the population. But these ideas would surely have been pressed on governments even if no crisis had occurred; what the crisis did was to make it harder for governments to resist them on purely ideological grounds. At least, this is the case for privatization and for user fees, ideas which most Latin American governments generally rejected before the 1980s, but which have subsequently been embraced with varying degrees of enthusiasm and desperation.

The peculiar case of Brazil

In some of the smaller countries, particularly those in Central America which are relatively dependent on foreign assistance and especially on help from USAID, policy change can be strongly pushed by a combination of financial need and external conceptual or ideological pressure. These pressures are less effective in larger and more self-sufficient countries, and what happens to policy can be correspondingly more complex. Brazil is probably the most studied example. As in other countries, there was a sharp reduction in central government health care spending at the beginning of the crisis (1983–94), and this provoked a search for "fat to burn" or opportunities to reduce waste and inefficiency (Piola and Vianna 1991). Partly for this reason, and partly for perceived equity reasons, there was also a push to curtail hospital services and expand ambulatory care. At the same time, Brazil shows some tendencies that were generated domestically and with little or no reference to the economic situation. These include the near-universalization of social security coverage, even to people not contributing to the system; the express inclusion of an unlimited "right to health" in the new Constitution of 1988; an *increase* in the public provision of care, at the expense of public finance for privately provided care through contracts with the social security system; and a devolution of both money and responsibilities, including the transfer of control over health facilities and the transfer of personnel, to states and municipalities. All these changes have much more to do with the democratization of the country in the 1980s than with anything else.

Brazil also illustrates the improvised, turbulent nature of health policy reform to an extreme degree, because of the struggles among levels of government, agencies of the federal government, and interest groups. The country has had three substantial efforts at reform in the last decade, and while they are consistent in some respects, there are also instances of reversal (Couttolenc 1991; Piola and Vianna 1991). Thus the decentralization of services under the 1988 SUDS (Unified and Decentralized Health Systems) operated through the states, which determined how much of their newly acquired federal money and facilities to turn over to municipalities, whereas the subsequent 1990 SUS (Single Health System) reform reasserted federal control and provided for the social security system to deal directly with municipalities.

Concluding Reflections

It is difficult to reach any substantial and defensible conclusions about the relation between economic crisis and health policy, so these final reflections are not so much a summing up as suggestions of other questions to contemplate.

How much does health policy matter?

Health policy responds to many factors, some of them political and some quite ideological, in addition to the economic circumstances that constitute a crisis or the adjustment to one. That alone makes it difficult for health policy to change quickly and sensibly if a crisis arises. Most "policy change", leaving aside the most general pronouncements of goals or wishes, involves a great deal of coping with adversity, improvisation, and struggle among competing interests. That means that what actually happens is unlikely to correspond exactly to declared policy, and generally has to sacrifice some objectives to satisfy others. Together these two arguments suggest that the importance of policy, and of changes in policy, is overrated. Perhaps the rhetorical component should be ignored altogether, and the real component judged simply by how much health improvement is obtained, relative to money spent. Good results mean, implicitly, good policy: bad results mean something needs to be changed.

The limitation of this view, of course, is that bad results by themselves do not tell one what needs to be changed. And if policy is (part of) what mediates between inputs and outputs, then one has to look at policy to see what is, or has gone, wrong. So the argument that "policy matters", and that good policy is preferable to bad policy, survives this skeptical view. What may not survive is any simple notion of a one-to-one correspondence from economic phenomena to health policy, and from there to health outcomes. There is similarly not much reason to believe in a relatively uniform, systematic response to economic crisis across countries or even across a few years in one country. From the scant empirical evidence, it is hard to say how much health policy has mattered recently in Latin America, and while much past and present policy can be roundly criticized on theoretical grounds, it is hard to tell how much better outcomes might have been with better policies.

Dealing with crisis and adjustment: are there any lessons?

There is no shortage of attempts to answer this question, in both theoretical and empirical terms (Bell and Reich 1988). Even if the economic crisis of the 1980s turns out to have had little impact on life and death in Latin America, it largely halted the expansion of public health coverage, probably reduced the quality and accessibility of care, and severely shook the public institutions which had to cope with it or adjust to it; so it is natural to try to derive lessons from the experience. Most of the lessons really amount to suggestions for *better* policy, which would be just as relevant if there had never been a crisis. To concentrate on cost-effective interventions, to favour the poor and those most at risk, to finance the system on a sound basis, to avoid duplication of effort, to use prices and fees both for internal efficiency and to steer demand in appropriate directions, to buy and use inputs in the right proportions—all this excellent advice may carry more weight when governments are broke and desperate, but it will make just as much sense if economic growth resumes and health budgets expand. There is even a potentially perverse effect, in that any public health sector which becomes lean and efficient will have no "fat to burn" if confronted with a future retrenchment. A little bit of waste in good times is a protection in bad times; how much waste ought to be tolerated depends, unfortunately, on the likely duration and severity of bad times, which are hard to predict.

This suggests that governments need policies not only for a point in time, but for a course over time. To have to change policy when budgets are cut—or to need to do so, but fail to come up with anything but panicky improvisation—indicates that the pre-crisis policy did not adequately contemplate the possibility of a crisis or spell out what to do about it. A medium-term policy should have built into it the "expansion path" of the sector, both when budgets are rising and when they are falling; it should already say what to cut and what to save, if resources drop by X percent. Like all plans, such a policy would need to be revised every year, because what to do depends on what one is already doing or has the capacity to do. But it should avoid the need to introduce entirely new policies purely under financial pressure, and it should forbid the kind of retrenchment which guarantees reduced efficiency because some inputs are protected while others are abandoned. It might even build in a counter-cyclical protection for health care. This kind of policy—actually a portfolio of contingent plans, of "what to do if" policies—seems to have been conspicuously lacking in Latin America at the beginning of the 1980s, and that, as much as the pressures of adjustment, may account for the reduction in effective health protection in the early years of the crisis.

References

Bell. D. E. and Reich, M. R. (eds.) (1988), *Health, Nutrition and Economic Crises: Approaches to Policy in the Third World.* Dover, MA: Auburn House.

Berk, D. A. (1992), personal communication, 19 May.

Carroll, L. (1865), *Through the Looking Glass,* Macmillan.

Cornia, B. A. (1989), "Investing in human resources: health, nutrition and development for the 1990s", *Journal of Development Planning, 19/159.*

Couttolenc, B. (1991), "Change in the Brazilian health system: key issues for SUS", Latin American Country Department 1, Human Resources Division, World Bank, Washington, DC.

Fox, L. (1992), *Romania: Human Resources and the Transition to a Market Economy,* World Bank Country Report, Washington, DC.

Fuenzalida-Puelma, H. and Scholle Connor, S. (1989), *The Right to Health in the Americas: a Comparative Constitutional Study,* Washington, DC: Pan American Health Organization.

Griffin, C. C. (1988), "User charges for health care in principle and practice", Seminar Paper 37, Economic Development Institute, World Bank, Washington, DC.

Grosh, M. E. (1990), *Social Spending in Latin America: The Story of the 1980s,* World Bank Discussion Papers 106, Washington, DC.

Jamison, D. T., Mosley, W. H., Measham, A. R., and Bobadilla J. L. (eds.) (1993), *Disease Control Priorities in Developing Countries,* New York: Oxford University Press for the World Bank.

Jimenez, E. (1987), *Pricing Policy in the Social Sectors: Cost-Recovery for Education and Health in Developing Countries,* Baltimore: Johns Hopkins University Press.

Musgrove, P. (1984), "Health care and economic hardship", *World Health,* October.

Musgrove, P. (1986), "Measurement of equity in health", *World Health Statistics Quarterly, 39.*

Musgrove, P. (1988), "Crisis Económica y Salud: la experiencia de cinco países latino-americanos en los años ochenta", unpublished study, Pan American Health Organization, Washington, DC.

Petrera, M. (1989). "Effectiveness and efficiency of Social Security in the economic cycle: the Peruvian case", In: Musgrove, P. (ed.), *Health Economics: Latin American Perspectives,* Pan American Health Organization, Washington. DC.

Piola, S. F. and Vianna, S. M. (1991), "Políticas e prioridades do sistema único de saúde–SUS", Latin American Country Department I, Human Resources Division, World Bank, Washington, DC.

Roth, G. (1987), *The Private Provision of Public Services in Developing Countries*, New York: Oxford University Press.

Task Force for Child Survival (1990), *Protecting the World's Children: A Call for Action*, Fourth International Child Survival Conference, Bangkok, 1–3 March.

World Bank (1987), *Financing Health Services in Developing Countries: An Agenda for Reform*, Washington, DC.

World Bank (1992), "Poland, health system reform: meeting the challenge". Report 9182-POL. Washington, DC (restricted circulation).

World Bank (1991), *Indonesia: Issues in Health Planning and Budgeting*, World Bank Country Report 7291, Washington, DC.

World Health Organization (1978), *Alma-Ata 1978: Primary Health Care*, Geneva.

Index

United Kingdom,
lifetime health care costs, 85
tax increases on tobacco, 96–97
United States
DRG payments, 63
Food Stamp Program, 339
health care reform, 62
height and protein availability, 353
lifetime health costs, 85
Medicare and Medicaid, 134–36
Presidential Commission studying
access to health care, 122
public expenditures for poor or
elderly, 199–200
tax increases on tobacco, 96, 97
teenage smoking, 81, 83–84
Women, Infants and Children
(WIC) Program, 338–39
United States Agency for International
Development (USAID), 108
health care in Central
America, 416
Urban-rural health care expenditures
compared, 370–73
Urban studies of height and weight of
young adults, 344–47
User fees for health services, 59, 408,
415–16
Utilization of offered services by
patients, 124

van der Gaag, 35
Vaccination, 144–45
cost-benefit analysis of system,
223–46
coverage, 112–14
effects of delay in, 242
vaccine administration costs,
231–32
vaccine costs, individual, 238
vaccine development costs,
225–27, 231–32
Valdés, Alberto, 297

Varejista, 278, 281–82, 288, 291
Vector control of disease, 41
Vehicular accidents, 149
Vertical equity in health care, 176–79,
183
Vitamin A deficiencies, 326–27,
330–32
Vitamin D supplementation, 333
Vulnerable groups, priorities for, 162

Wagstaff, Adam, xvii–xviii
Walton, Michael, 77
Welfare function in state-provided
public health, 123–25
WHO. *See* World Health
Organization.
Women, Infants and Children (WIC)
Program, 338–39
Workplace smoking bans, 92
World Bank, 164, 247, 260
colleagues at, 77, 297
disease control priorities, 326
policy paper on health in China,
344–45
reports, 350
World Bank Development Report, 187
World Bank Institute, 167
World Children's Conference, 1990,
223
World Development Report 1979, 350
World Development Report 1993, 153,
160, 163–64
World Health Organization (WHO),
157, 341
Member States' expenditures on
health, 375–76

Yazbeck, Abdo, 15
Young, Dennis, 203
Yurekli, Ayda, 77

Zeramdini, Riadh, 375
Zschock, Dieter, 203